LECTURE NOTES ON UROLOGY

Lecture Notes on Urology

John Blandy
MA, DM, MCh, FRCS, FACS
Professor of Urology
in the University of London
at The London Hospital Medical College,
and Consultant Urologist,
St Peter's Hospital, London

FOURTH EDITION

OXFORD
BLACKWELL SCIENTIFIC PUBLICATIONS
LONDON EDINBURGH BOSTON
MELBOURNE PARIS BERLIN VIENNA

Editorial Offices:
Osney Mead, Oxford OX2 0EL
25 John Street, London WC1N 2BL
23 Ainslie Place, Edinburgh EH3 6AJ
3 Cambridge Center, Cambridge
Massachusetts 02142, USA
54 University Street, Carlton
Victoria 3053, Australia

Other Editorial Offices:
Arnette SA
2, rue Casimir-Delavigne
75006 Paris
France

Blackwell Wissenschaft
Meinekestrasse 4
D-1000 Berlin 15
West Germany

Blackwell MZV
Feldgasse 13
A-1238 Wien
Austria

First published 1976
Second edition 1977
Reprinted 1979
Third edition 1982
Reprinted 1984, 1986, 1988
Fourth edition 1989, 1991

Spanish edition 1979
Portuguese edition 1980

Set by Times Graphics, Singapore
Printed and bound in Great Britain
at The Alden Press, Oxford

DISTRIBUTORS

Marston Book Services Ltd
PO Box 87
Oxford OX2 0DT
(*Orders*: Tel: 0865 791155
Fax: 0865 791927
Telex: 837515)

USA
Mosby–Year Book, Inc.
200 North LaSalle Street
Chicago, Illinois 60601
(*Orders*: Tel: 312 726-9733)

Canada
Mosby–Year Book, Inc.
5240 Finch Avenue East
Scarborough, Ontario
(*Orders*: Tel: 416 298-1588)

Australia
Blackwell Scientific Publications
(Australia) Pty Ltd
54 University Street
Carlton, Victoria 3053
(*Orders*: Tel: 03 347-0300)

British Library
Cataloguing in Publication Data

Blandy, John P. (John Peter)
Lecture notes on urology.—4th ed.
1. Man. Urogenital system. Diseases
I. Title
616.6

ISBN 0–632–02492–5

Contents

Preface to the Fourth Edition

In the six years since the previous edition there have again been so many major advances and changes in urology that it has been necessary not merely to revise, but entirely to rewrite this book. I have taken the opportunity to leave out a good deal of material that has become obsolete, and to add as much as possible of the new advances. The former section on operative urology has been omitted, each operation now being described, where it seems to be most appropriate, in the main text. Once more, however, it should be pointed out that these descriptions are not intended for the use of the would-be specialist in urology, but merely to make his day-to-day experience in the wards and operating theatre more interesting for the medical student.

J.P.B.

Preface to the First Edition

This book has been written for the undergraduate medical student. About a quarter of all the operations of surgery concern the genitourinary system: about 15% of all doctors suffer at some time or other from a stone in the urinary tract: one in ten of all males has to have an operation on his prostate before he reaches the end of his days. The management of haematuria, of impotence, of infertility, and of urinary tract infections: the investigation of hypertension, and the evaluation of albuminuria — no doctor, however recondite his specialty, is not at some time touched by one or other of these common problems. Of all diseases in the world, in prevalence second only to malaria, schistosomiasis affects more human beings, and those more miserably, than any other. The author makes no apology therefore for the claim that the specialty of urology encompasses some of the most important, and arguably the most fascinating of all the topics of medicine and surgery. My object has been to communicate my own interest and enthusiasm to my students, for unlike some topics which they have to learn, there ought to be nothing boring or dull in this, the oldest and most vigorous of all the specialties. It is for this reason that the solemn minded reader may not approve of some of my pictures, or my omission of the customary protracted dissertation about body fluids and electrolytes for which he will have to consult those of his textbooks which deal with them in a way which I could not imitate even if I understood. Sexually transmitted diseases are not covered in this book, not because I find them tedious, but because they are too important to be dealt with by other than an expert. On the other hand I found it impossible not to trespass from time to time on the ground normally and correctly assigned to my colleagues in nephrology from whom I crave forgiveness if, in an attempt to make an understandable and unified presentation of the subject, my ignorance has led me into too many and too barbarous errors concerning the esoteric mysteries of nephritis and hypertension. The last chapter about the operations of urology is there simply to make the students' visits to the operating theatre more interesting: they should not attempt to learn surgical technique — though I hope they may find watching operations helps in the understanding of living pathology. For the same reason the little glossary of jargon, eponyms and gobbledegook is added for fun, not because students need learn any of it.

J.P.B.

1 History and Examination

Begin at the beginning — how old is your patient, and what is his or her occupation? If he is retired, what did he do before? Could he ever have been in contact with rubber, chemicals, plastics, tar, pitch or any other occupational hazard known to affect the urinary tract? Do not accept vague terms like 'company director' or 'process worker' — the company he directed may have been manufacturing naphthylamine or the process the mixing of raw rubber with noxious antioxidants. If your patient is female ask when she was married, how many and how old are her children, and whether there was any complication during pregnancy or delivery that may have necessitated the passing of a catheter, e.g. the use of forceps in delivery or the suturing of a perineal tear.

Turn to the trouble which brings the patient to your clinic. Try to determine when the symptoms began and what they were like to start with, before any treatment was given. As you listen — and listening is the key to taking a useful history — try to make clear in your own mind how the pattern of the illness has developed over the years. At the end, be sure you understand what it is that bothers the patient right now, and never end your enquiry without asking whether the patient has noticed blood in the urine: haematuria is the most important symptom in the whole of urology.

Note-taking (Fig. 1.1)

Although you must set down all the relevant facts in the history, it is no good writing down a host of irrelevant twaddle in the hope that somebody, sometime, will be able to make sense out of it. Try to keep your notes as brief and as clear as possible. You are not writing them down only for your own benefit, but also so that your successor can understand the problem, and take up the care of the patient where you have left off. So do write legibly and if you cannot write clearly, teach yourself to use a typewriter. Whatever you write down may later be vital evidence in a law court so in addition to being accurate and clear, be circumspect and never allow yourself to be tempted to write down anything that could be construed as criticism of a colleague.

A drawing may save lines of prose, e.g. a sketch noting where the pain starts and radiates to and a word or two to specify the type of pain — sharp, colicky, dull, etc.

THE LONDON HOSPITAL
UROLOGY HISTORY SHEET
PROFESSOR BLANDY

UNIT No. 235678.81
SURNAME (Block Letters) DOE
FIRST NAMES JOHN

DATE	CLINICAL NOTES (Each entry must be signed)
25.5.81	Referred by Dr Richard Roe (See letter)
	Aged 71 Retired foreman, mixing plant Imported Carcinogens Company x 25 yrs
	Smokes 30 cigs/day
	C/o "blood in my water" for 3 wks: no pain. Clots ++ at end of stream. No fever. No backache. D = 6, N = 1
	PH. Malaria and dysentery 1942. Served Egypt, N. Africa. Denies V.D. Appendix '49.
	OE. Lean wiry old man BP 160/90
	Lump: not fixed; Appendix 1949; L hydrocele
	P.R. 45 gram benign prostate
	Urine Frank blood
	Urgent IVU; Urine culture; Pap'; Hb; Group; Urea
	Admit urgently for Cystoscopy ? Right retrograde
	JPB

Fig. 1.1. Keep your notes as brief as possible.

Avoid phoney Greek and Latin terms unless they are clear, short, and unambiguous: never use them to decorate your work with pretentious respectability. Shun the word *dysuria* which can mean pain or difficulty or both: say which you had in mind. *Micturition* is a tiresome euphemism for passing urine and in most languages in most parts of the world this physiological function is expressed by *p* — or if your prefer *pee*. Frequency is more clearly expressed by writing down how often your patient pees by day and by night, and the notation D=6 N=3 is used when he passes urine 6 times by day and thrice at night. Avoid *polyuria, nocturia, pollakiuria* and *enuresis* — these terms are all open to misinterpretation: if you mean the patient *wets the bed*, say so.

Blood in the urine is allowably and more briefly noted as *haematuria* but even this can be confusing, since blood found in the urine on microscopy is no less an indication for investigation. Whether the blood was well mixed with the urine, had formed clots, or appeared at the beginning or end of urination is of little importance. Blood that trickles away between the acts of urination is usually coming from the urethra itself. Do not be put off by a history of taking anticoagulants: haematuria on anticoagulation therapy always needs to be investigated.

Previous history

Ask if your patient has lived in a hot climate, especially in Africa and those parts of the world where schistosomiasis is common. Ask about rheumatism and arthritis, for which analgesics may have been taken — analgesic nephropathy is surprisingly common and will not be disclosed unless you ask indirectly about the possibility of overconsumption of pain-killing tablets. Direct questions on this topic will seldom be answered truthfully.

In women, enquire about the menstrual history, not only because of the obvious possibility of confusing menstrual loss and haematuria, but also because X-rays must be avoided if there is the slightest possibility of the patient being pregnant. Note the date of the last menstrual period on the X-ray request form.

Students often feel awkward when asking about venereal disease. In fact a man is usually secretly flattered at the suggestion that he may once have been a Don Juan and tactful questions referring to youth are seldom taken amiss.

Do not waste time: even as you are listening to the patient's story it will be obvious that certain investigations are going to be needed. Unobtrusively filling the relevant forms will not stop you listening politely but will save time, and more importantly, prevent you writing down too many irrelevant details. *Listening is far more important than writing.*

PHYSICAL EXAMINATION

Physical examination begins as the patient comes into the room: does he look ill; has he obviously lost weight; does he walk in a way that suggests pain, Parkinsonism or ankylosing spondylitis? Does he bring with him that scent of urine that suggests uraemia, or perhaps wet trousers? As you rise to shake his hand, remember this is not mere politeness, but may give useful information. Never forget that you are a doctor first, and a urologist second: your first task is to look at the patient as a whole. In an ideal world, where no doctor was ever pushed for time, and no patient ever in a hurry to get back to his work or her children you could spend all day over one case, getting to know the patient in depth and making a thorough and complete physical examination of every system. Such a thorough clerking will of course apply to a patient who is admitted to the ward, but in the clinic such a method of working would be cruelly slow, and unfair to the many others who are waiting. Of course, if you notice something that draws attention to a disorder in another system by all means examine that system as well.

In most patients who attend the urological clinic you will be looking for enlargement of a kidney or bladder, disorders in the inguinal region and genitalia, hypertension, swellings in the pelvis that may be detected by internal examination per rectum or per vaginam, and it is to these features that your attention will be mainly directed.

Abdominal examination

The physical signs of an *enlarged bladder* (Figs 1.5, 1.6) can be a rounded lump in the loin, bimanually palpable, that moves on respiration, above which one can get the hand between the lump and the edge of the costal margin, and in front of which there is resonance from gas in the bowel (Fig. 1.3). In practice these supposedly classical signs are notoriously misleading and should never be trusted. On the right side the supposed 'kidney' may turn out to be the gall-bladder or the liver; on the left it may prove to be the spleen despite your being able to slide your hand under the costal margin. A large mass may displace the colon and so there will be no resonance in front of the kidney, or it may in fact be arising from the colon. The notorious 'kidney punch' is never required (Fig. 1.4).

The physical signs of an *enlarged bladder* (Figs 1.5, 1.6) can be equally misleading. Classically a rounded swelling arising from the pelvis that is dull to percussion ought to be the bladder. In practice a floppy, over-distended bladder may feel soft and does not always rise up in the

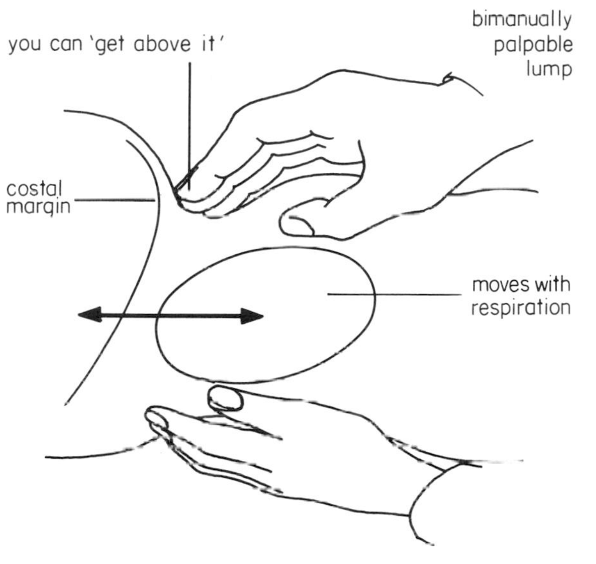

Fig. 1.2. Physical signs of an enlarged kidney.

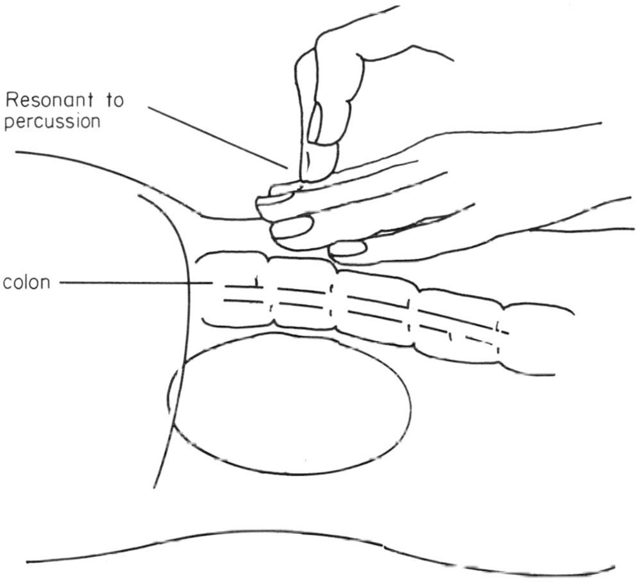

Resonant to percussion
colon

Fig. 1.3. A band of resonance may be found in front of the kidney.

midline but it may be more on one side than the other (Fig. 1.7). The most useful physical sign here is when the swelling goes away after the urine has been let out with a catheter.

Examination of the *inguinal regions* is concerned with three hernial orifices on each side (Figs 1.8, 1.9). Each one must be felt both in the supine and erect positions, with and without the patient coughing. An *inguinal hernia* may be direct or indirect — the difference between them is that the hernial orifices are separated by the line of the inferior epigastric vessels. In practice also the *indirect hernia* in a male slides indirectly and obliquely along the line of the spermatic cord towards the scrotum whereas the *direct hernia* pushes out anteriorly and seldom enters the scrotum. Never be surprised to find your pre-operative diagnosis proved wrong when the hernia is exposed at operation. It is common to find a direct sac accompanied by an indirect one — the so-called 'saddlebag' or 'pantaloon' hernia.

Do not forget to feel for a *femoral hernia*. The neck of the sac is always rather narrow, and its fundus is surrounded by layer upon layer of fat, like an onion. The hernia pushes out below the inguinal ligament and medial to the femoral vein, and then it bulges out through the fossa ovalis — the gap in the deep fascia where the saphenous vein dives down to enter the femoral vein. In practice, unless a femoral hernia is strangulated, it feels quite like a lipoma and a cough impulse is very hard

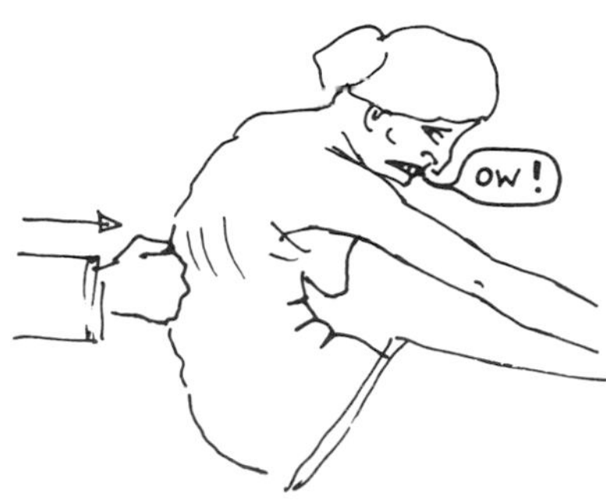

Fig. 1.4. The notorious kidney punch—gentle palpation is just as informative.

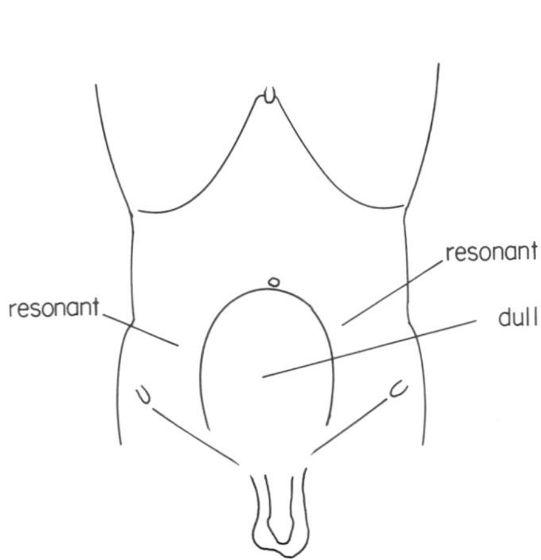

Fig. 1.5. An enlarged bladder is dull to percussion while the flanks are resonant.

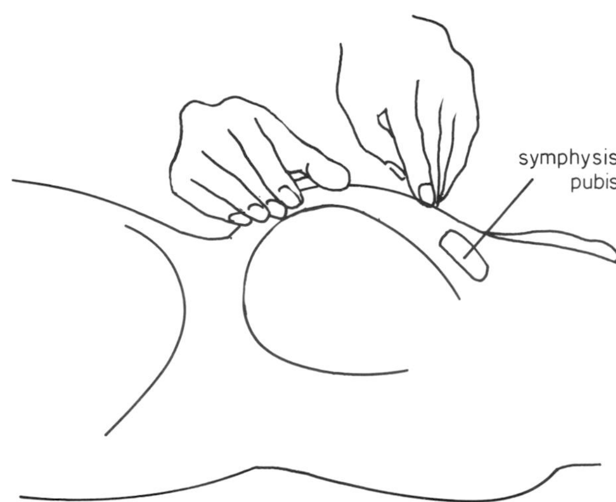

Fig. 1.6. Bimanual examination may show the fluid-filled bladder even when it is atonic and floppy.

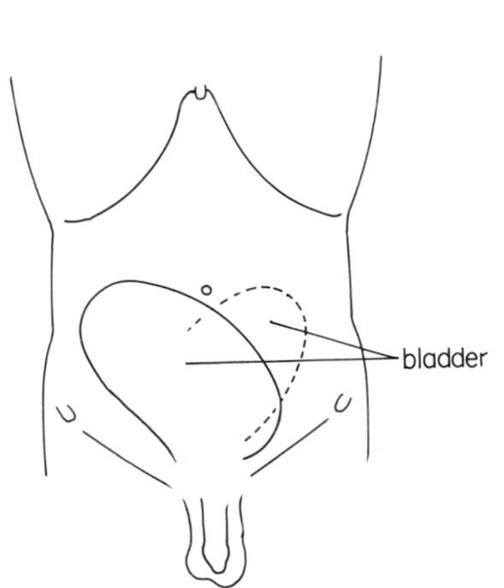

Fig. 1.7. The bladder may not enlarge in the midline, but lean over to one side or the other.

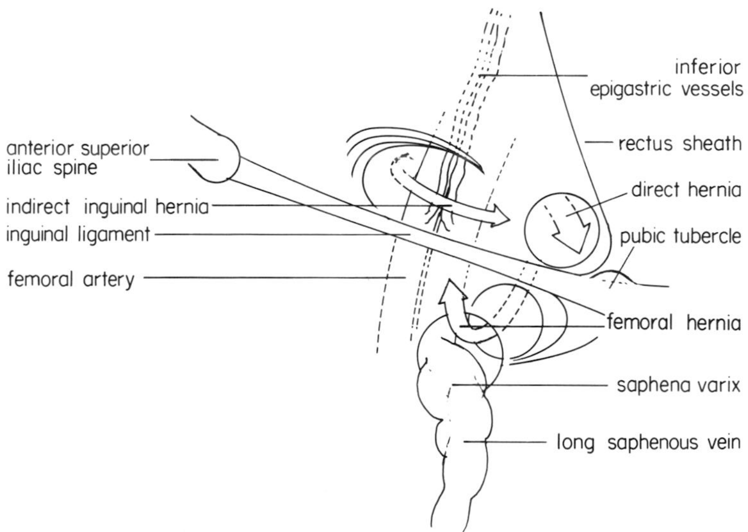

Fig. 1.8. Landmarks in the groin showing the anatomy of the three important types of hernia, indirect and direct inguinal and femoral.

to elicit. In the standing-up position a *saphena varix* can mimic a femoral hernia, but will vanish when the patient lies down, and usually feels 'thin' rather than the fatty lump so typical of a femoral hernia. A saphena varix has a very obvious cough impulse which coincides with the impulse and thrill running down the rest of the saphenous vein.

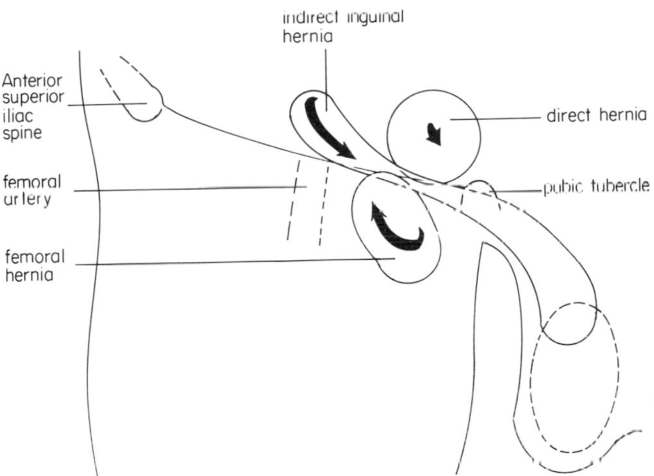

Fig. 1.9. The indirect inguinal hernia slides obliquely down the course of the spermatic cord towards the scrotum; the direct hernia pushes straight out in front; the femoral hernia rises upwards and laterally, and is covered by several layers of fat.

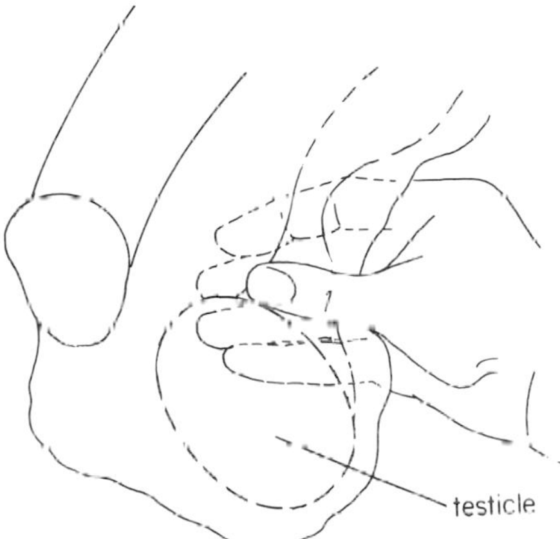

Fig. 1.10. First step in examination of a scrotal swelling: can you get above it?

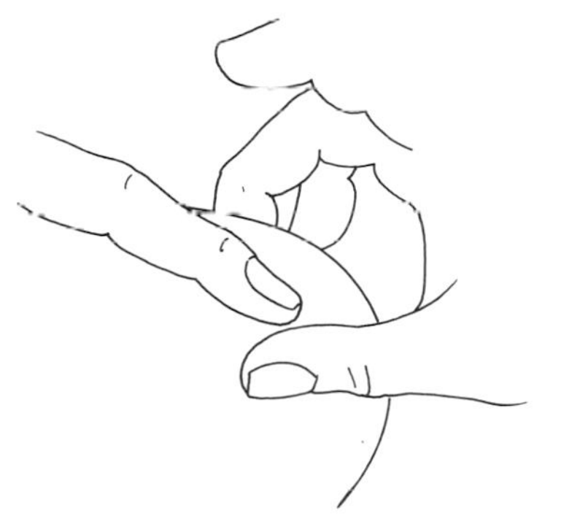

Fig. 1.11. Second step in examination of a scrotal swelling: is it fluctuant or solid? Fluctuation is determined in two planes as shown.

The scrotum and its contents

By tradition the term 'testicle' is taken to include both testis and epididymis. When examining the scrotum, the first thing to make sure is that the swelling is not a hernia, i.e. coming down along the cord from above. If you can 'get above' the swelling, then you know it is arising from the testicle (Fig. 1.10).

The second step is to ascertain whether the swelling is solid or fluctuant (Fig. 1.11). If the swelling is fluctuant it must either be made up of fluid in the sac of the tunica vaginalis around the testis (i.e. a hydrocele) or fluid in one or more cysts of the epididymis. The epididymis lies behind the testis (Fig. 1.12) and its cysts lie behind the body of the testis. A *hydrocele* envelopes the testis, making it difficult to feel clearly, but when the testis can be distinguished, it lies posteriorly (Fig. 1.13). In practice, *cysts of the epididymis* often coexist with hydroceles and again it is not at all uncommon for a confident pre-operative diagnosis to be disproved at operation. Traditionally it is usual to shine a light through a hydrocele or an epididymal cyst. If the wall of the cyst or the hydrocele has become thickened, or if the contents have been rendered opaque by haemorrhage or the accumulation of debris, it will no longer be translucent.

If the lump is not fluctuant, but solid, the next step is to decide whether it is in the testis or the epididymis. If it is in the testis (Fig. 1.14) then it is malignant until proved otherwise. If there is a solid lump in the

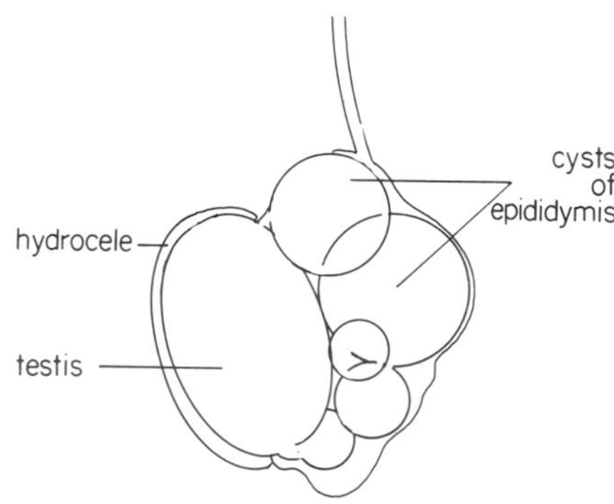

Fig. 1.12. Cysts of the epididymis are multilocular, fluctuant swellings behind the testis. There may be an associated hydrocele.

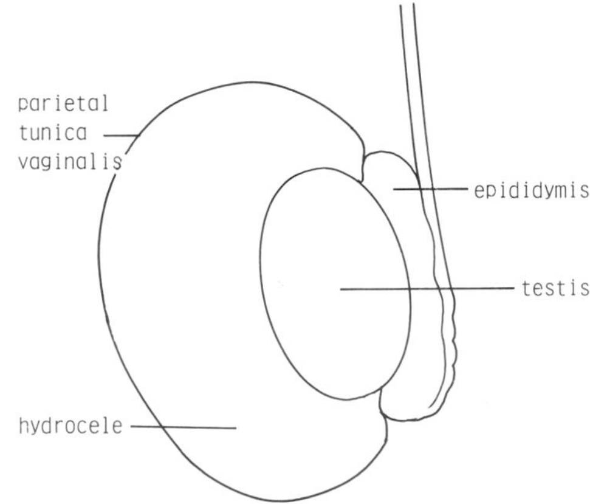

Fig. 1.13. Hydroceles tend to surround and hide the testicle: when it can be found, it lies behind the hydrocele.

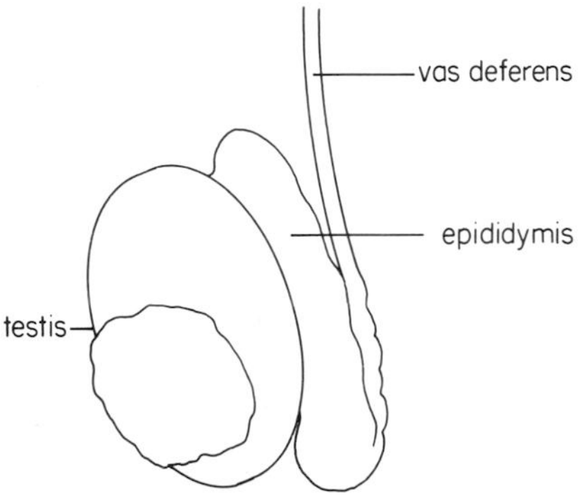

Fig. 1.14. Non-fluctuant (solid) swellings in the testis are usually due to malignant tumour, and always demand to be explored.

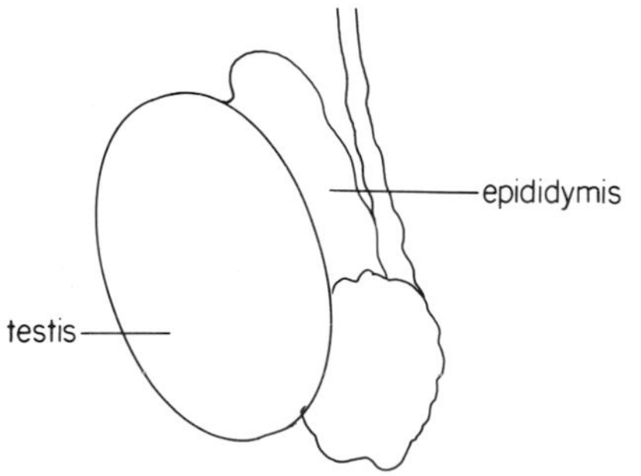

Fig. 1.15. Solid lumps in the epididymis are usually due to chronic inflammation.

epididymis (Fig. 1.15) then it is a granuloma either arising in reaction to extravasated sperm (sperm granuloma) or tuberculosis, or one of the very rare tumours that arise in the epididymis itself.

Swellings in the spermatic cord

The veins draining the testicle may become varicose and distended — a *varicocele*. By tradition a varicocele is said to feel like a 'bag of worms' (Fig. 1.16). Like the reader, the author has never actually felt a bag of worms but that does not stop him from knowing what one would feel like, and it is certainly a very apt description.

The vas deferens lies posterior to the cord. If the vas is inflamed or has been operated on, e.g. by vasectomy, one may feel nodules along its course. Multiple knotty swellings are typical of tuberculosis (Fig. 1.17). Inflammatory swellings in the cord are seen in the tropical conditions of schistosomiasis and filariasis.

Rectal examination

Rectal examination in either sex may be carried out either in the supine position, the knee-elbow position, or the left lateral position. It is important to introduce the finger slowly and gently. Everyone will have experienced the discomfort of passing a constipated stool and should appreciate the need to introduce the finger slowly. Once inside the rectum, feel the prostate and the rest of the wall of the rectum carefully (Fig. 1.18). Occasionally you will detect an unexpected cancer of the

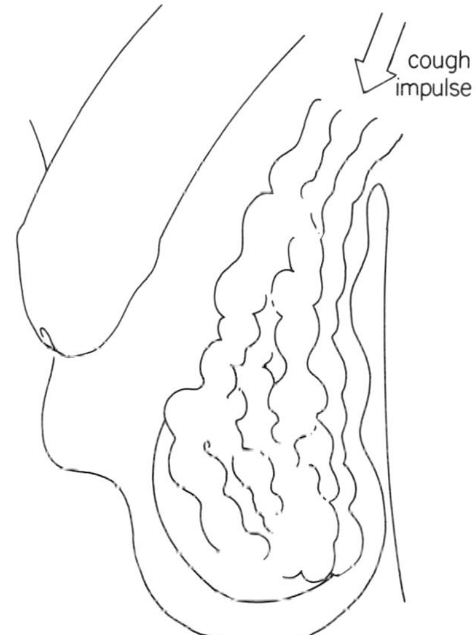

Fig. 1.16. A varicocele is formed by enlarged and tortuous spermatic veins. It feels like a 'bag of worms'. There is usually a cough impulse.

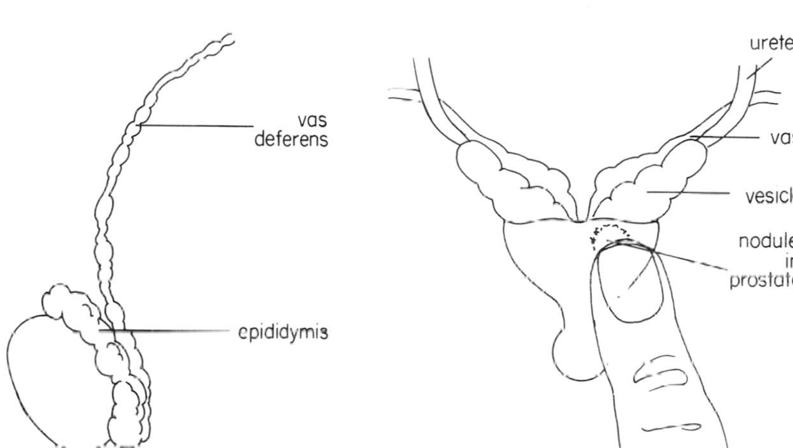

Fig. 1.17. Multiple, knotty swellings along the course of the vas deferens are typical of tuberculosis.

Fig. 1.18. Anatomical landmarks that may be felt per rectum.

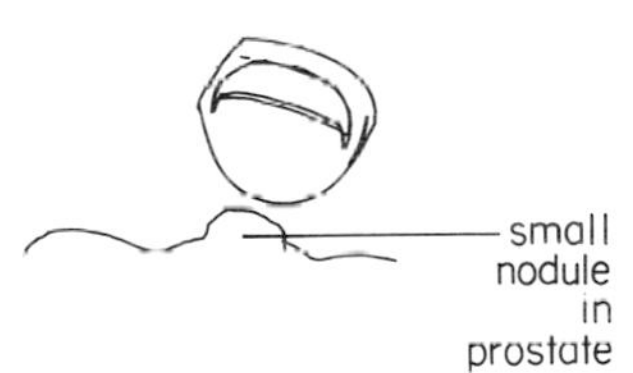

Fig. 1.19. Small nodules protruding from the surface of the prostate may be caused by cancer, and call for biopsy.

rectum. In men you will usually feel the prostate bulging backwards either because the bladder is full or because the prostate is enlarged.

More important is to feel for any hard nodules in the prostate for these may signify carcinoma (Fig. 1.19). A clinical suspicion of prostatic carcinoma will need confirmation by biopsy.

The most experienced surgeons make mistakes in rectal examination: it is notoriously fallible and the beginner should always take the opportunity to learn what the normal and abnormal prostate feels like in the anaesthetized patient.

FURTHER READING

Blandy JP (Ed) (1976) *Urology*. Blackwell Scientific Publications, Oxford.

Gillenwater J, Grayhack JT, Howards S & Duckett J (1987) *Adult and Pediatric Urology*. Wolfe & Year Book Publications, London.

Gosling JA, Dixon JS & Humpherson JR (1982) *Functional Anatomy of the Urinary Tract*. Gower Medical Publishing, London.

Lloyd-Davies RW, Gow JG & Davies DR (1983) *A Colour Atlas of Urology*. Wolfe, London.

Mundy AR (1988) *Scientific Basis of Urology*. Churchill Livingstone, Edinburgh.

Murphy LJT (1972) *The History of Urology*. Charles C Thomas, Springfield, Illinois.

Whitfield HN & Hendry WF (Eds) (1985) *Textbook of Genitourinary Surgery*. Churchill Livingstone, Edinburgh.

2 Investigations

TESTING THE URINE

For centuries the physician has learned much by careful examination of the patient's urine. In times past he would look at it, measure it, smell it and taste it: today he need not taste it. Crystal clear urine is rarely infected. There are many occasions when the diagnosis rests, not upon sophisticated tests, but upon the simple recording of the time and the volume of urine passed on each occasion — *the fluid chart* (Fig. 2.1).

pH

Two indicator dyes are impregnated on a paper test strip giving a measure of pH which is sufficiently accurate for most purposes: a very acid urine should make one consider uric acid stone formation, and a very alkaline one usually signifies infection with a urea-splitting organism such as *Proteus mirabilis*.

Protein

Paper impregnated with tetrabromphenol blue usually turns blue in the pH range found in normal human urine, but the presence of protein alters

7·30 am	300	cc	Tuesday
8·15 "	150	cc	
11·10 "	100	cc	
12·35 pm	150	cc	
2·00 "	150	cc	
4·30 "	150	cc	
6·30 "	175	cc	
8·00 "	175	cc	
11·00 "	150	cc	
7·00 am	250	cc	Wednesday

Fig. 2.1. Fluid chart.

this reaction — turning it more yellow the more protein is present. Because the dye is essentially an indicator, it is unreliable in the extremes of acidity or alkalinity. An alternative test for protein is to add 25% salicylsulphonic acid to the urine: protein is precipitated as a cloud unless it is exceptionally dilute. One can still test for protein without special apparatus by boiling it, checking with a drop of a dilute acid that the first cloud thrown down by boiling is not phosphatic. When protein has been discovered in the urine and there is good reason to want to know whether the quantity is significant or not, the urine is collected over a 24 hour period and the protein measured accurately in the laboratory. More than 150 mg protein per 24 hours is abnormal and calls for further investigation.

Glucose

The paper strip is impregnated with glucose oxidase, which converts glucose to gluconic acid and hydrogen peroxide. The paper also contains peroxidase, which catalyses the reaction of hydrogen peroxide and a potassium iodide chromagen to give a green–brown colour. If these strips are not available one may boil the urine up with Fehling's or Benedict's solution — glucose and other reducing substances will precipitate orange copper oxide.

Red cells in the urine

Several commercial 'stix' tests for urine rely on the oxidation of tetramethylbenzidine by cumene peroxidase which is catalysed by haemoglobin to give a green–blue colour. This test detects free haemoglobin, and its sensitivity is adjusted to the haemoglobin that is present in as few red cells as 10 per high power field — this is twice the number found in normal urine, i.e. it is a significant amount and always calls for a thorough investigation (see p. 187). This begins by microscopy to make sure whether intact red cells (haematuria) are present or just haemoglobin (haemoglobinuria). False positive tests may be found if the urine is slightly contaminated with povidone iodine or hypochlorite.

Microscopic examination of the urine

In busy clinical practice one often needs to know if there is blood or pus in the urine. Never forget how useful it can be to examine a drop of urine on a microscope slide covered with a cover-slip: significant amounts of pus and blood can easily be seen without the need to centrifuge the urine

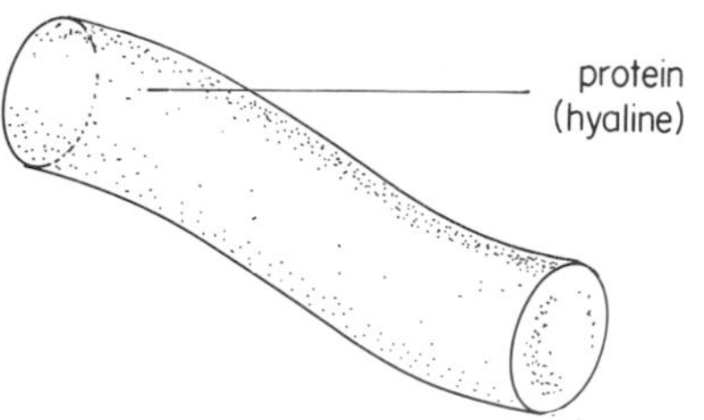

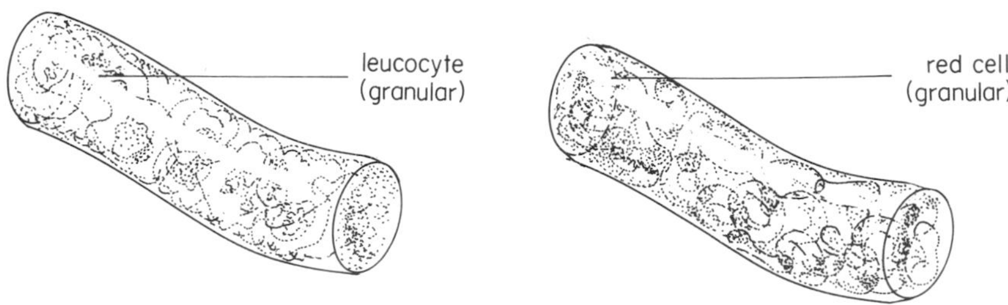

Fig. 2.2. Casts in the urine are extrusions from collecting tubules and may contain protein, pus, or blood.

or use special stains. Even more information may be gained by gently centrifuging the urine and placing a drop of the sediment on a slide under a cover-slip: you may see casts, crystals, pus cells and bacteria.

Casts are the squeezed-out contents of the collecting tubules of the kidney: they may be clear or granular. Clear (hyaline) casts are formed of protein. Granular casts are made of cells — red, white or both (Fig. 2.2).

Crystals are common, and can give a useful lead in diagnosis: the octahedral diamonds of calcium oxalate and the dodecahedrons of triple phosphate are found in normal urine when it cools down, but the rare hexagonal plates of cystine may make the diagnosis in an otherwise difficult case (Fig. 2.3).

In cases of urinary infection bacteria will be seen in the centrifuged deposit, and the Gram stain may help identify the responsible organism. In searching for *Mycobacterium tuberculosis* the urine is stained with the *Ziehl–Neelsen* method and at least three specimens of the first urine passed in the morning are sent to the laboratory.

In searching for cancer cells any specimen of urine may be sent *except* that passed first thing in the morning (when the cells may be autolysed from being in the bladder overnight) after being fixed by adding about an equal volume of 10% formalin. It is then centrifuged and stained with the *Papanicolaou* stain (Fig. 2.4). The ova of *Schistosoma haematobium* may be found in the urine of people who have visited Africa (Fig. 2.5) and for the same reason it is easier to find them in urine that has not been in the bladder overnight.

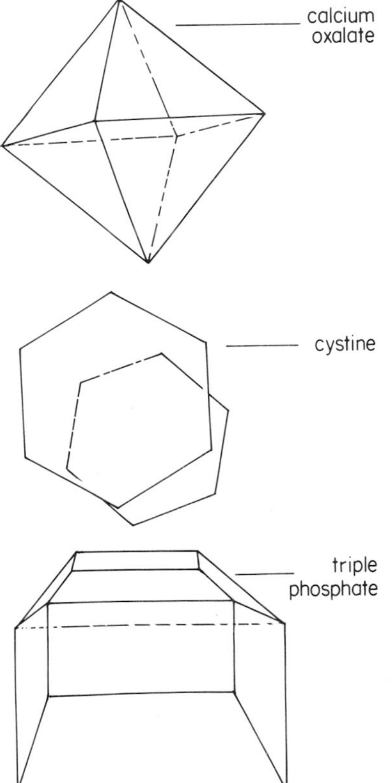

Fig. 2.3. Crystals have characteristic shapes in the urine of which oxalate, cystine and triple phosphate are some of the more common types.

Culture of the urine

Urine is readily contaminated from the wall of the urethra, prepuce or vulva, and by air-borne dust entering the specimen bottle. Urine is an excellent culture medium: indeed it was chosen by Pasteur for this reason in his classical experiments. At room temperature air-borne contaminants will grow rapidly so that specimens of urine should either be plated out at once, or if there is to be any delay, kept in a refrigerator. Infection

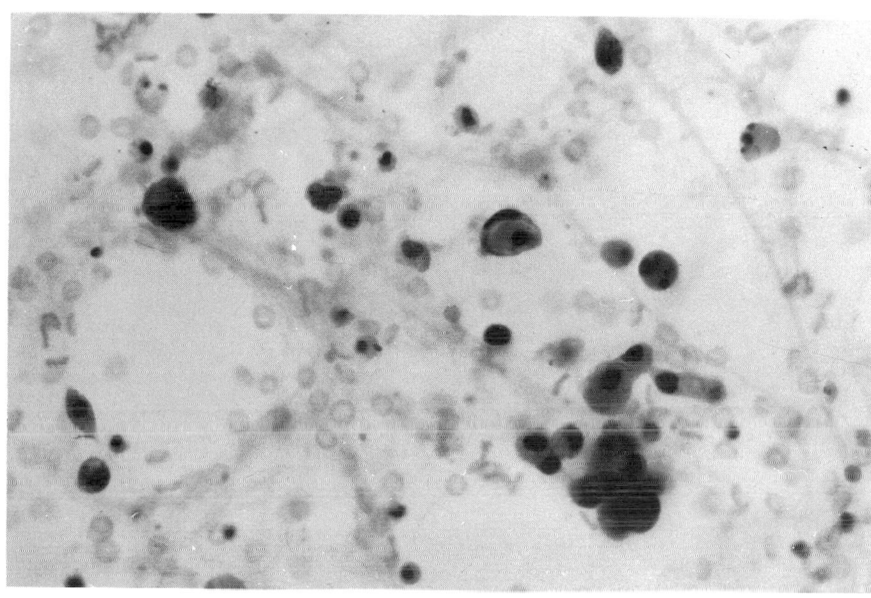

Fig. 2.4. The urine is fixed, centrifuged and stained with Papanicolaou's stain. Cancer cells have large hyperchromatic nuclei.

may be mistakenly diagnosed if urine has been allowed to stand around at room temperature for several hours before it gets to the laboratory.

Even if cultured promptly, some of the organisms that appear in the urine will be contaminants. If urine is mixed up with a culture medium, every organism will produce a single colony, and counting the colonies makes it possible to distinguish between 5×10^5 per ml, the number that signifies real infection, from the lesser number that is likely to be caused by contamination (Fig. 2.6).

Inspection of the freshly passed urine is still exceedingly useful: clear urine the colour of white wine is almost never infected. This can be verified by looking at the urine with the microscope: in infected urine myriads of bacteria can easily be seen under the high power.

In the busy practitioner's surgery a useful way to make a reasonably accurate 'colony count' is to use the 'dip-slide' method (Fig. 2.7). Cheap plastic slides coated with culture media are dipped in the fresh urine, drained off and placed in a sterile sealed bottle which is put in a warm place (e.g. an incubator or near a radiator). Within 12 hours a glance at the chart supplied with the dip-slides shows with tolerable accuracy whether there is a significant infection or more likely only contamination.

When it is really important to know if there is urinary infection urine may be obtained directly from the bladder by suprapubic puncture (Fig. 2.8) using a fine needle: this is almost painless and quite safe.

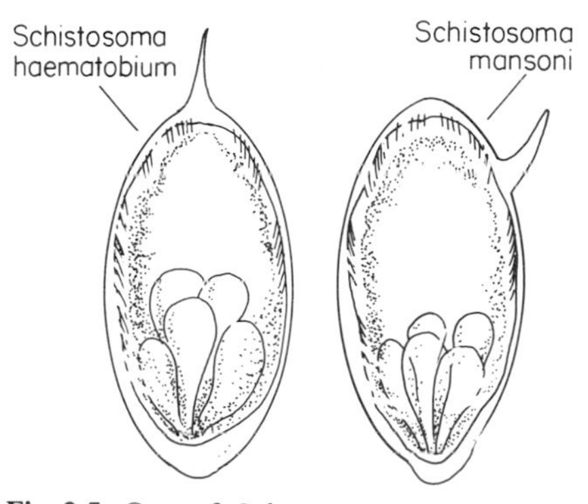

Fig. 2.5. Ova of *Schistosoma* contain live *Miracidia* which will hatch out in fresh-water. A terminal spine is typical of *S. haematobium*, a lateral spine of *S. mansoni*.

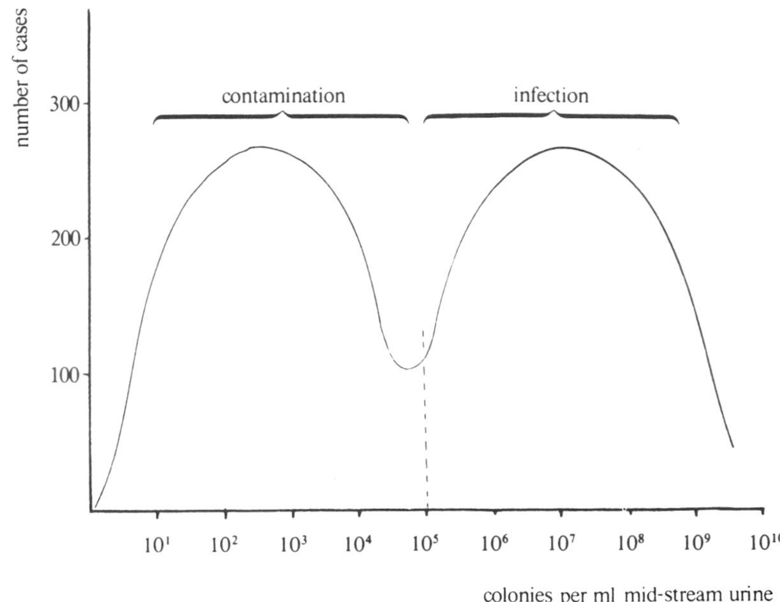

Fig. 2.6. Quantitative differences between urinary contamination and infection.

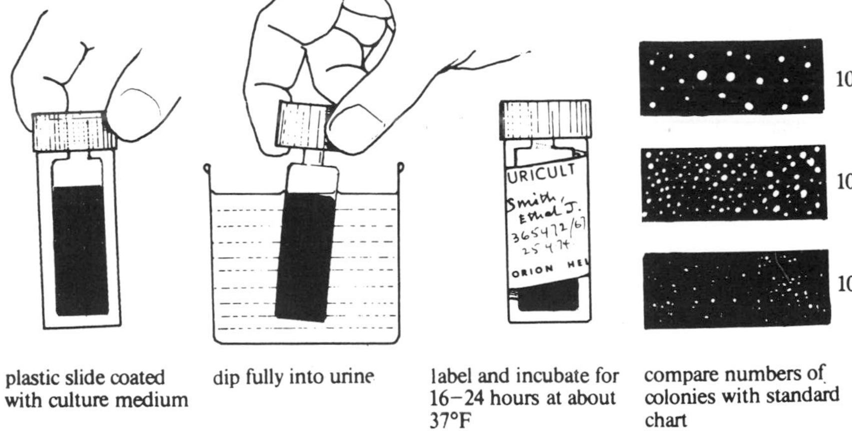

Fig. 2.7. Use of the dip inoculum slide.

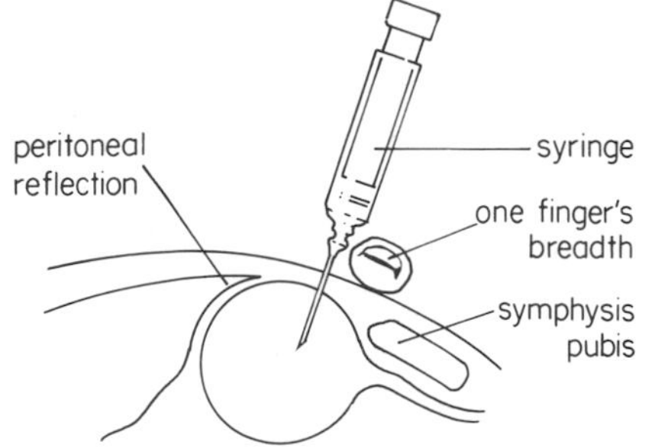

Fig. 2.8. Method of obtaining urine from the bladder by direct suprapubic puncture. This avoids errors due to contamination. *Any* colonies, however few, obtained from this specimen are significant.

IMAGING OF THE URINARY TRACT

The plain abdominal radiograph ('scout film': KUB)

Radiological examinations begin with a plain radiograph before any contrast medium is injected: this can be very informative. The interpretation of the KUB film starts with the 'four Ss': side, skeleton, soft tissues, stones (Fig. 2.9).

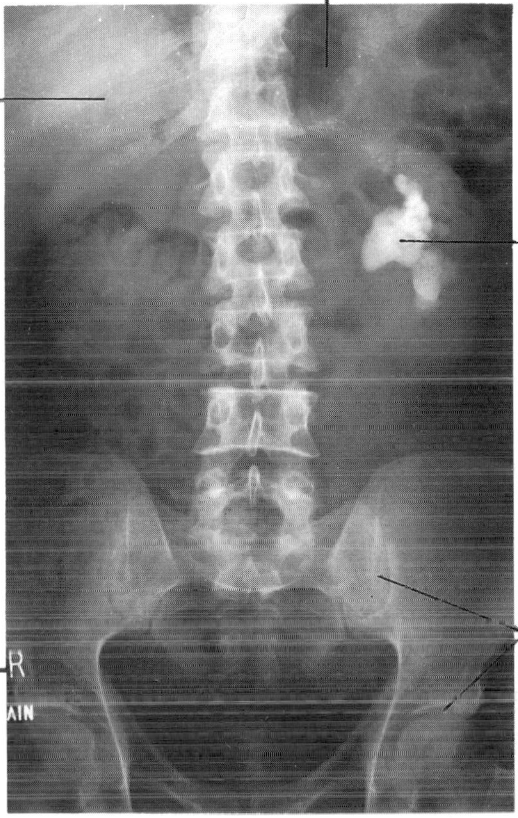

Fig. 2.9. The plain film: check the 4 Ss. Is the *side* correctly marked (look for the liver and gastric air-bubble as well as the radiographer's sign)? Is the *skeleton* normal? Is there any obvious abnormality in the *soft tissue* shadows? Are there any radio-opaque shadows that might be *stones*?

Side

Radiographers are only human and can easily put the wrong letter on the film: always check that the soft tissue shadow of the liver is on the right side and the gastric air bubble on the left.

Skeleton

Examine the spine, ribs, hips and sacroiliac joints: watch out for osteoblastic and osteoclastic metastases, ankylosing spondylitis and disease in the hip joints which may have forced the patient to take analgesics in excess.

Soft tissues

Especially in a fat person, when the kidneys are surrounded by radiolucent adipose tissue, one can make out the renal outlines, but these should always be checked carefully against the nephrogram phase of the urogram. Look for the soft tissue shadows of a distended bladder or an enlarged uterus and note Riedel's lobe of the liver and an enlarged spleen.

Stones

Any radiodense shadow in the line of the urinary tract raises the suspicion of a calculus. If there is doubt, when the shadow lies in front of the soft tissue shadow of the kidney, films are taken in inspiration and expiration to move the kidneys up and down: adjacent tissues containing calcified material such as the costal cartilages will change position relative to the kidney. Watch out for gall-stones, calcified fibroids, and the presence of phleboliths in the pelvis — often a cause of confusion with calculi in the line of the ureter. Calcified nodes are common in the mesentery.

Ultrasound

Sonar, as used to map the sea floor to find shoals of fish or enemy submarines, has become a most useful, almost universal investigation in urology. It provides a picture of structures deep in the abdomen: it is safe, painless, uses no ionizing radiation and requires neither needles nor contrast media. For these reasons it has become almost an extension of the palpating fingers of the clinician.

Everyone will remember how one could irritate the teacher at school by making the chalk squeak on the blackboard. This is the simplest reminder that sound may be produced from crystals by applying force. It also reminds us that the higher the pitch of the sound the more penetrating it can be. The force that is applied to a crystal can be an electric one, and with an appropriate current, the sound waves may be of an ultrasonic frequency that penetrates soft tissues of the body but is reflected from bone and the interface between tissues of different density, e.g. the calices and the parenchyma of the kidney, or the adenoma and capsule of the prostate (Fig. 2.10).

To get a picture the returning echoes are received by a crystal which (by the reverse process) transforms the sound impulse into an electrical one which is processed as an image of a cross-section through the body (Fig. 2.11).

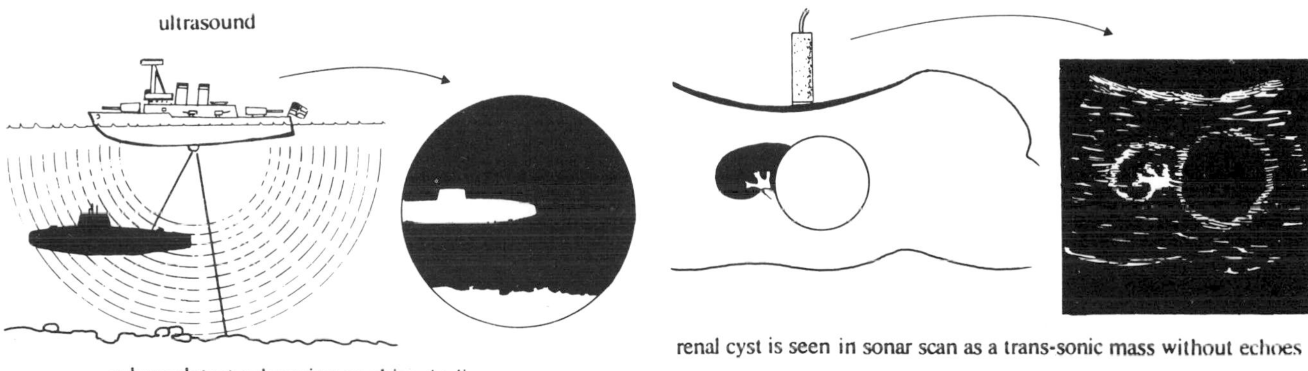

Fig. 2.10. Ultrasound.

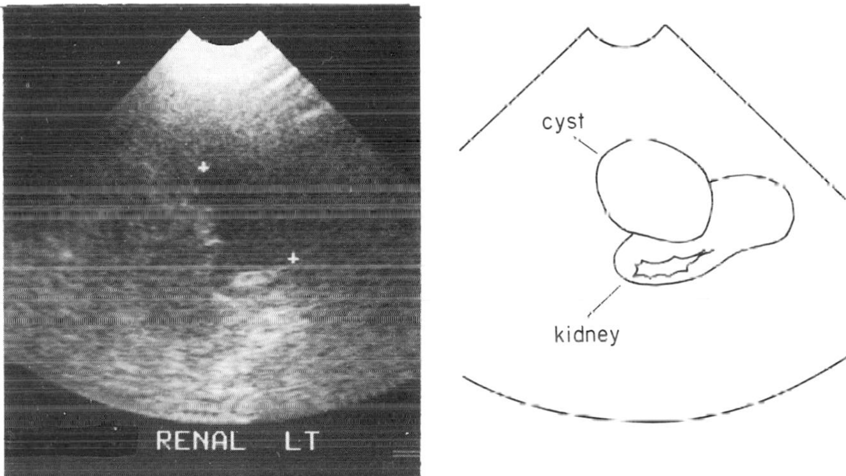

Fig. 2.11. Ultrasound picture of a kidney containing a renal cyst: white crosses mark the edges of the cyst to measure it.

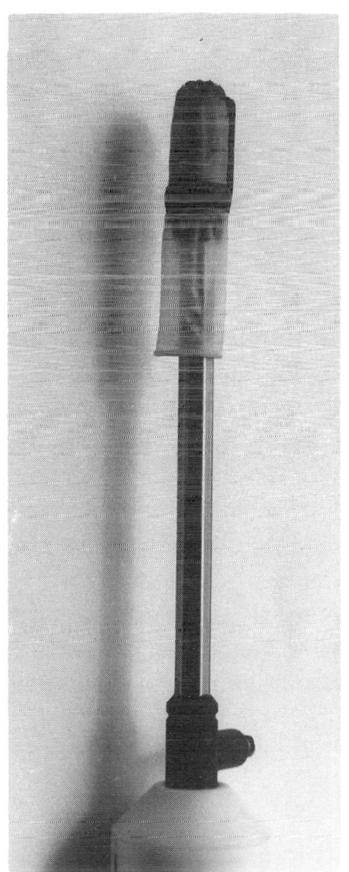

Fig. 2.12. Ultrasound rectal probe used to give an image of the prostate, vesicles and bladder.

The piezo-electric crystals which emit and receive the ultrasound waves are mounted in various convenient forms: some are mounted in 'sector arrays' which give a slice like a wedge of cheese through the tissue, others are placed on rotating heads on the tips of probes that can be put into the bladder or the rectum (Fig. 2.12). The images vary in quality and all suffer from the drawback that they are quite easy to understand when seen moving on the screen, but difficult to interpret from a still picture. For this reason, when the surgeon has to make the decision whether or not to operate, unless he performs the ultrasound examination himself,

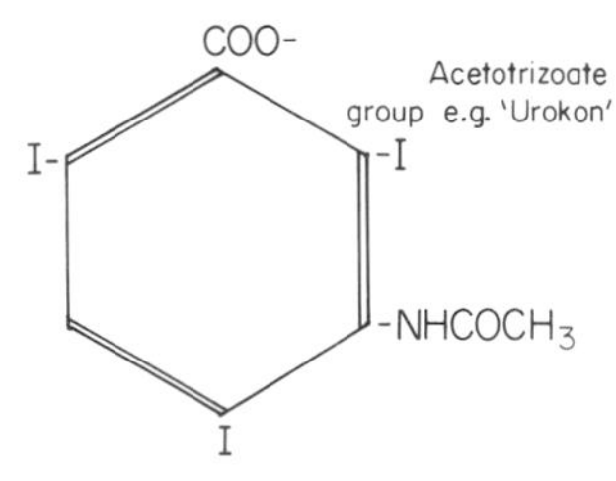

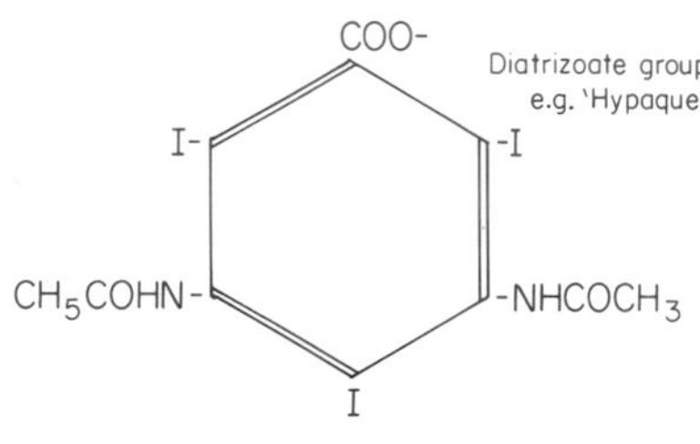

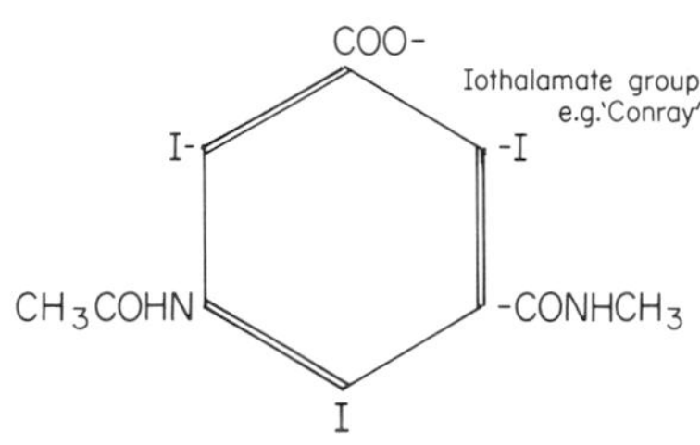

Fig. 2.13. All the commonly used contrast media employed for urography are based on benzoic acid.

he is likely to insist on the older methods of imaging that use X-rays with the addition of contrast media. Of these the most common and most important investigation is the intravenous urogram.

The intravenous urogram (IVU, IVP)

Iodine is relatively opaque to X-rays because of its high atomic number but free ionic iodine is very toxic. To make it possible to give it intravenously the iodine atoms are attached to benzoic acid in one of a family of compounds (Fig. 2.13) which are given as sodium or methylglucamine salts. A large dose is given — usually containing about 300 mg of iodine/kg body weight, or 1 ml/kg of the usual commercial preparations. In this concentration the fluid is very hypertonic and may irritate the vein causing pain along the arm and shoulder, and sometimes actual thrombosis of the vein (often misinterpreted as infection). When the contrast medium gets into the systemic circulation there is often a feeling of nausea and flushing. Neither of these side-effects is serious. If the hypertonic contrast medium gets into the tissues outside the vein it will give rise to some inflammation.

Much more serious are the effects that follow from allergy to the contrast medium. These can cover the complete spectrum from a trivial urticarial rash which clears with an antihistamine, to angioneurotic oedema of the glottis and trachea, widespread vasodilatation, hypotension and cardiac arrest. These are manifestations of allergy to the whole iodobenzoate molecule, not to free iodine and it is useless to perform skin testing with iodine beforehand, and of little value to give the first few millilitres of the injection slowly. The important thing is to realise that a mild allergic reaction can be a warning of a more serious one next time. In all cases where contrast medium is to be injected intravenously make sure that the essentials for treating an allergic response are readily available, e.g. adrenaline, hydrocortisone, oxygen, a face mask, an airway and a 'minitracheostomy' kit. The emergency telephone number to summon the cardiac arrest team should be known to the X-ray staff. Fatal reactions occur in 1:200 000 IVUs — but millions of IVUs are performed every year.

Handling of the contrast medium by the kidney

It takes 15–20 seconds for the intravenously injected contrast medium to reach the kidney so that films taken in the first minute will catch the contrast lying in the glomeruli and proximal tubule. Most of the tubular reabsorption of water takes place in the proximal tubule so this first film

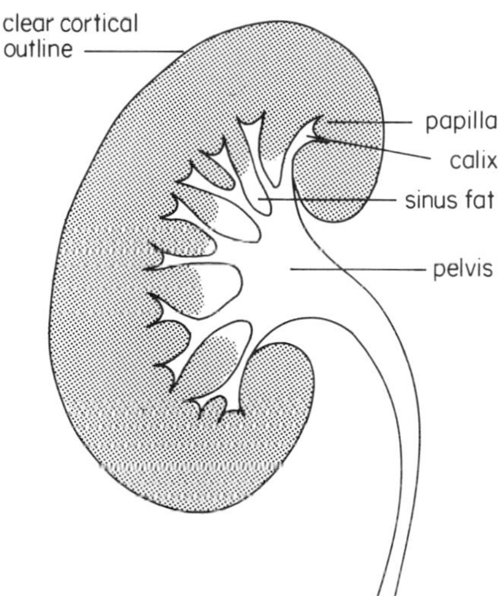

Fig. 2.14. The 'nephrogram phase' of the IVU. The contrast medium has just reached the glomeruli and proximal tubule.

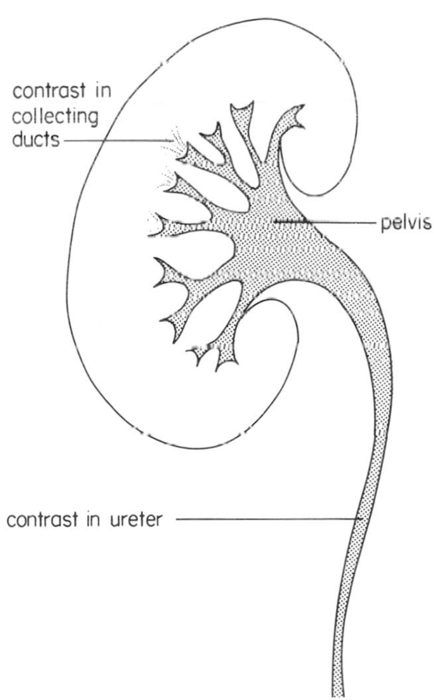

Fig. 2.15. The 'pyelogram phase' of the IVU. Most of the contrast has now reached the calices and pelvis.

of the IVU series gives a good image of the renal parenchyma — the *nephrogram* (Fig. 2.14) and when it is particularly important to get a clear picture of the renal outline, e.g. when scarring or a tumour are suspected, these nephrogram pictures are supplemented by tomograms to eliminate unwanted shadows from gas in the bowel.

In obstruction the rate at which the filtrate flows down the tubule is slowed up and the nephrogram is more pronounced, more dense, and longer lasting. When a stone is stuck in the ureter the nephrogram may persist for up to 24 hours after the original injection of the contrast medium.

In a normal patient the flow of filtrate containing the contrast medium quickly reaches and fills the calices and pelvis to give the *pyelogram* (Fig. 2.15). To distend the calices many radiologists prefer to compress the ureters by tightening a band around the abdomen for the first 10 to 15 minutes. Films are taken after the band has been released to depict the whole length of the ureter and to include the bladder (Fig. 2.16).

The patient is then asked to empty the bladder, and if it is appropriate to show the urethra, oblique films are taken as the patient passes urine (the *voiding urethrogram*). In suspected obstruction to the outflow from the bladder a *post-micturition film* is taken which gives a very accurate and useful measure of the volume of residual urine.

A good radiographic image of the kidney does not necessarily mean good renal function. When one kidney is very small and scarred most of the solute load will be eliminated by the good kidney, but in the contracted kidney the small amount of filtrate that passes slowly along its convoluted tubules is well-concentrated and gives a clear radiographic image.

Preparations for the IVU

It is common practice to deprive the patient of fluid for 6 hours before an IVU. This gives a slight increase in the concentration of contrast in the filtrate and hence in the quality of the radiograph but it is a measure which should be used with great care: it is futile in patients whose impaired renal function makes it impossible for them to concentrate urine anyway; it can be dangerous in diabetes; in myeloma it may lead to fatal sludging of protein in the tubules.

In many centres it is still the practice to purge the patient before an IVU to get rid of unwanted gas shadows. The removal of the shadows caused by faeces and gas in the colon seldom justifies the discomfort of the colic caused by the purgative, and to postpone a badly needed urogram merely because 'the patient is not properly prepared' is seldom justified.

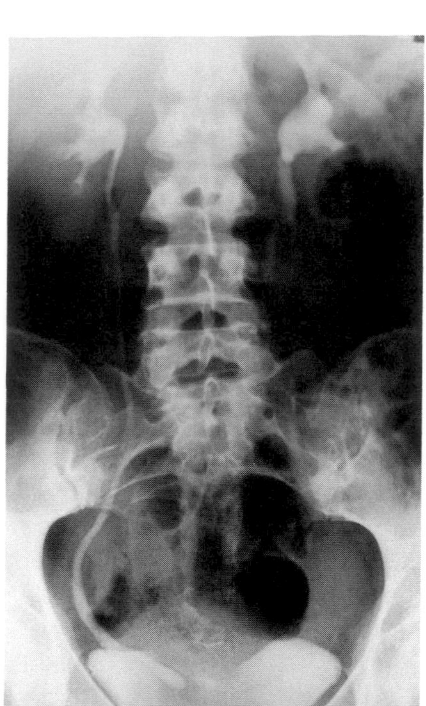

Fig. 2.16. The entire length of the ureter is depicted when the compression band is released. In this case it shows a round swelling at the lower end of the right ureter — a 'ureterocele'.

Retrograde urography

A fine ureteric catheter may be inserted into the ureteric orifice via a rigid or flexible cystoscope (see p. 161) and contrast medium is injected through the catheter to outline the upper tract. This is particularly useful when exact detail is needed in the calices (e.g. when a small filling defect is suspicious of a tumour) and when attempting to discover the cause of obstruction in a ureter. There are two types of ureteric catheter: one is passed right up into the renal pelvis (Fig. 2.17), the other has a bulb shaped tip which is placed in the ureteric orifice through which contrast is injected along the length of the ureter — *ureterogram* (Fig. 2.18). Retrograde ureterograms and pyelograms are nowadays performed under fluoroscopic control using the image intensifier.

Antegrade or descending urography

The renal pelvis is punctured with a fine needle under ultrasound control or after giving a dose of intravenous contrast medium. A fine flexible guide-wire is passed along the needle which is then withdrawn, and over the guide-wire is slipped a narrow cannula. This is the so-called *percutaneous nephrostomy* (Fig. 2.19). It is the first step in the whole range of percutaneous operations on the kidney which have wrought a major revolution in the treatment of stones and other lesions of the kidney within the last 5 years. Contrast injected into the cannula is used to define lesions inside the kidney and ureter, and is of great help when the ureter is obstructed (see p. 141). The cannula can also be used to measure the pressure inside the renal pelvis when saline is infused — a test employed in the diagnosis of upper tract obstruction (the *Whitaker test*).

Cystogram

For most purposes the image of the bladder provided towards the end of the standard IVU is sufficiently clear to reveal diverticula or large tumours of the bladder (Fig. 2.20), but in the diagnosis of vesicoureteric reflux and incontinence it is necessary to fill the bladder with diluted contrast medium and watch the patient passing urine on the fluoroscope. In the investigation of neuropathic lesions of the bladder the cystogram is combined with measurements of the pressure inside the bladder and of the urine flow rate — the *micturating cystometrogram* (see p. 156).

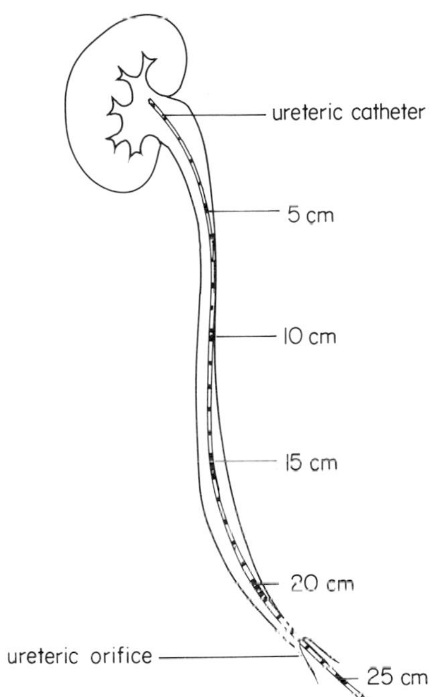

Fig. 2.17. Retrograde urography: a ureteric catheter is passed by means of the operating cystoscope up the ureter to the kidney. Urine may be aspirated from the kidney and examined for TB or malignant cells, and contrast injected to give a clear radiograph.

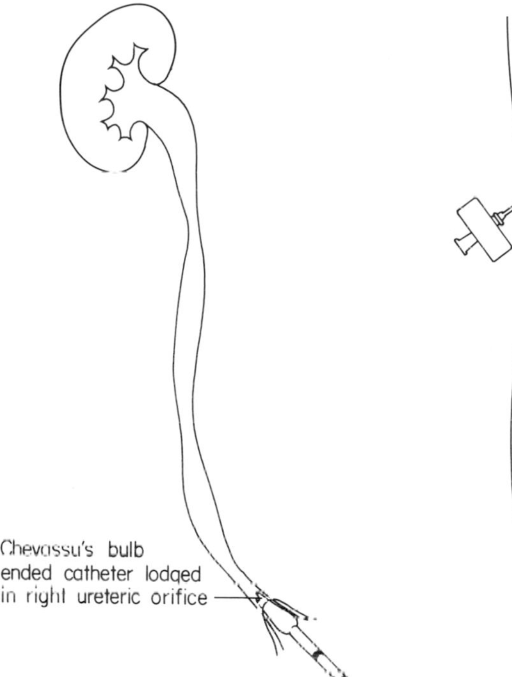

Fig. 2.18. Contrast medium is injected up the ureter to display the entire upper urinary tract.

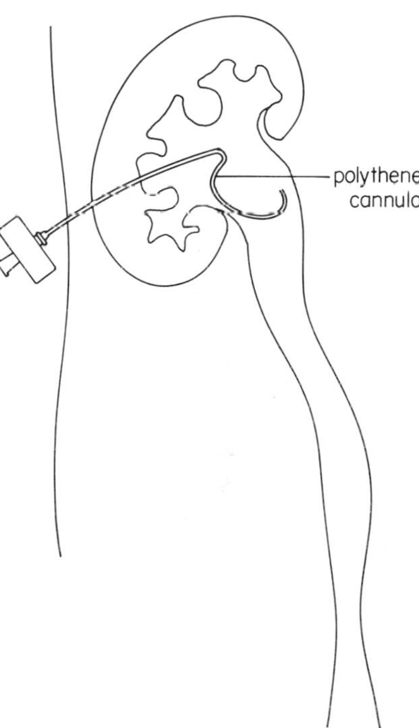

Fig. 2.19. Antegrade urography and the 'medical nephrostomy'; the cannula may be left in the kidney to keep it decompressed.

Urethrography

The descending urethrogram at the end of the IVU is often clear enough to define a urethral stricture, but in planning an operation more clear definition may be needed, and this is provided by injecting water-soluble contrast medium into the urethra through a small catheter — the *ascending urethrogram* (see p. 243).

Angiography

A fine flexible guide-wire is passed through a needle into the femoral artery, and a cannula with a curved tip is slid over the guidewire and directed under X-ray control until it slips into the opening of the renal artery, when contrast is injected into the renal artery to obtain an arteriogram (Fig. 2.21). This is used when stenosis of the renal artery is suspected of being the cause of hypertension (see p. 113), or in the diagnosis of renal parenchymal cancers (see p. 101).

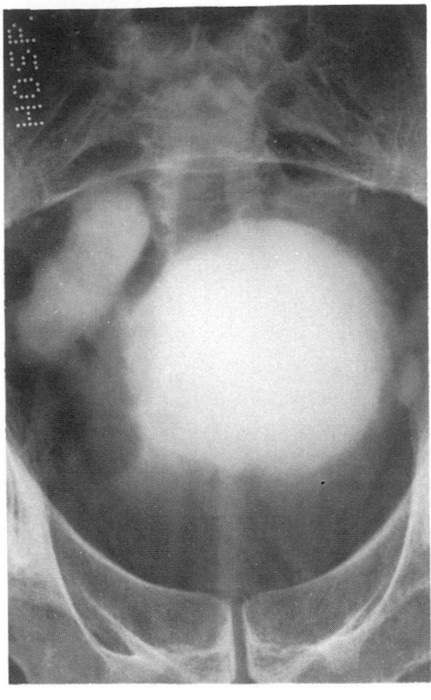

Fig. 2.20. The cystogram film taken at the end of the IVU series. There is a filling defect on the right of the bladder as well as a diverticulum. Cystoscopy showed an invasive carcinoma involving the far wall of the diverticulum.

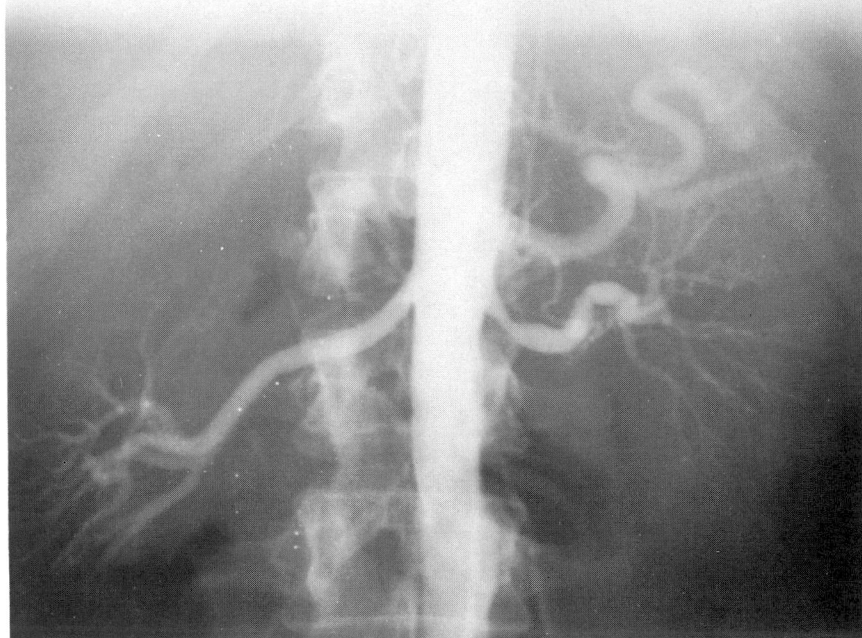

Fig. 2.21. 'Flush' arteriogram showing both renal arteries and the splenic artery. There is a narrowing about 1 cm from the origin of the left renal artery. The patient had hypertension.

Similar studies of the vena cava are performed when it is thought that there may be extension of a renal cell carcinoma into the vena cava — *cavography* (Fig. 2.22).

Subtraction angiography

In any of these angiographic studies the finer vessels are often confused by shadows of bones and gas bubbles in the adjacent bowel. To remove these unwanted shadows a plain X-ray is taken just before giving the contrast medium: a positive print is made of this, which is then photographed against the film taken after the contrast has been injected. By this trick the bones and gas shadows are 'subtracted' leaving only the blood vessels showing (Fig. 2.23).

This trick can now be performed by a computer which produces *digital vascular imaging* (DVI) — this has the additional advantage of needing much smaller doses of the contrast medium which can therefore be given through a much finer arterial catheter or even given intravenously.

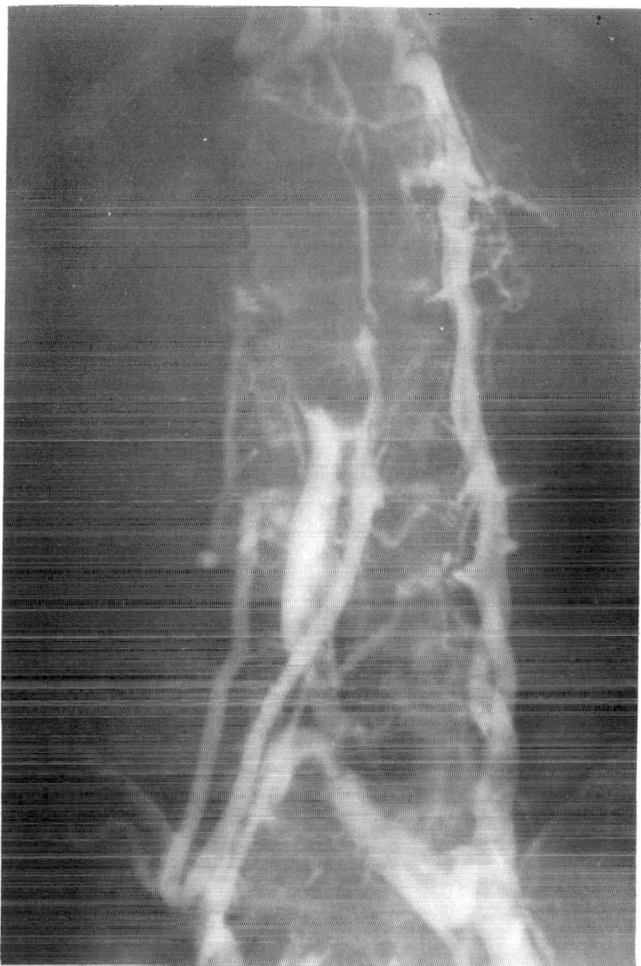

Fig. 2.22. Cavogram obtained by injecting contrast up the right femoral vein. The vena cava is blocked by extension of a carcinoma of the kidney, and the contrast finds its way back to the heart through collateral veins.

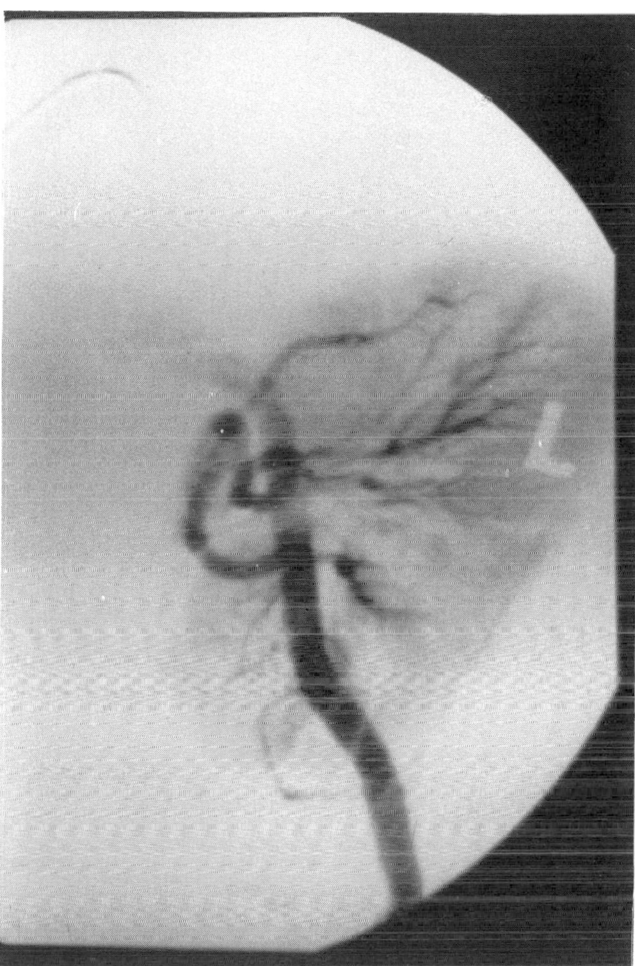

Fig. 2.23. Subtraction angiogram of a renal transplant. The transplant has been put into the left iliac fossa. The contrast has been injected into the left common iliac artery. The donor renal artery is anastomosed to the internal iliac artery.

Lymphangiography

Patent blue violet is injected into the first two web spaces of the dorsum of the foot. After about an hour the blue dye has been taken up into the lymphatics. Under local anaesthesia one of these lymphatics is cannulated and an oily contrast medium is very slowly injected so that it runs up the lymphatics of the leg and by the next day has been taken up by the lymph nodes, first of the groin and then of the pelvis and para-aortic region (Fig. 2.24). The test is still used occasionally in diagnosis and planning treatment of tumours of the penis and testis, but has very largely been superseded by computer assisted tomography scanning.

Computer assisted tomography — CT scan

In conventional X-ray imaging the picture is a contact photograph made from a screen which glows (like a television screen) when it is bombarded by X-rays (Fig. 2.25). The screen and the silver emulsion which responds to its glow are not sufficiently sensitive to detect fine shades of grey — the small differences in radiodensity that exist between one soft tissue and another. But there are electronic crystals which are a hundred times more capable of detecting these small differences. In the CT scanner a battery of these crystal detectors is mounted in a large ring through which a couch can be slid by centimetre steps (Fig. 2.26). A computer receives the information provided by the ring of detectors and processes it in the form of a slice that shows not only the bones, but also the soft tissues (Fig. 2.27).

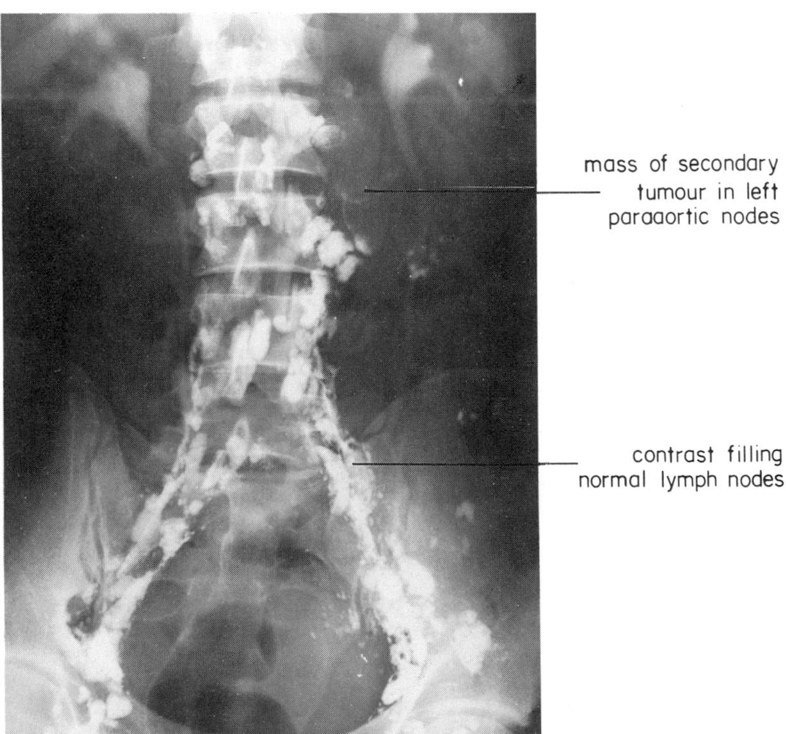

Fig. 2.24. Lymphangiogram used to reveal abdominal metastases from testicular tumour. Here the large mass of growth has displaced the lymphatics.

Godfrey Hounsfield, wartime radar expert and designer of the first chip computer, invented the CT scanner. He devised an arbitrary scale of values (the Hounsfield numbers) for the radiodensity of the different tissues: 0 is the density of water, +1000 for bone, −1000 for air. Fat is about −100. Intravenous contrast medium will make tissues such as the

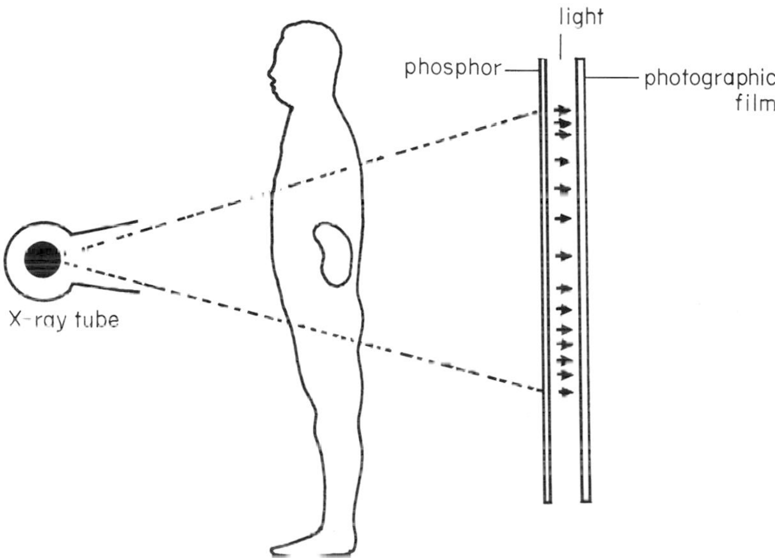

Fig. 2.25. The principle of a conventional X-ray: the cassette contains a phosphor which, when struck by X-rays, emits light which activates the silver halide emulsion in the photographic film.

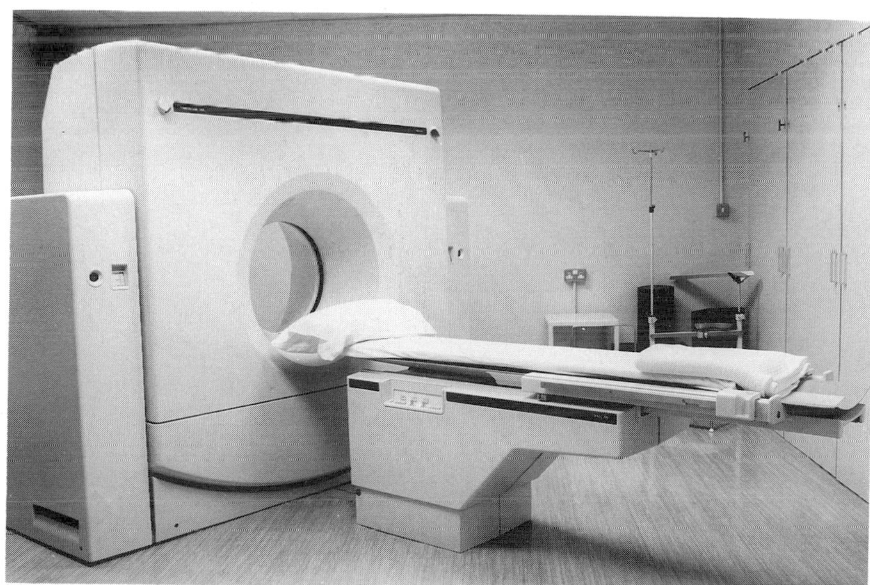

Fig. 2.26. Computer assisted tomography. The patient lies on the couch and is moved centimetre by centimetre through the doughnut containing the sensors.

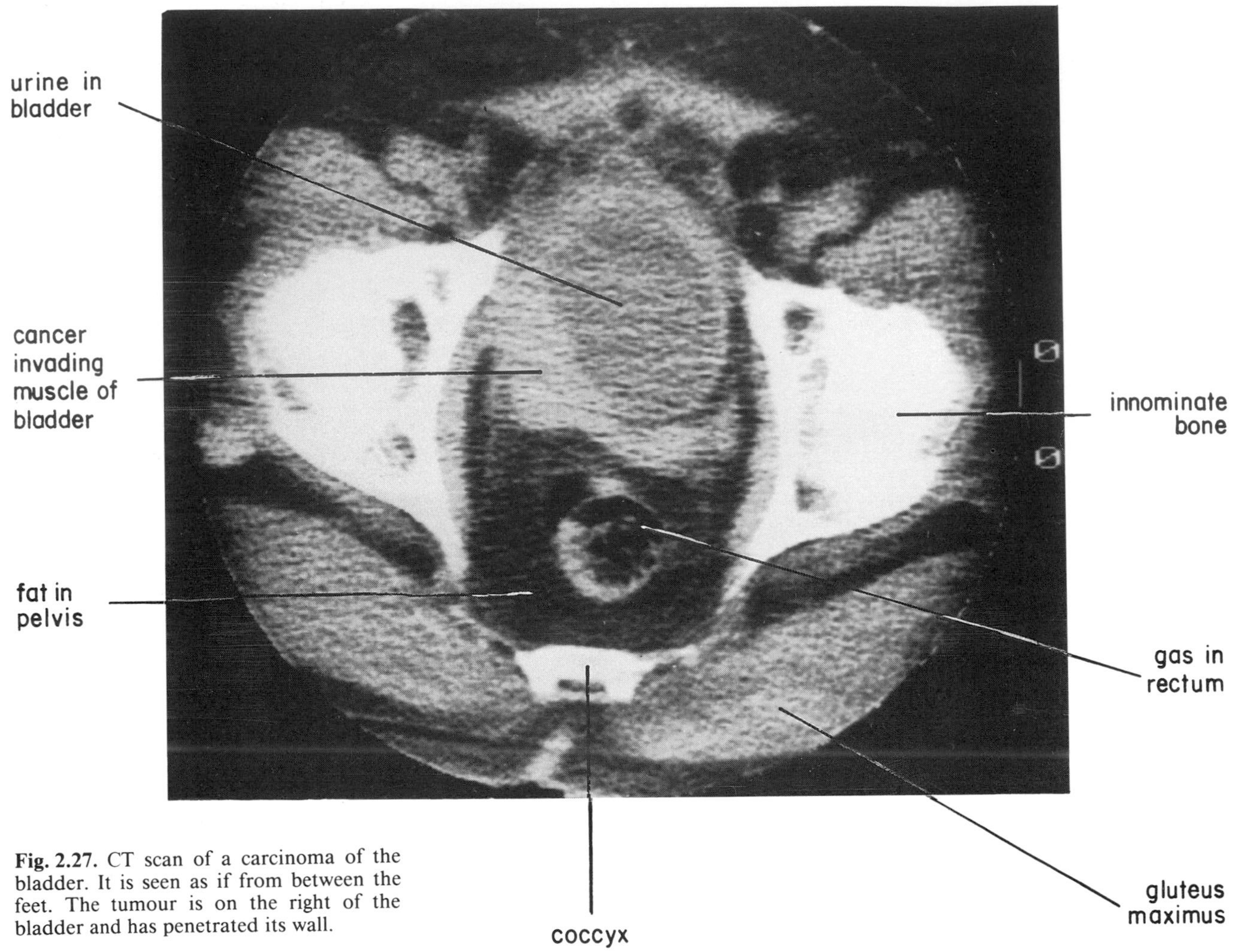

Fig. 2.27. CT scan of a carcinoma of the bladder. It is seen as if from between the feet. The tumour is on the right of the bladder and has penetrated its wall.

kidney even more dense (enhancement) and dilute barium will outline the bowel so that in this way the extent of a tumour can be mapped, lymph node metastases can be defined, and surgical excision or radiotherapy may be planned with accuracy.

Magnetic resonance imaging (MRI)

Images which at first glance resemble those of the CT scanner can be obtained by an even newer method which does not use X-rays. It relies upon a wonderfully simple effect. Everyone remembers playing with a toy gyroscope: its axis could be tilted but it would remain spinning. Every atom in every tissue of the body behaves like a minute gyroscope

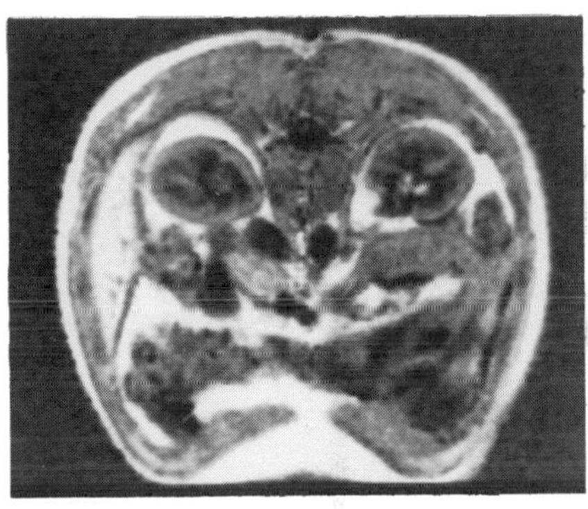

Fig. 2.28 Magnetic resonance image at the level of the kidneys. Note that the bones of the vertebrae and ribs do not obtrude, and the maximum contrast is between the parenchyma of the kidneys and the surrounding fat. Courtesy of Dr. G. Bidder.

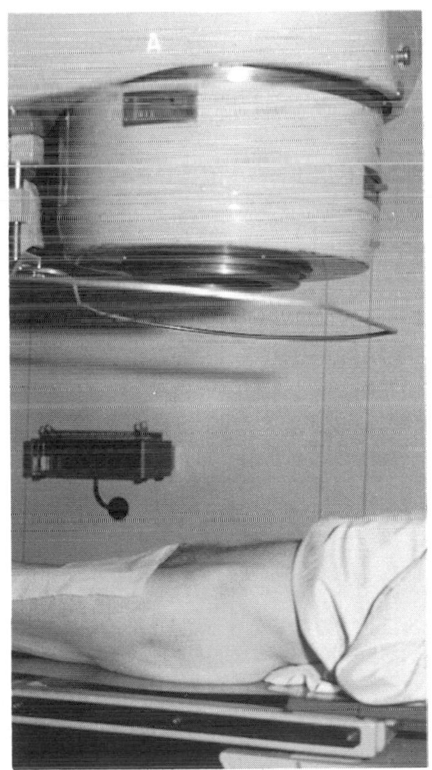

Fig. 2.29. Patient undergoing a scan with the gamma camera.

spinning on its axis. A very strong magnetic field will tilt these axes. When the magnetic field is turned off, the little gyroscopes return to their normal position and as they do, they emit a tiny pulse of electromagnetic energy (magnetic resonance) which can be detected by suitable electronic sensors. When these sensors are built into a ring a computer can make a picture from the information supplied to it much as with the CT scan (Fig. 2.28).

Magnetic resonance can be used to study different atoms: usually the instrument is adjusted to the hydrogen, i.e. the water content of the body, but it can be set to other atoms and so provide not only anatomical information but also physiological changes, e.g. ischaemia. In the nervous system MRI can detect areas affected by an infarct or changed by multiple sclerosis. As a method of imaging MRI has hardly touched urology, but there is no doubt that it will become a most useful way of mapping the spread of tumours. The slices that the MRI computers can provide need not only be coronal — they can be sagittal or oblique.

At the time of writing MRI machines are being rapidly improved and are all exceedingly expensive but the writer predicts that by the time this little book appears in another edition MRI (like CT scanning) will have become a routine investigation.

Isotope studies

Radionuclides are not only used for imaging, but also to measure various aspects of renal and other body functions. The most simple apparatus consisted of a pair of Geiger counters pointing at each of the kidneys, which measured how much isotope was accumulated in each kidney — this was the original *'isotope renogram'*. Today the instrument is a battery of Geiger counters mounted in a dish — *the Gamma Camera* (Fig. 2.29) — which can not only give an image of the tissue at which it is pointed (Fig. 2.30), but also a measure the rise and fall of the radioactivity as the isotopes are handled by the tissue under study (Fig. 2.31).

In the kidney two main types of radionuclide are used: one (diethylene triamine pentacetic acid — DTPA) is used to measure glomerular filtration and to study the rate at which this flows through the kidney, and is extremely useful in the investigation of obstruction. The other (dimercaptosuccinic acid — DMSA) is taken up and excreted by the renal tubules — and is used to give an image of the renal parenchyma and a measure of tubular function.

^{99m}Tc MDP is taken up by bone is proportion to its blood flow and detects areas where the bone is more vascular, e.g. because of metastatic tumour, fracture, or osteoarthritis (Fig. 2.32). It is valuable in the

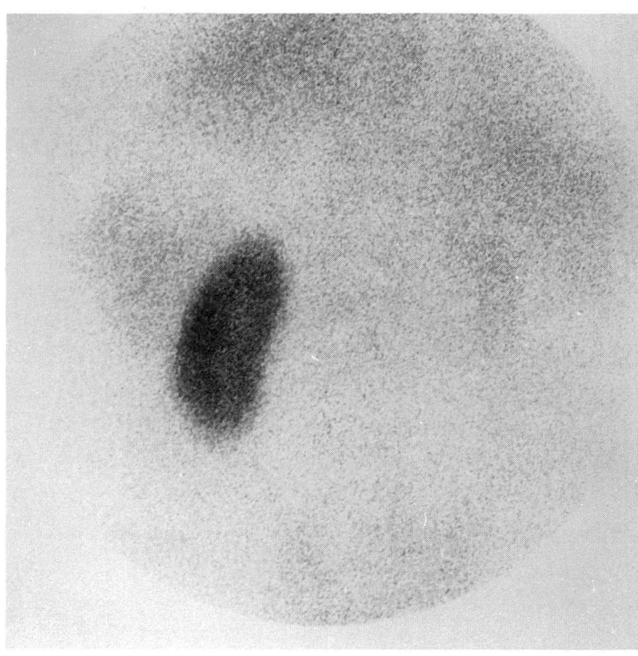

Fig. 2.30. Gamma camera scan showing a normal kidney on the right side but almost no isotope on the left. The patient had a tiny left kidney almost destroyed by scarring.

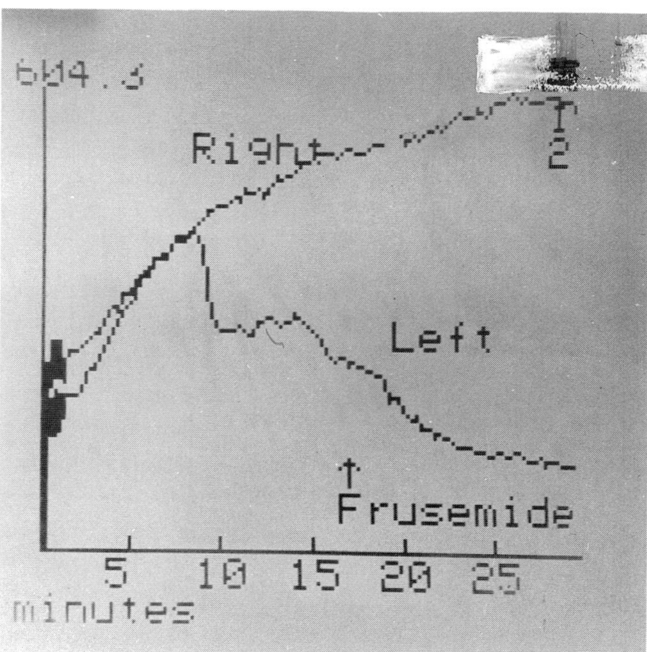

Fig. 2.31. Isotope renogram. On the left the isotope accumulates in the renal pelvis but as soon as frusemide is given it is washed out of the system. On the right side it continues to accumulate showing obstruction. At operation there was a fibrous stenosis at the junction of the renal pelvis and ureter.

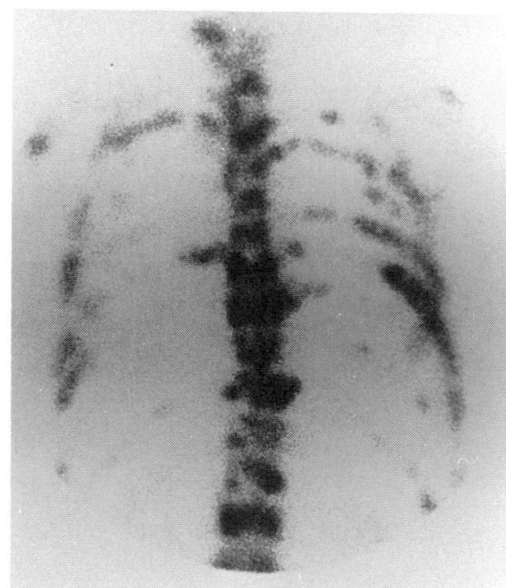

Fig. 2.32. The ^{99m}Tc MDP is taken up according to the blood flow to the bone. Where there are deposits of prostatic cancer, there are 'hot spots' showing widespread metastases.

diagnosis and follow-up of cancer of the prostate but it is necessary to keep in mind that there is more than one reason for a 'hot spot' in the bone and that, when necessary, the bone scan should be supplemented by appropriate X-rays.

FURTHER READING

Arm JP, Peile EB, Rainford DJ, Strike PW & Tettmar RE (1986) Significance of dipstick haematuria 1. Correlation with microscopy of the urine; 2. Correlation with pathology. *British Journal of Urology* **58**, 211–23.

Britton KE (1985) Radionuclide studies. In: Whitfield HN & Hendry WF (Eds) *Textbook of Genitourinary Sugrery*. Churchill Livingstone, Edinburgh. pp. 67–103.

Cotes PM (1988) Erythropoietin: the developing story. *British Medical Journal* **296**, 805–6.

Dent TL, Strodel WE & Wurcotte JG (1985) *Surgical Endoscopy*. Year Book Publications, Chicago.

Foster MA (1984) *Magnetic Resonance in Medicine and Biology*. Pergamon Press, Oxford.

Lee JKT, Sagel SS & Stanley RJ (1983) *Computed Body Tomography*. Raven Press, New York.

Lote CJ (1987) *Principles of Renal Physiology*. 3rd Ed. Croom Helm, London.

Mundy AR (Ed) (1988) *Scientific Basis of Urology*. Churchill Livingstone, Edinburgh.

Reidy JF (1988) Reactions to contrast media and steroid pretreatment. *British Medical Journal* **296**, 809.

Ritchie CD, Bevan EA & Collier StJ (1986) Importance of occult haematuria found at screening. *British Medical Journal* **292**, 681–3.

Sherwood T (1985) Basic uroradiological investigations. In: Whitfield HN & Hendry WF (Eds) *Textbook of Genitourinary Surgery*. Churchill Livingstone, Edinburgh. pp 5–21.

Shirley IM, Blackwell RJ, Cusick G, Farman DJ & Vicary FR (1978) *A User's Guide to Diagnostic Ultrasound*. Pitman Medical, Tunbridge Wells.

Thompson IM (1987) The evaluation of microscopic hematuria: a population-based study. *Journal of Urology* **138**, 1189–90.

3 The Kidney — Structure and Function

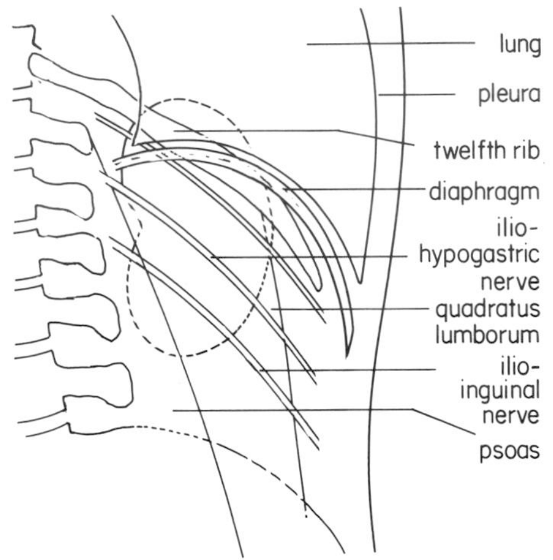

Fig. 3.1. Posterior relations of the kidney.

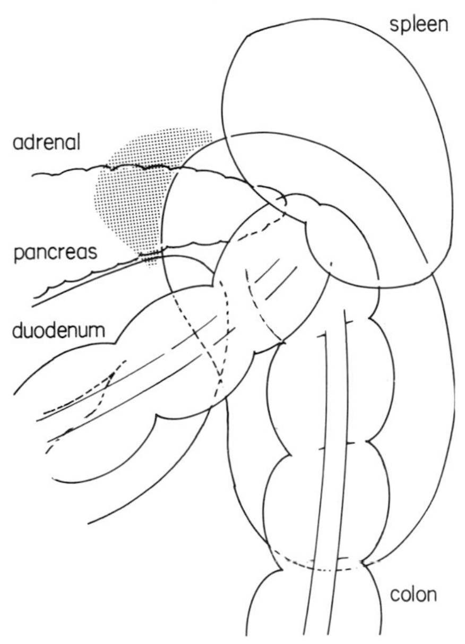

Fig. 3.2. The left kidney lies behind the colon, duodenum, pancreas and spleen.

SURGICAL RELATIONS OF THE KIDNEY

Behind each kidney lie the 12th rib, diaphragm, pleura and lung (Fig. 3.1). Below the rib the kidney lies upon the quadratus lumborum and psoas muscles. The ilioinguinal and hypogastric nerves traverse the quadratus lumborum muscle and are easily injured in operations on the kidney. The hilum of the kidney moves with respiration up and down around the level of the second and third transverse processes of the lumbar vertebrae.

In front of the left kidney are the spleen and tail of the pancreas, the duodenojejunal flexure and the descending colon, any of which may be densely stuck to the kidney by inflammation or cancer and injured at operation (Figs 3.2, 3.3).

In front of the right kidney are the ascending colon, the second part of the duodenum and the common bile duct (Figs 3.4, 3.5).

Medial to the left kidney is the aorta and medial to the right the vena cava: above and medial to each kidney lies the suprarenal gland. These surgical relations govern the choice of surgical approach and determine what complications are likely to be seen after operations on the kidney.

SURGICAL APPROACHES TO THE KIDNEY

Posterior incisions

Twelfth rib approach

Most operations on the kidney are performed through an incision through the bed of the 12th rib which skirts the pleura (but sometimes opens it) and is carried forward in the gap between the 11th and 12th subcostal neurovascular bundles, cutting the latissimus dorsi and the external and internal oblique muscles, and splitting the transversus in the line of its fibres (Fig. 3.6).

Vertical lumbotomy

One may also reach the kidney through a vertical incision along the lateral border of sacrospinalis, freeing the attachments of the abdominal

muscles from the lumbar fascia (Fig. 3.7). This incision gives rather limited access and is mainly used for relatively simple operations on small kidneys.

Anterior incisions

When it is necessary to perform a wide resection of the kidney, e.g. in carcinoma, the anterior transperitoneal approach is used, with a transverse or long midline incision according to the build of the patient (Figs 3.8, 3.9). The colon and duodenum are reflected medially to give access to the renal vessels (Figs 3.10, 3.11).

The surgical relations of the kidney explain most of the common postoperative complications. They all give rise to postoperative pain on breathing and coughing, so *atelectasis* of the basal segments of the lung is common: it is even more common if the pleura has been opened in the

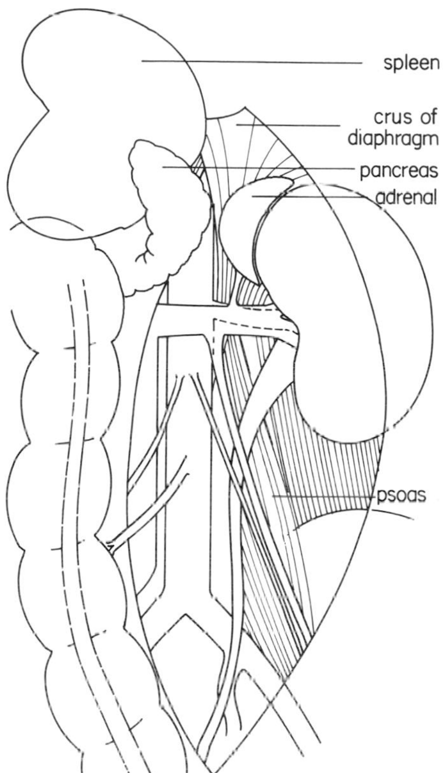

Fig. 3.3 By mobilizing the colon medially, and detaching the spleen from the diaphragm, the kidney can be exposed completely.

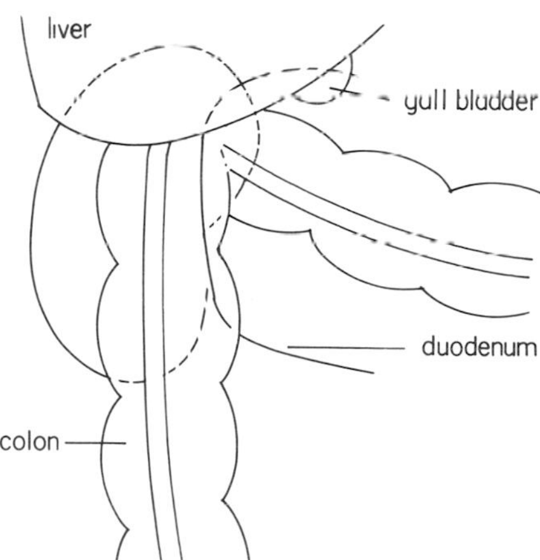

Fig. 3.4. The right kidney is hidden behind the ascending colon and hepatic flexure and the second part of the duodenum.

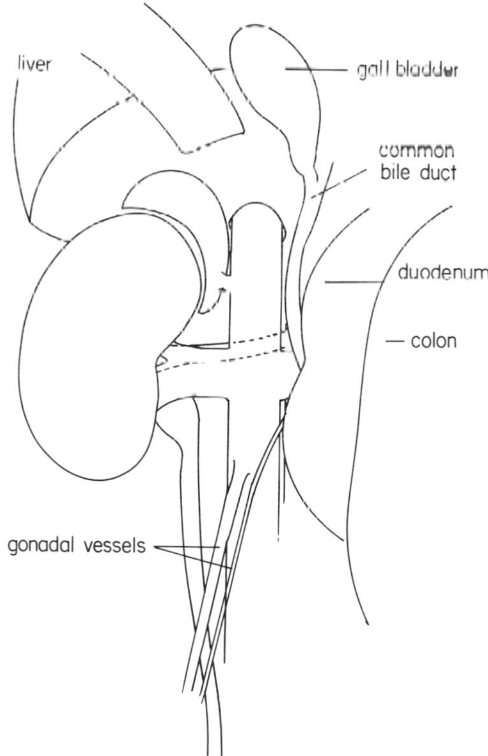

Fig. 3.5. When the right colon and hepatic flexure are mobilized medially the right kidney is exposed.

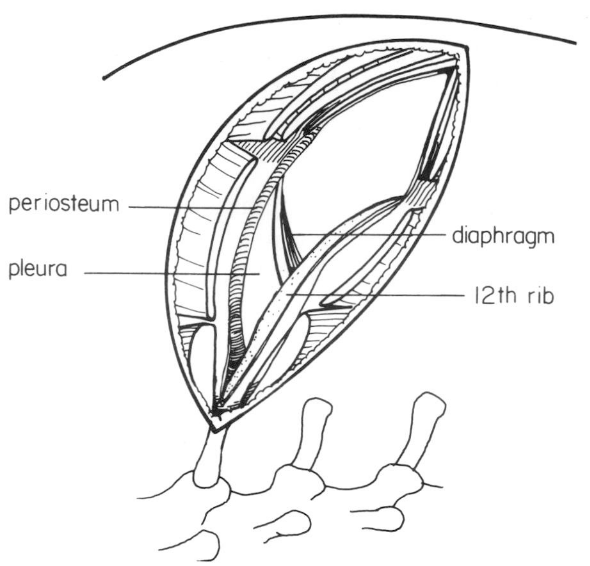

Fig. 3.6. Twelfth rib-bed exposure of the right kidney through the periosteum of the rib. Note the close relationship to the pleura.

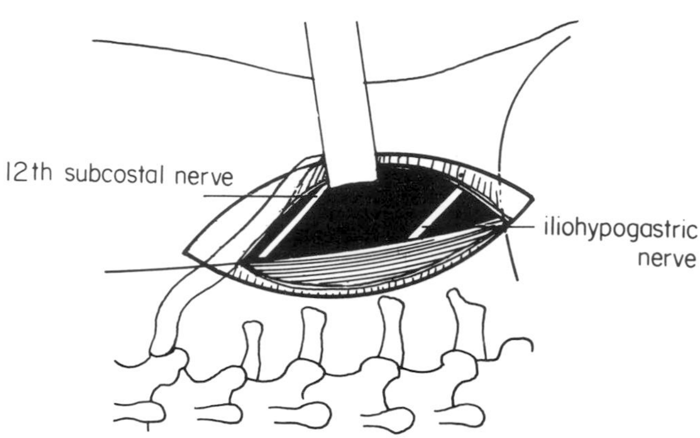

Fig. 3.7. Vertical lumbotomy approach to the right kidney.

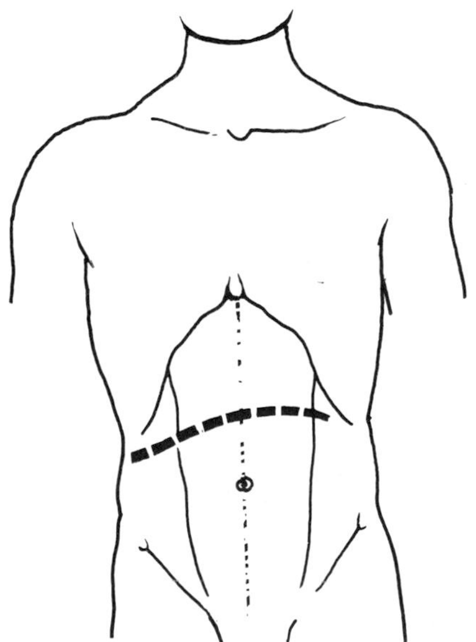

Fig. 3.8. Transverse approach to the right kidney for transabdominal nephrectomy.

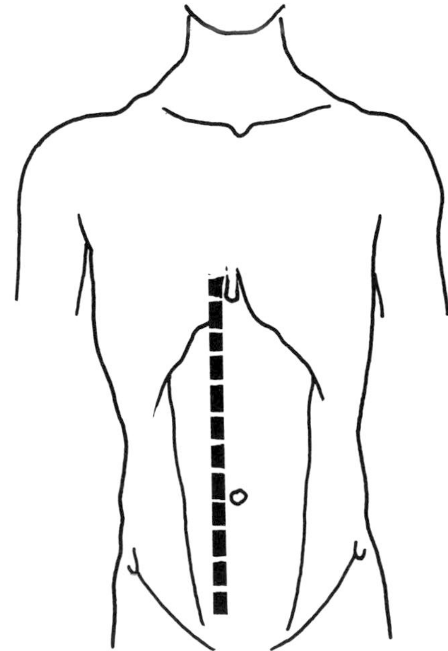

Fig. 3.9. Long paramedian approach to the right kidney in a long, thin patient.

12th rib approach, when a *pneumothorax* may need to be aspirated or drained with an underwater system. Most operations involve mobilizing the colon or duodenum to give access to the kidney, so there is often a short-lived disturbance of intestinal transport — *paralytic ileus.*

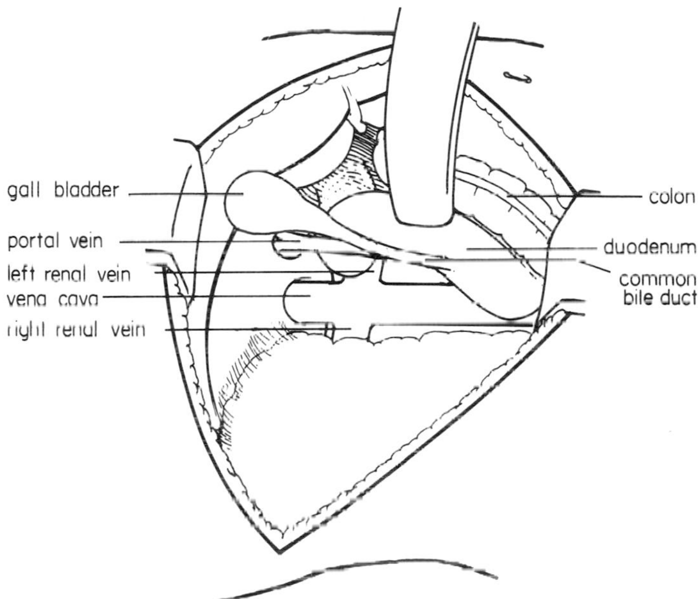

Fig. 3.10. Right kidney displayed through transverse incision after mobilizing the colon and duodenum.

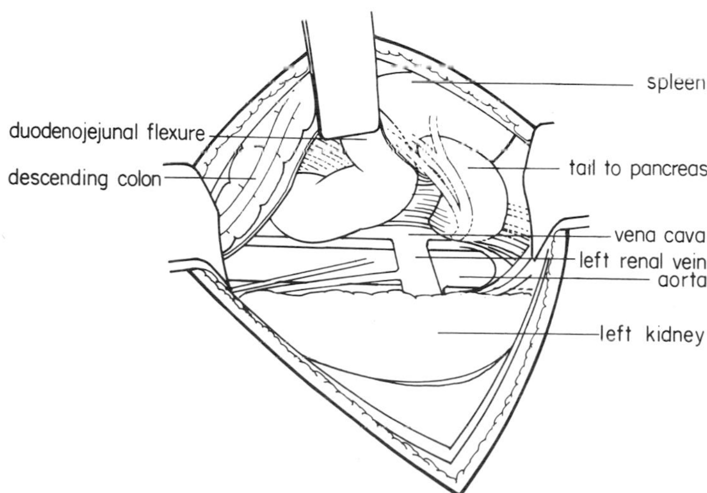

Fig. 3.11. Exposure of left kidney through transverse incision after mobilizing the colon and the tail of the pancreas medially.

STRUCTURE OF THE KIDNEY

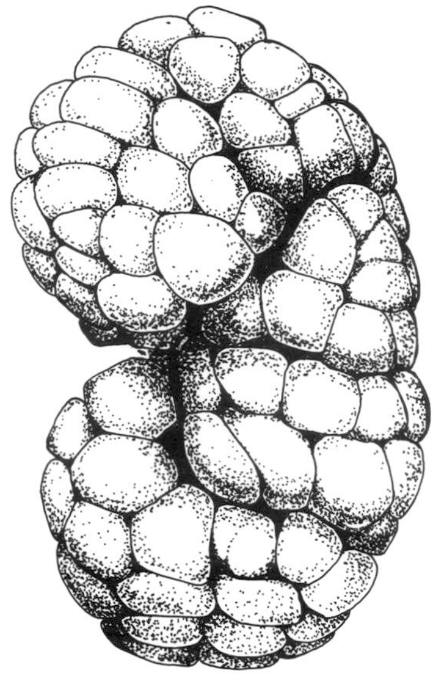

Fig. 3.12. The kidney of a common seal. In marine mammals, otters, bears and some other animals, the kidney resembles a bunch of grapes — there are 5–8 main lobules and many smaller lobules each with its own arterial and venous drainage and a single calix. (Redrawn, with permission, from Harrison R. J. & Tomlinson J. D. W. 1956. Observations on the venous system in certain *Pinnipedia* and *Cetacea*. *Proc. Zool. Soc. Lond.* **126**: Part 2; 205–233.)

The renal pyramid

The basic building block of the kidney is the *pyramid*. In some animals (e.g. porpoises and bears), the renal pyramids remain separate — like a bunch of grapes (Fig. 3.12). In man, these pyramids are squeezed together, but the kidney is made up of about a dozen pyramids (Fig. 3.13) each of which is made up of a bundle of collecting ducts, arranged like a bunch of flowers in a vase (Fig. 3.14) — the flowers are the glomeruli, the stems the collecting ducts of Bellini (Fig. 3.15), the vase is the calix.

The collecting ducts open onto the papilla obliquely so that when pressure increases in the calix the ducts are closed (Fig. 3.16). Sometimes children are born with these papillae more or less fused together so that the ducts open into a kind of crater on the summit of the 'compound papilla' (Fig. 3.17). When this happens the valve mechanism is ineffective and when there is obstruction or reflux of urine from the bladder, infected urine may be forced up the collecting tubes into the renal parenchyma where it causes inflammation followed by subsequent scarring.

The main collecting ducts of Bellini gather smaller collecting tubules which fan out into the renal cortex where they receive the straight

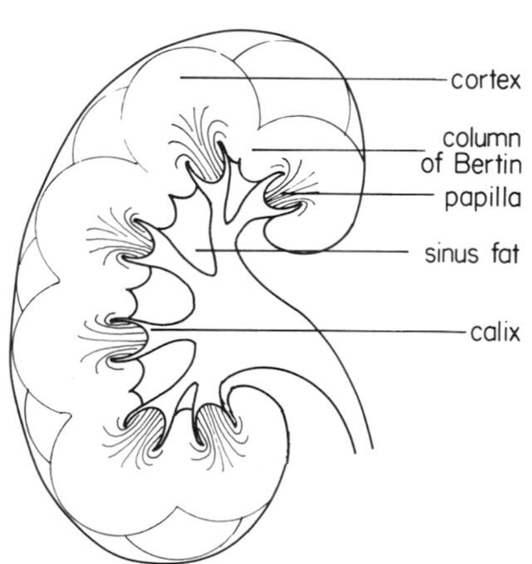

Fig. 3.13. The kidney is formed of a collection of renal pyramids, each draining its collecting ducts into a papilla. Where the pyramids come together they merge into a column of Bertin. A packing of fat separates the pyramids from the calices and pelvis.

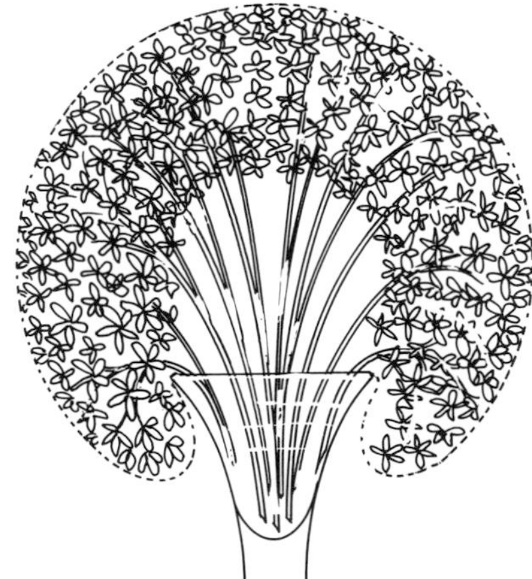

Fig. 3.14. Each pyramid has the structure of a bunch of flowers in a vase: the stems are the ducts of Bellini, the flowers the glomeruli, and the vase the papilla.

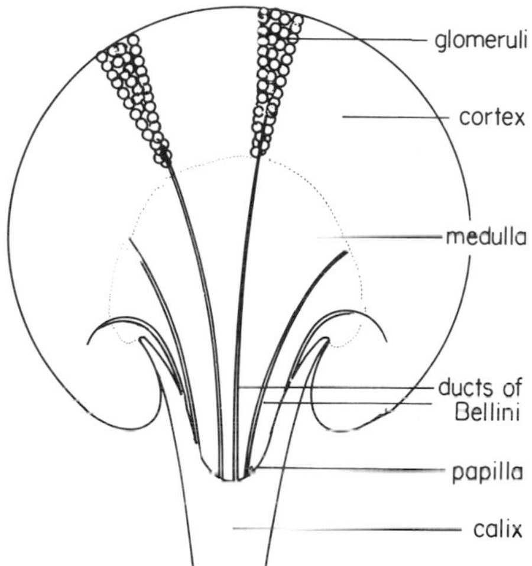

Fig. 3.15. The collection of glomeruli form the 'cortex', the colecting tubes the medulla. The collecting tubes open onto the papilla obliquely so that increased pressure inside the calix will close them by valve action.

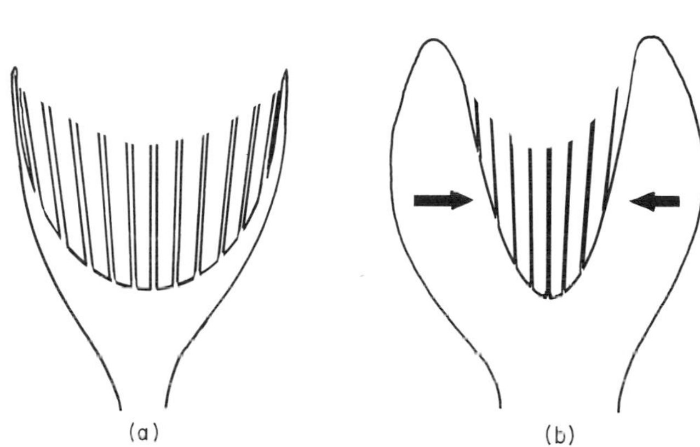

Fig. 3.16. The valvular arrangement of the normal papilla. (a) The collecting ducts open obliquely on the sides of the papilla. (b) When there is obstruction and the pressure rises inside the calix the ducts are squeezed shut to prevent urine refluxing into the renal parenchyma.

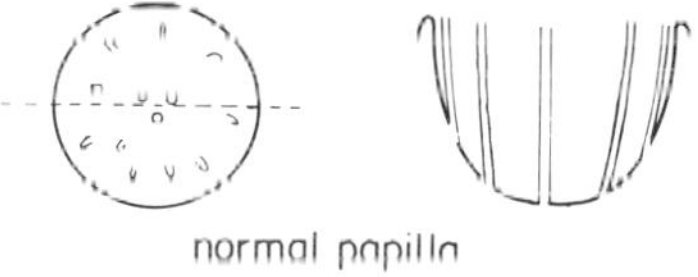

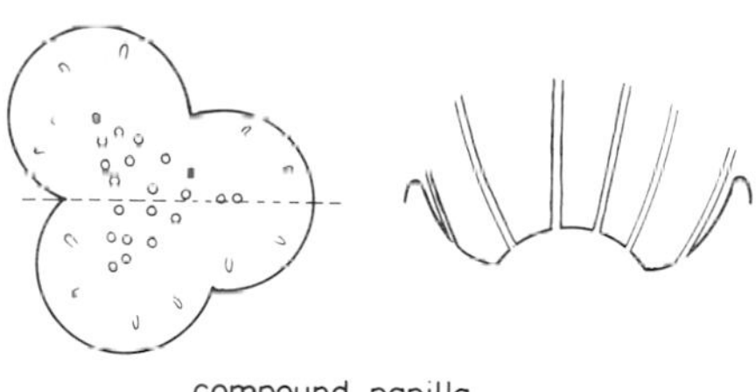

Fig. 3.17. In a normal papilla (above) most of the ducts of Bellini will be closed when the pressure inside the calix is increased, but in a compound papilla (below) those that open into the hollow of the crater, formed where the papillae fuse together, have no protective valves.

connecting segments from the *nephrons* which are arranged rather like clusters of flowers, or corn on the cob (Fig. 3.18). Each nephron consists of two elements — a filtering plant and a processing system.

The glomerulus

Each *glomerulus* is made up of a coiled arteriole looking like a ball of wool, invaginated into a hollow balloon — *Bowman's capsule* — whose stem forms the proximal tubule (Fig. 3.19). The glomerular arteriole is unusually permeable: its endothelial wall is impressed with innumerable dimples to increase its porosity. The endothelium rests on a basement membrane which, like filter paper, is supported on a grid formed by the epithelial cells of Bowman's capsule which are like little octopuses whose tentacles interlock like a zip-fastener (Fig. 3.20). The spaces between the tentacles are the 'slit-pores' (Fig. 3.21) which are bridged over by a thin and rather permeable membrane. It is possible to measure the size of the proteins which can escape through these slit-pores by using peroxidases of known molecular size: protein molecules up to 40 000 molecular weight can escape but those of 160 000 are too big. Filtration is not merely a matter of the size of the molecule: the proteins that make up the glomerular basement membrane are negatively charged and repel negatively charged protein molecules (e.g. albumin) while accepting positively charged ones.

The arteriole of the glomerulus is 50 times more permeable than any other small vessel (e.g. in muscle). As a result enormous volumes of fluid pass through the basement membrane every day: the plasma water is filtered every half-hour, and the entire body water is 'processed' four times over every day.

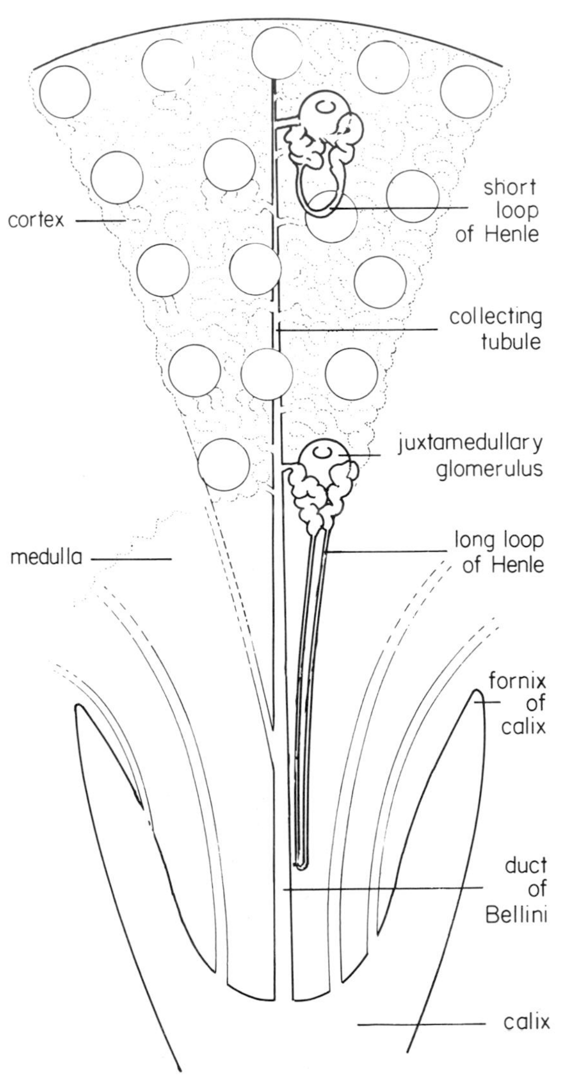

Fig. 3.18. The nephrons are arranged on their collecting tubes like corn on the cob. Those nearest to the medulla have long, hairpin loops of Henle.

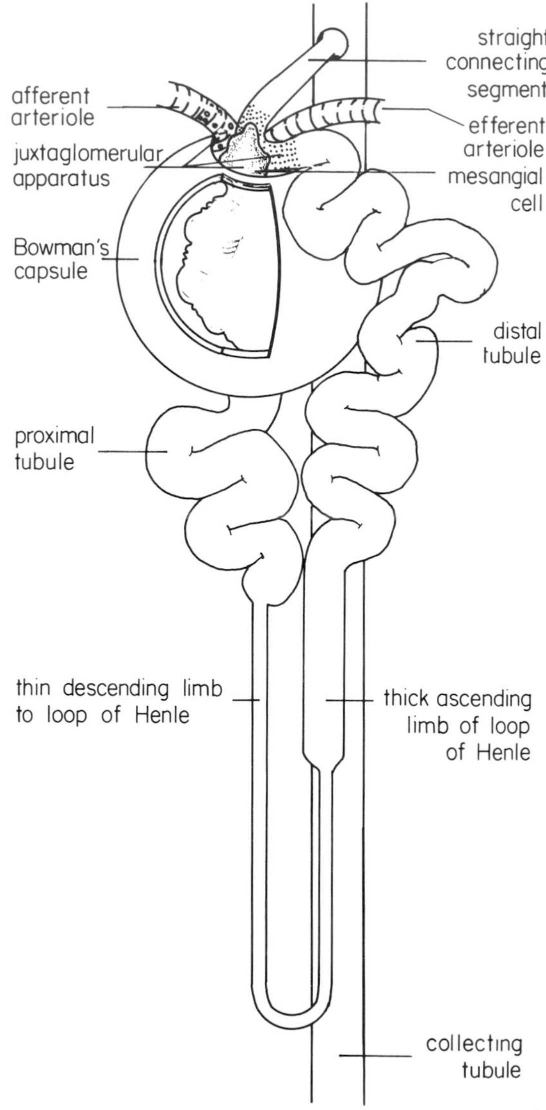

Fig. 3.19. The nephron.

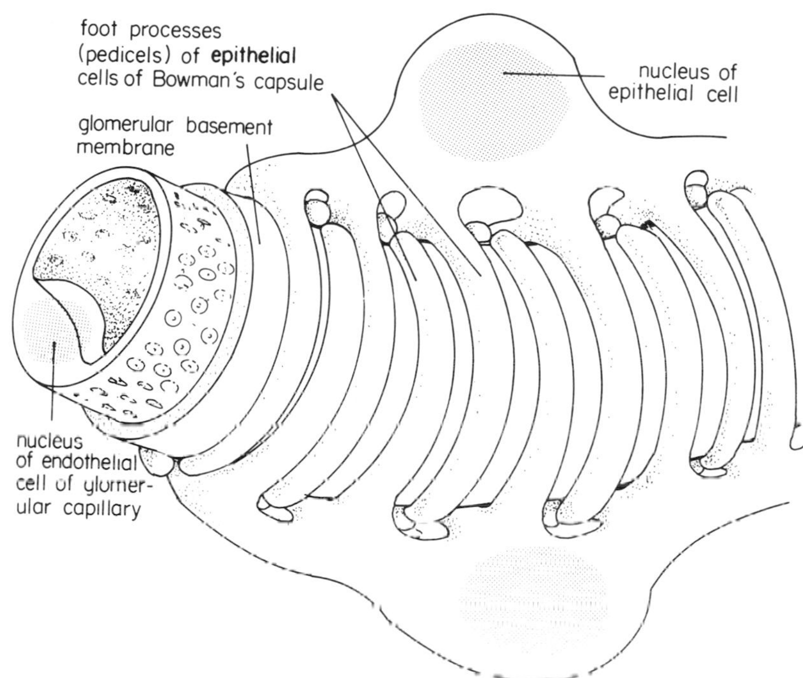

Fig. 3.20. Structure of the glomerular filter.

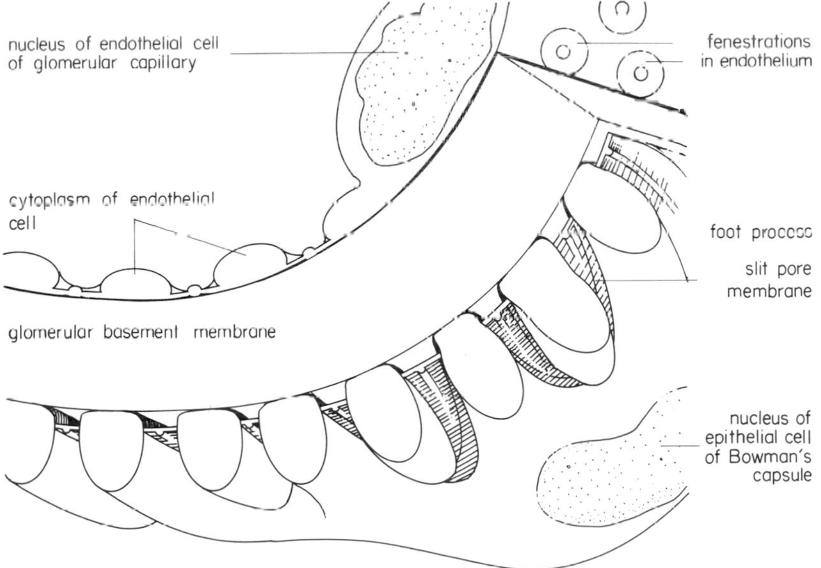

Fig. 3.21. A closer view of the glomerular filter.

The pressure inside the glomerular capillary is about 60 mmHg. The plasma oncotic pressure is 25 mmHg, so that there is a filtration pressure of 35 mmHg to push against the pressure inside Bowman's capsule which is usually about 10 mmHg. The first task in the processing plant is to recapture the excessive and wasteful volume of water that is squeezed out in the glomerulus.

Tests of glomerular filtration

The classic test of glomerular filtration is the *creatinine clearance*. To be accurate it demands an exactly timed collection of urine — usually over a 24 hour period. This can be difficult in a busy surgical ward. The plasma creatinine is measured at a convenient time during the period of collection of the urine. Clearance is given by the formula UV/P where U=urine creatinine mg/100 ml, V=urine volume ml/minute and P=plasma creatinine mg/100 ml, and the answer is expressed in ml/minute. In fact the level of plasma creatinine is a sufficient guide to the normality of glomerular function for most purposes.

In view of the practical difficulty of getting a really accurately timed urine collection, isotope studies using ^{99m}Tc-labelled DTPA are today used to measure the glomerular filtration rate either with a gamma camera over the kidney, or by measuring the rate at which an injected dose of the tracer disappears from the arm.

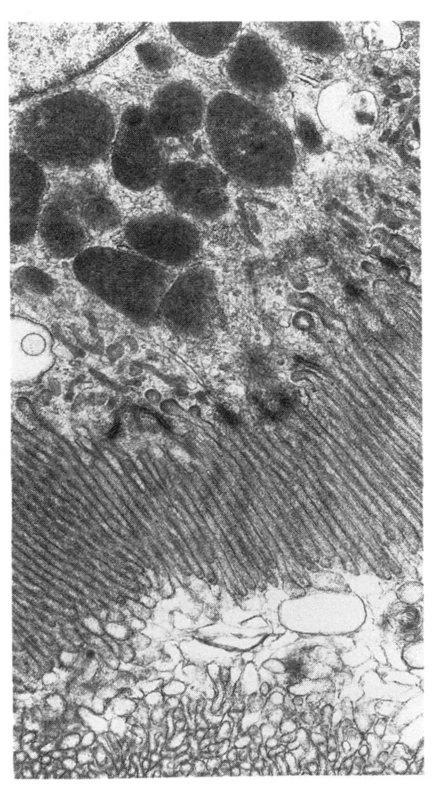

Fig. 3.22. Photomicrograph showing the brush border of the proximal renal tubule. ×12 000. (Courtesy of Dr Jo Martin, The London Hospital Institute of Pathology.)

The renal tubule

Most (about 75%) of the excess water is reabsorbed in the *proximal* tubule which is formed of thick active cells whose absorptive surface area is augmented by numerous bristles — the *brush border* (Fig. 3.22). As well as water, these metabolically busy cells recover glucose, phosphate and most of the amino acids that escape in the glomerular filtrate.

The filtrate now passes through the *loop of Henle* which in most nephrons is quite short. In about one in eight of them, in the inner part of the kidney, the loop dips down like a hairpin into the renal papilla. The loops of Henle are made of thin cells which allow osmosis to act on the glomerular filtrate and withdraw more salt and water.

The filtrate then rises up into the *distal convoluted tubule*, whose cells are again thick and metabolically active (but have no brush border). Here sodium is exchanged for potassium and hydrogen to regulate the acid-base balance of the body. Disease of the distal convoluted tubule prevents the kidney from forming an acid urine — so called renal tubular acidosis.

When it leaves the distal convoluted tubule the filtrate enters the *collecting tubule* and passes through the concentrated tissue of the renal papilla where the last fine adjustment to the reabsorption of water takes place under the influence of the pituitary antidiuretic hormone.

Tests of tubular function

Clinical tests of tubular function are so difficult and unreliable that they have largely been replaced by measurements of the renal handling of radionuclides such as ^{99m}Tc DMSA which is taken up and held in the renal tubules.

There are two classical tests: the response to an acid load and the urine concentration test. The *response to acid load* tests the function of the distal tubule: after collecting two specimens of urine over a period of 2 hours, the patient is given an acid load in the form of NH_4Cl (as gelatin-coated capsules 0.1 g/kg body weight) in a litre of water over a one hour period. Three hours later a one hour collection of urine is made. Healthy distal tubules should be able to handle this acid load by secreting urine with a pH < 5.3 and a titratable acidity > 25 mEq/minute and > 35 mEq/minute of ammonium.

The *urine concentration* test measures the ability of the proximal tubule to respond to antidiuretic hormone. One may deprive the patient of water, or give pitressin tannate (5 units s.c.) and follow the specific gravity of each specimen of urine passed thereafter. The test must never be used in patients in renal failure.

BLOOD SUPPLY OF THE KIDNEY

No surgeon who has had to operate on the renal parenchyma can forget how rich is its blood supply. Between them the kidneys receive one-fifth of the entire cardiac output, and the first step in any operation on the kidney is to get control of the *renal artery*.

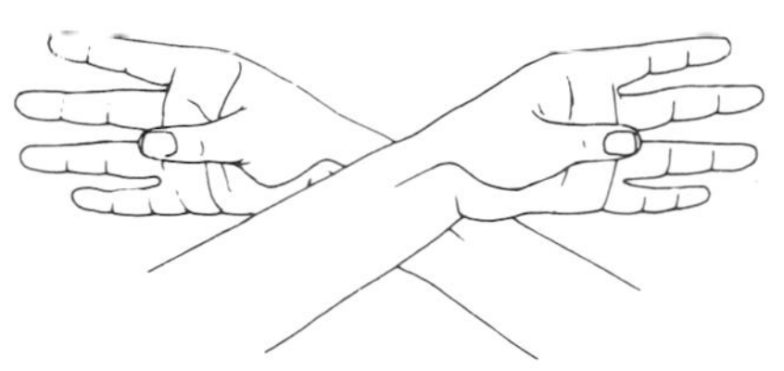

Fig. 3.23. To remember the branches of the renal arteries cross your hands in front of you: the thumbs remind you of the single posterior segmental branch, the four fingers represent the four main arterior segmental arteries.

As a rule there is only one renal artery on each side, but one or more of the five main branches may have a separate origin from the aorta. The five main branches are arranged like the fingers of your hand (Fig. 3.23): each supplies its own geographical part of the parenchyma and there is no anastomosis between them (Figs 3.24, 3.25).

There is no neat correspondence between the segmental arterial territories and the arrangement of the pyramids so that in planning an open operation that requires an incision into the renal parechyma, e.g. removing a stone, one makes the incision between the main segmental vessels — if necessary first locating them with a Doppler probe.

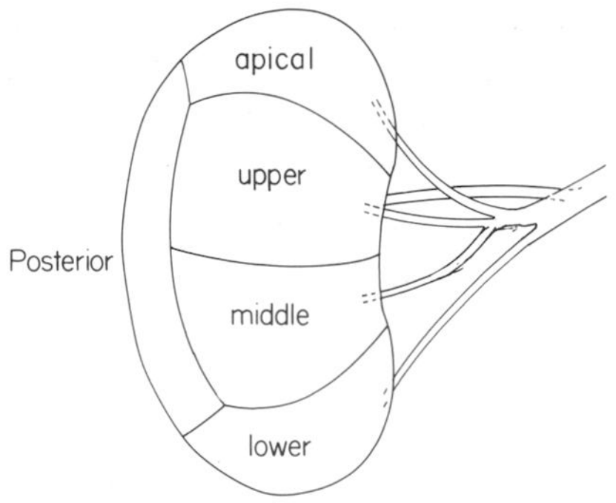

Fig. 3.24. Arrangement of the segments of the kidney; each one is supplied by one of the five main segmental arteries.

Entering its proper zone, each segmental artery divides into smaller *arcuate* arteries which curve out in the boundary between cortex and medulla. From each arcuate artery scores of branches run up along the stems of the collecting tubules which make up the pyramid (Fig. 3.26), giving off afferent arteries to each glomerulus.

Just before the afferent artery enters the glomerulus it runs close to the junction of the loop of Henle and the distal convoluted tubule. Here the cells of the tubule are darkly stained (*macula densa*) and the muscle cells in the wall of the artery contain conspicuous cytoplasmic granules believed to be the precursors of renin: this little system — the *juxtaglomerular apparatus* — is like a thermostat which constantly monitors the pressure in the afferent arteriole and plays a key role in the regulation of blood pressure (see p. 113).

Renal veins

Unlike the neatly compartmented system of the renal arteries, the veins communicate freely with each other (Fig. 3.27) so one can safely ligate

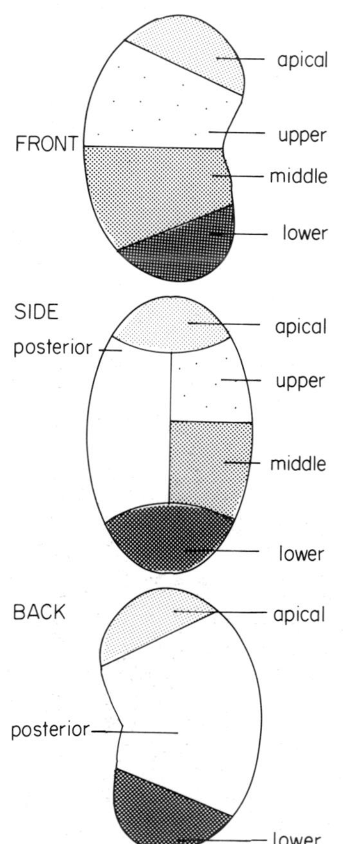

Fig. 3.25. Diagrammatic representation of the five segments of the kidney.

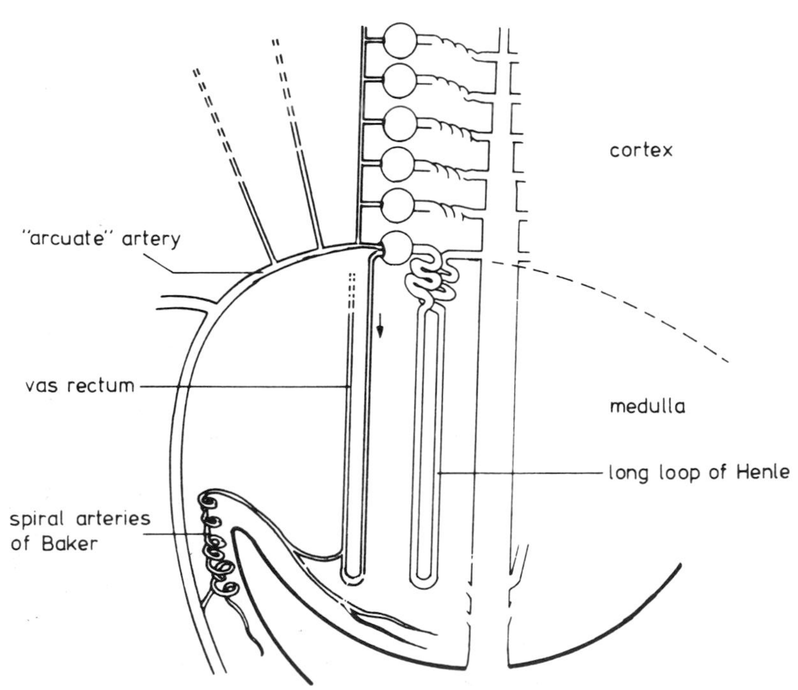

Fig. 3.26. Blood supply of the renal papilla.

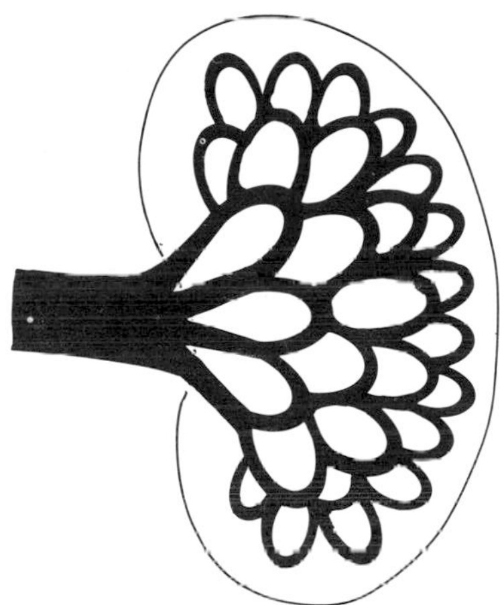

Fig. 3.27. The veins of the kidney are arranged in arcades which communicate freely with each other.

several venous branches without risking infarction of the kidney. Often the main left renal vein splits into two — one part running in front of the aorta, the other behind — an unpleasant trap for the surgeon unaware of this possibility. On the left side the renal vein is about 5 cm long, but on the right side it is right up against the vena cava — one reason for choosing the left kidney in live-donor transplantation.

The collecting system

The renal papillae are covered with a thin cubical epithelium perforated like a pepper pot with the openings of the collecting ducts of Bellini: but the remainder of the pelvis and calices is lined by transitional epithelium just like that of the bladder and ureters. The transitional epithelium is surrounded by a strong muscular wall made of smooth muscle cells joined to each other by jig-saw connections — nexuses — (Fig. 3.28) which transmit the wave of peristaltic contraction from the calices down

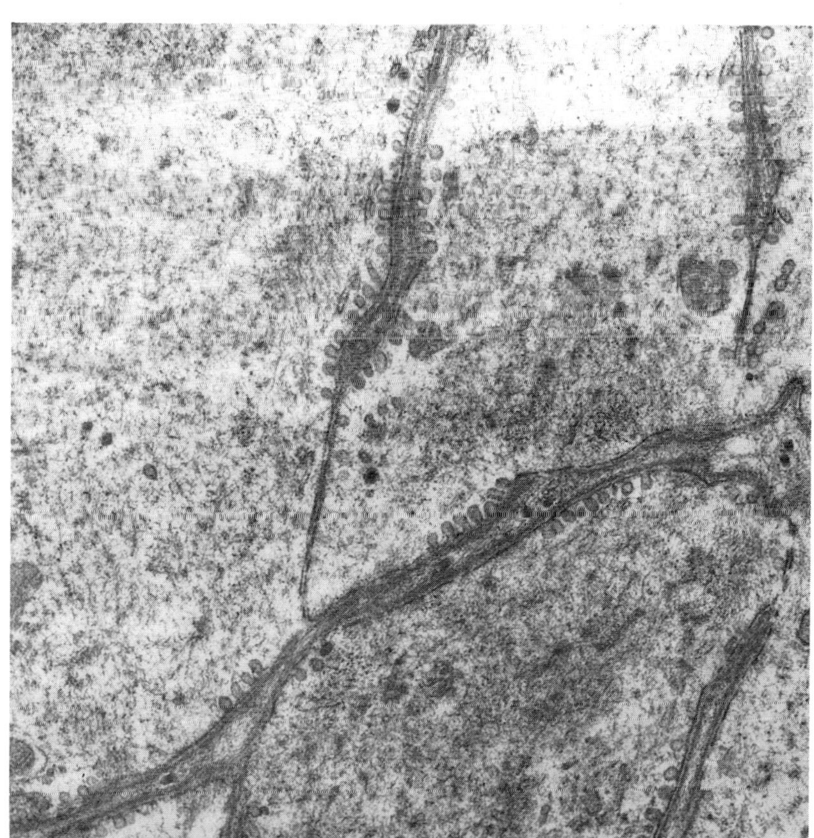

Fig. 3.28. Electron micrograph showing the border between two adjacent ureteric smooth muscle cells. They fit together like a zip-fastener or the pieces of a jigsaw: these are the nexuses through which the contractile impulse is transmitted. ×40 000. (Courtesy of Mr R G Notley.)

the pelvis into the ureter. This peristaltic activity is slower than that of the bowel but has the advantage that it needs no nerve supply and so a transplanted kidney continues to pump out its urine perfectly well (Fig. 3.29).

To allow the calices to pump freely they are separated from the parenchyma by a packing of *sinus fat* which is fluid at body temperature (Fig. 3.30).

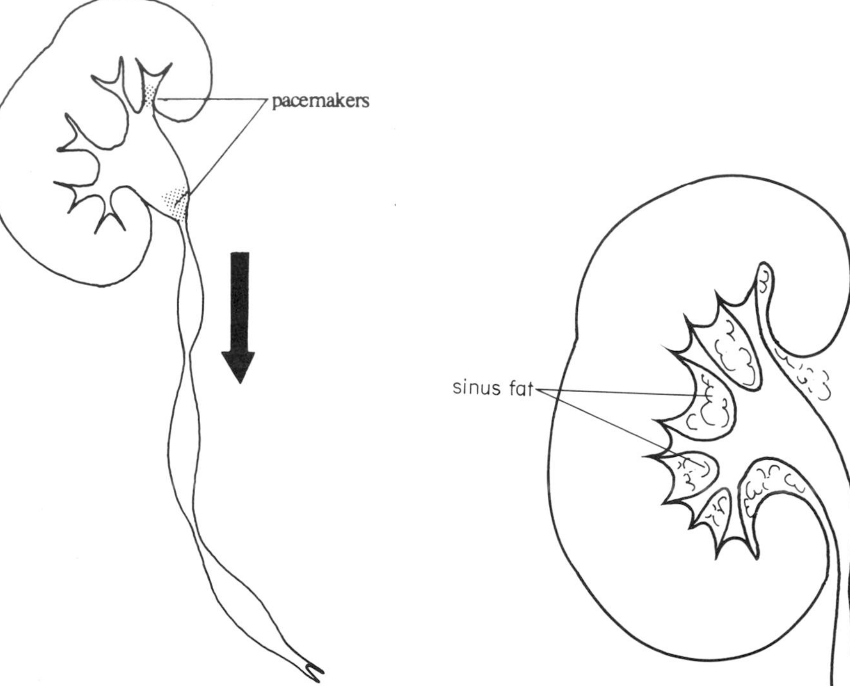

Fig. 3.29. Co-ordinated peristalsis passing discrete compartments full of urine down the ureter.

Fig. 3.30. There is a packing of fat between the calices and the renal parenchyma. It is fluid at body temperature and permits free movement of the calices in all directions.

FURTHER READING

Baker SB de C (1959) The blood supply of the renal papilla. *British Journal of Urology* **31**, 53–9.

Brenton DP (1985) Tubular function and its disturbance in disease. In: Marsh FP (Ed) *Postgraduate Nephrology*. Heinemann Medical Books, London. pp 151–79.

Upsdell SM, Leeson SM, Brooman PJC & O'Reilly PH (1988) Diuretic-induced urinary flow rates at varying clearances and their relevance to the performance and interpretation of diuresis renography. *British Journal of Urology* **61**, 14–18.

4 The Kidney — Congenital Disorders

The most primitive of all vertebrates had one set of nephrons for each somite of the body from head to tail draining along a single duct. They fell into three groups: the most cranial of these — the *pronephros* — is only an evolutionary curiosity, purported to be found in certain fish embryos, but it figures nowhere in human embryology. The next set — the *mesonephros* — corresponds to the functioning kidney of fish and frogs whose *mesonephric* or *Wolffian duct* empties into their cloaca. In man the mesonephros has disappeared, and the human kidney is derived from a yet more caudal set of nephrons — the *metanephros* which drain into a duct that buds out from the caudal end of the mesonephric duct (Fig. 4.1) to form the ureter.

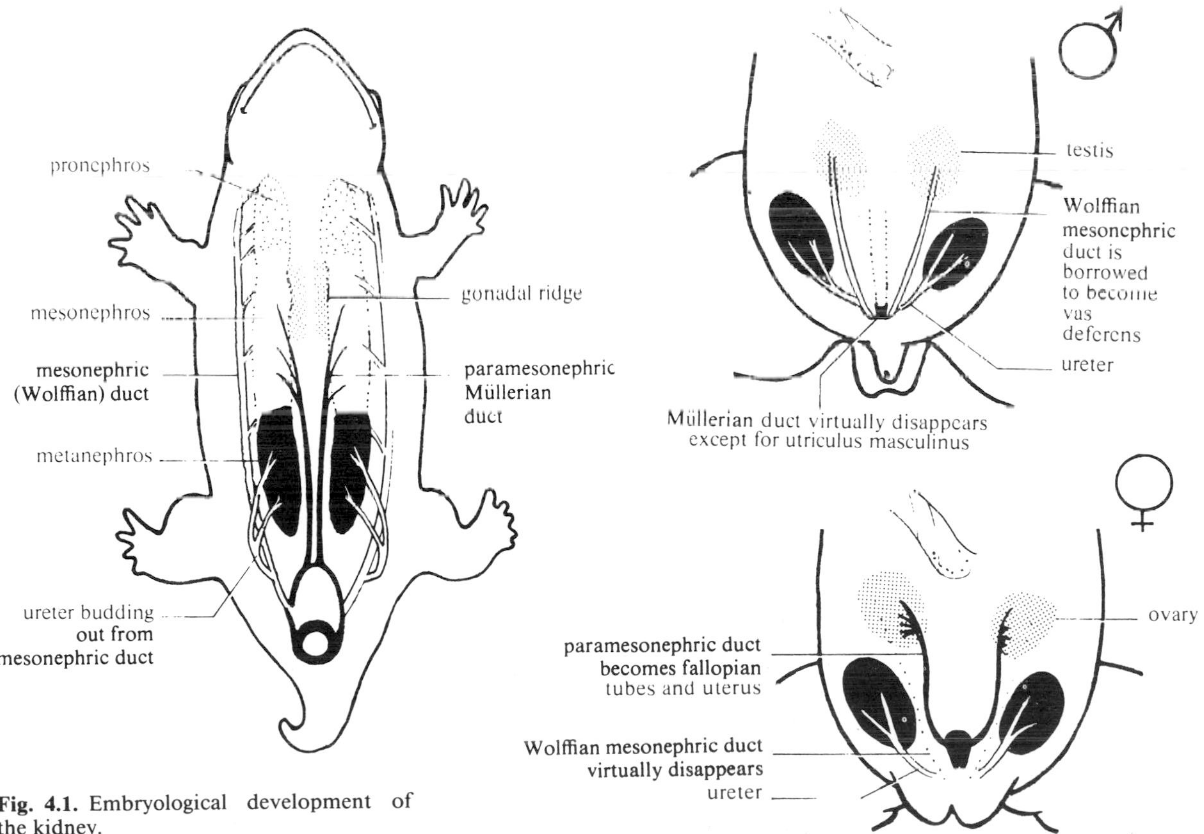

Fig. 4.1. Embryological development of the kidney.

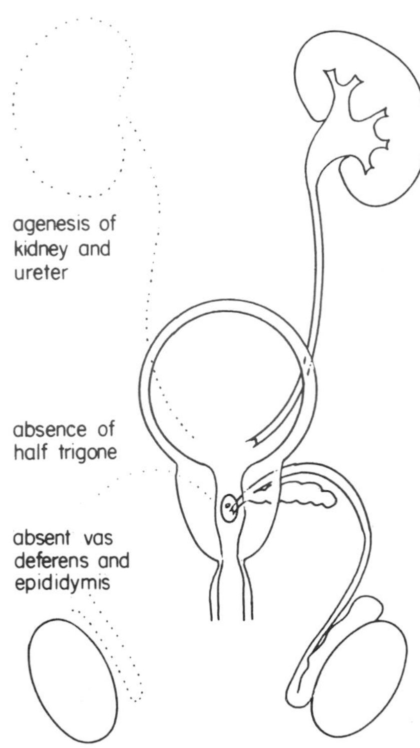

Fig. 4.2. Agenesis of the kidney.

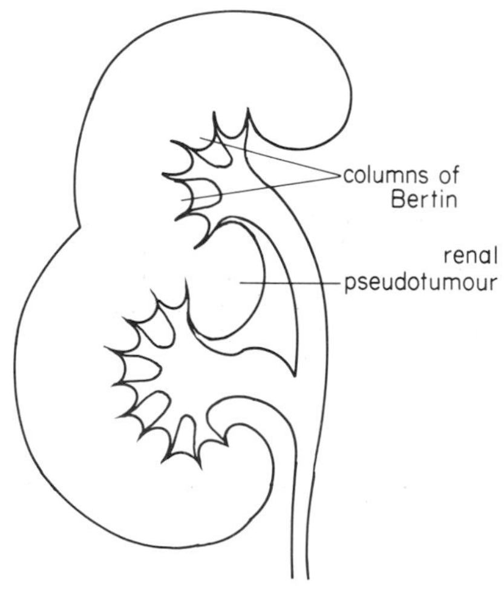

Fig. 4.3. Pseudotumour of the kidney—a particularly big column of Bertin.

The mesonephric Wolffian duct persists in males as the vas deferens. If the mesonephric Wolffian duct fails to develop altogether, there is neither ureter, kidney nor vas deferens on that side — renal agenesis (Fig. 4.2).

There is a second pair of ducts which run parallel to the mesonephric Wolffian ducts — the *paramesonephric* or *Müllerian ducts.* In women they form the Fallopian tubes which fuse in the midline to form the uterus. In men they persist as two tiny vestiges — a pit on the verumontanum in the prostatic urethra called the utriculus masculinus — and a tiny cyst attached to the upper pole of the testis — the appendix testis — which sometimes causes trouble by becoming twisted on its stalk (see p. 298).

Duplex kidney and ureter

After budding out from the lower end of the mesonephric Wolffian duct, the ureter usually begins to branch only when it gets near the metanephros, but it often begins to divide earlier to produce a double system of renal pelves and calices. The overlying kidney parenchyma is never completely separated into two parts though there is often a distinct 'waist' demarcating the upper from the lower half kidney and where the two halves meet there may be a prominent bulge in the parenchyma — an exaggerated column of Bertin or *pseudotumour* which may be mistaken for a carcinoma by the unwary (Fig. 4.3).

As a rule the upper half-kidney has two main calices, the lower part has three and makes more urine: sometimes where the ureters join together urine is squirted from the larger lower half up into the upper one — the so called see-saw (Fig. 4.4).

In a duplex kidney the ureter from the upper half enters the bladder caudal to the ureter from the lower half-kidney. This is the Weigert-Meyer law, and it arises in the course of the development of the human bladder from the ancestral cloaca at a stage when the primitive metanephros is forming in the tissues in the tail end of the embryo. While the ureters are budding out towards the metanephros (Fig. 4.5) a shutter of tissue (the urogenital septum) is growing down to separate the cloaca into an anterior part — the bladder, and a posterior part — the rectum. The Wolffian duct and its buds are carried down by this shutter to form a loop (Fig. 4.6) and then the lower part of the Wolffian duct is absorbed into the trigone of the future bladder (Fig. 4.7). The upper part of the Wolffian duct (borrowed to form the vas deferens in the male) swings down with the migration of the testis (Fig. 4.8).

In most patients with duplex kidney the anomaly is innocent and symptomless but it can be associated with three important conditions that cause trouble — ectopic ureter, reflux and ureterocele.

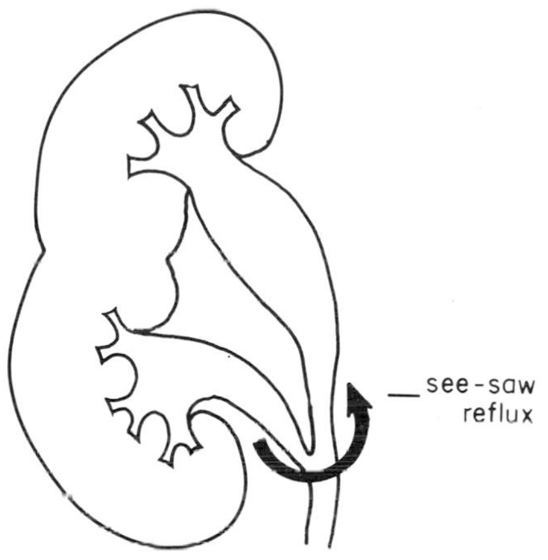

Fig. 4.4. See-saw reflux.

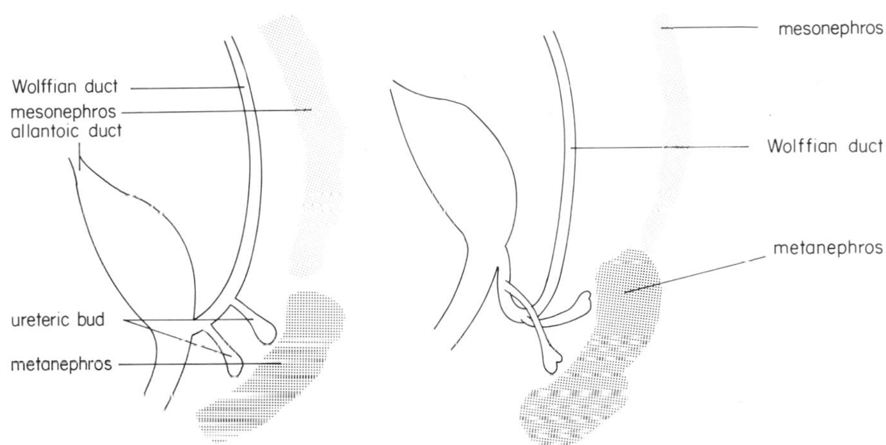

Fig. 4.5. Duplex kidney: two ureteric buds sprout from the Wolffian duct towards the metanephros.

Fig. 4.6. As the Wolffian duct forms its hairpin bend, the ureteric buds are carried with it.

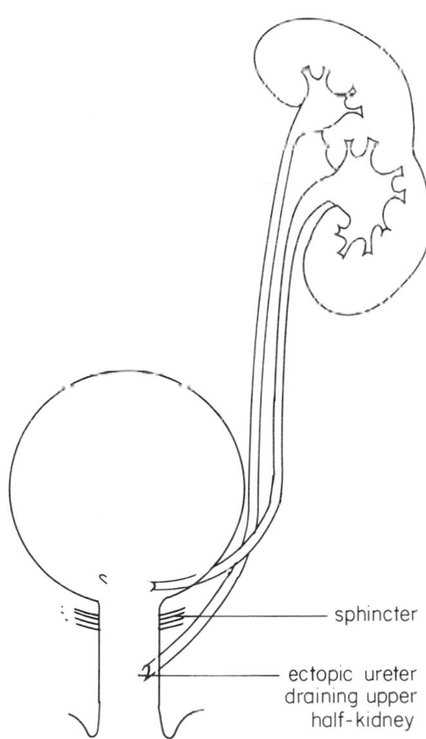

Fig. 4.9. If the more caudally opening ureter is placed downstream of the sphincter it causes incontinence.

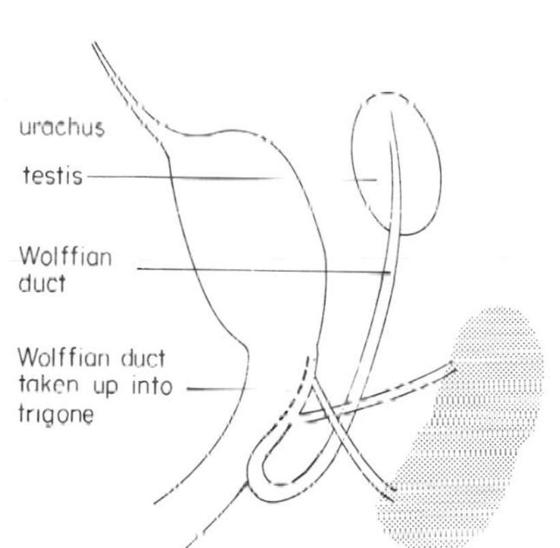

Fig. 4.7. The inner wall of the Wolffian duct is taken up into the developing trigone. The upper part of the Wolffian mesonephric duct is borrowed by the testis.

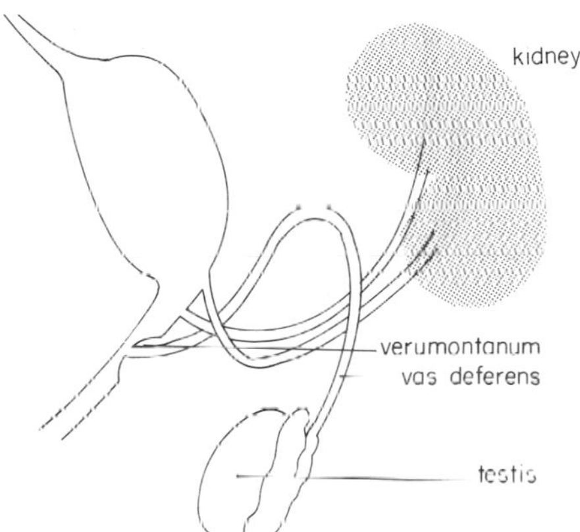

Fig. 4.8. In the end, the ureter from the upper half of the kidney comes to enter the trigone below that belonging to the lower half, and the entry of the Wolffian duct that is now borrowed to form the vas deferens, is even further caudal.

Ectopic ureter

The ureter draining the upper half-kidney may open in the vagina of girls caudal to the sphincter so that urine leaks away constantly (Fig. 4.9).

Reflux

Because the ureter from the lower half-kidney has a relatively short

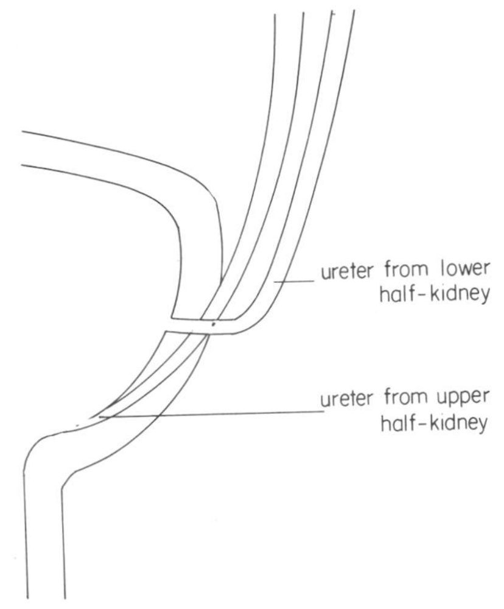

Fig. 4.10. The ureter draining the lower half-kidney may have such a short tunnel through the bladder that it has no protective valve and permits reflux of urine from the bladder to the lower half-kidney.

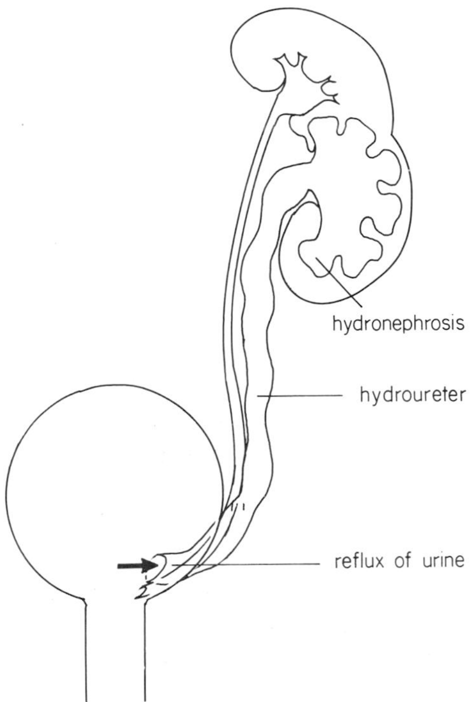

Fig. 4.11. Reflux giving rise to hydronephrosis in the lower half-kidney.

course through the wall of the bladder (Fig. 4.10) it has a less efficient flap-valve and urine may reflux from the bladder up to the kidney (Fig. 4.11).

Ureterocele

The inner part of the Wolffian duct may be incompletely absorbed into the trigone and may persist as a balloon (ureterocele) just where the ureter enters the trigone. This may be found in a normal single ureter, or at the lower of the two ureteric orifices in duplex (Fig. 4.12). In girls the ureterocele may be pushed right out of the urethra and appear as a painful, translucent 'cyst' associated with acute retention of urine (Fig. 4.13).

Errors of position of the kidney

Rotated kidney

It is common for a kidney to face forwards rather than sideways. The outline is then an ellipse and some of the calices point medially (Fig. 4.14): it is of no consequence but may present a confusing radiographic appearance.

Horseshoe kidney

Here both kidneys are rotated and their lower poles fuse together in the shape of a horseshoe (Fig. 4.15). It is thought that this happens because the two metanephroi get fused together in the fetal pelvis, but nobody knows why. They join in front of the aorta and the isthmus may have to be divided in operations on the aorta (Fig. 4.15). One congenital anomaly tends to be associated with others, so that in horseshoe kidney it is common to find reflux, ureterocele and hydronephrosis from congenital obstruction at the pelviureteric junction (see p. 140). Most horseshoe kidneys are found by chance, cause no trouble, and need no treatment.

Crossed renal ectopia

Instead of being united in the midline, both kidneys may come to be fused together on one side although their ureters always arise on their own proper side. As with horseshoe kidneys it is believed that the trouble arises from fusion of the fetal metanephroi and as with horseshoe kidney the condition is only important when it is associated with some other anomaly such as reflux or obstruction (Fig. 4.16).

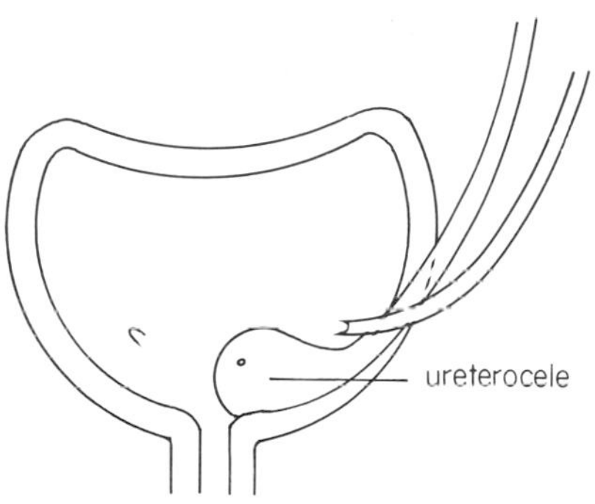

Fig. 4.12. The upper half-kidney draining into the lower of the two ureteric orifices may open into a ureterocele where the inner wall of the Wolffian duct has not been completely absorbed.

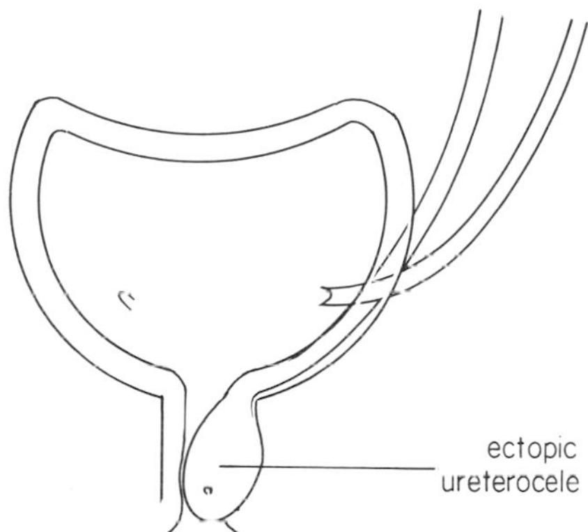

Fig. 4.13. The ureterocele may occur in an ectopic ureter, and so present as a 'cyst' near the external meatus in a girl.

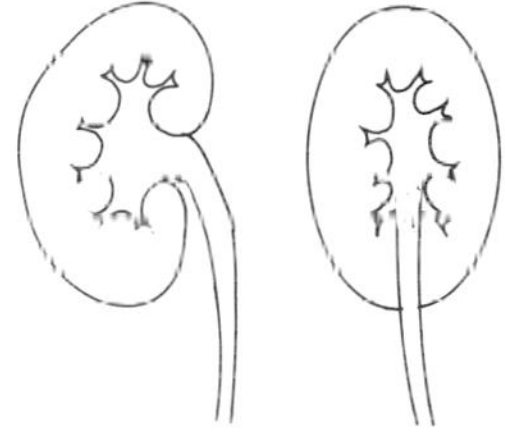

Fig. 4.14. Diagram of a rotated kidney: note the medially pointing calices.

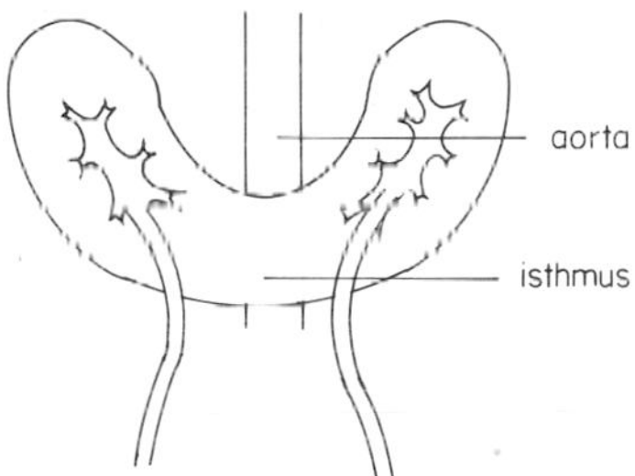

Fig. 4.15. Two rotated kidneys may fuse together in the midline in front of the aorta to form a 'horseshoe kidney'.

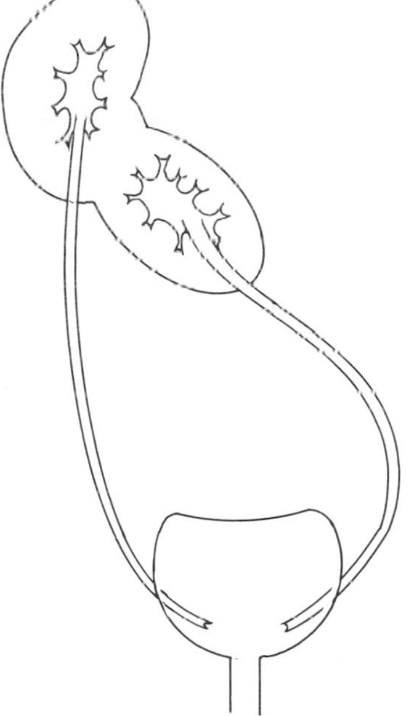

Fig. 4.16. Crossed renal ectopia. Note that the ureter enters the trigone in the right place but the metanephros has crossed over to become stuck to the other side.

Pelvic kidney

Here the metanephros remains in the pelvis. One might expect it to get in the way of the baby during childbirth, but it hardly ever does. It is usually detected by chance and seldom needs any treatment unless associated with hydronephrosis. There is, however, one major hazard with a pelvic kidney: it may be discovered at laparotomy for abdominal pain, and not be recognized. Since these pelvic kidneys have their proper number of segmental arteries which may arise separately from the aorta, common and internal iliac arteries, they can cause confusion especially if the surgeon mistakes this innocent anomaly for a tumour and tries to remove it (Fig. 4.17).

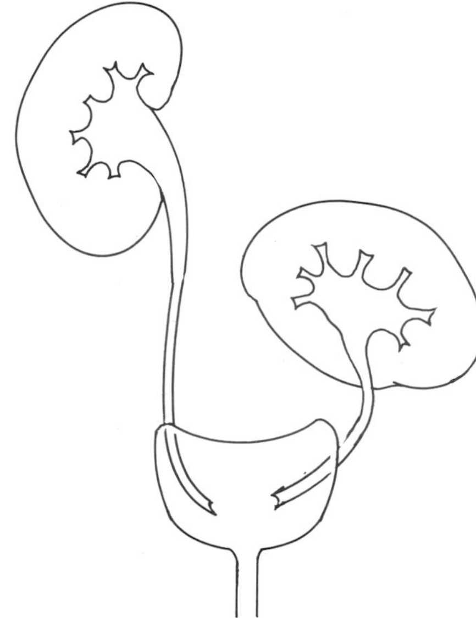

Fig. 4.17. Pelvic kidney. Lying in front of the sacrum the contrast in the IVU may easily be overlooked.

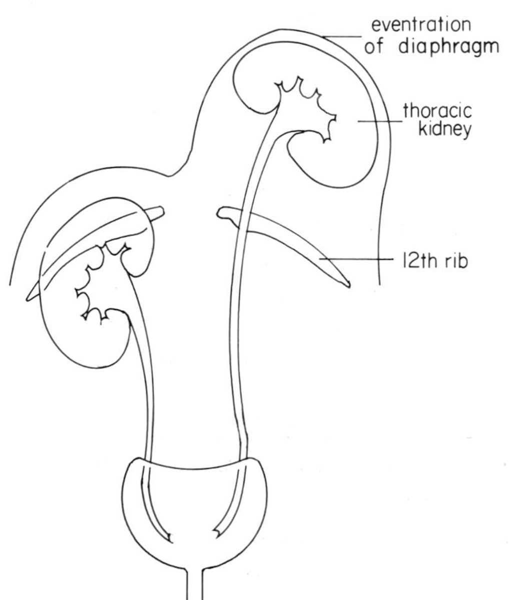

Fig. 4.18. When the diaphragm fails to develop properly, the kidney, along with other viscera, may be displaced into the thorax.

Thoracic kidney

This is not so much an error of development of the kidney as of the diaphragm. There is a congenital failure of development of the diaphragm and one kidney is carried up into the chest along with other viscera. Such a *thoracic kidney* may be found by chance in a chest radiograph or an IVU. The kidney is not really in the thorax: there is always a thin layer of diaphragm and pleura separating it. It needs no treatment (Fig 4.18).

Errors of development of the kidney

In *agenesis* the entire mesonephric Wolffian duct fails to develop so there are neither ureter, trigone, kidney nor (in boys) vas deferens (see Fig. 4.2). The mesonephric Wolffian duct may develop properly, but the ureteric bud may wither. The metanephros needs the ureter to develop properly. As a result the metanephros is either not differentiated at all — *aplasia* (Fig. 4.19) or it develops poorly with odd looking tissue including cartilage and little cysts — *dysplasia* (Fig. 4.20). *Hypoplasia* is a term to avoid: it implies that the kidney is small but otherwise normal. This is hardly ever the case: most small kidneys are either dysplastic or have been scarred by acquired disease.

CYSTIC DISORDERS OF THE KIDNEY

Not all cysts are of congenital origin, but it may be helpful to consider them all together. Cysts are very common in the kidney. They arise from

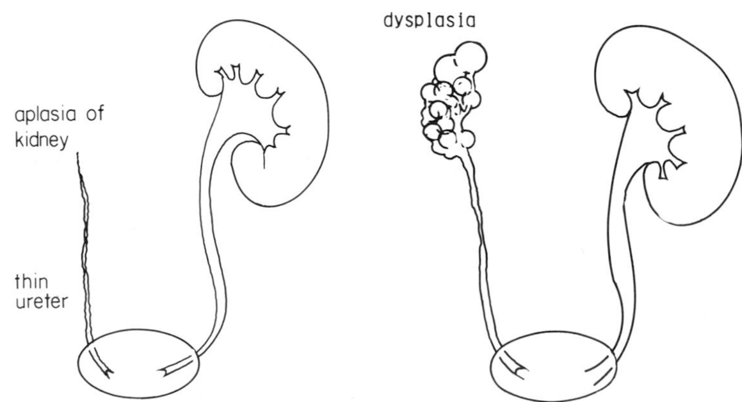

Fig. 4.19. Aplasia.

Fig. 4.20. Dysplasia.

the collecting tubules, by dilatation, obstruction or as outpouches — diverticula.

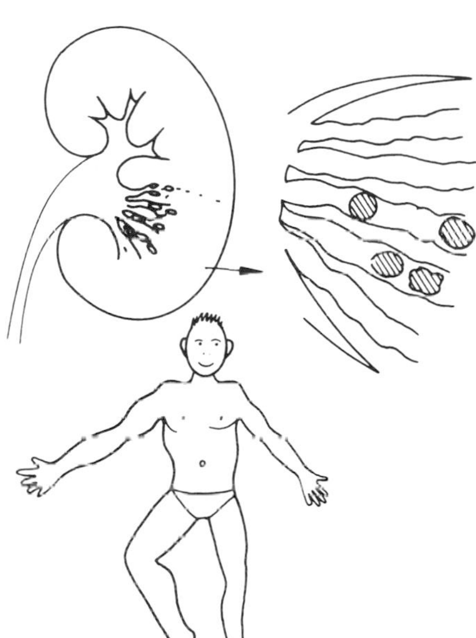

Fig. 4.21. Medullary sponge kidney. Congenital 'ectasis' of the collecting tubules which lead to stone formation and eventually to renal failure. This is associated with unilateral hemihypertrophy of the limbs—so ask about odd sizes of shoes and gloves!

Medullary sponge kidney

In this condition the collecting ducts are dilated and baggy (Fig. 4.21). It affects the kidney either in part or entirely, and it may be unilateral or bilateral. It is usually noticed in young adults and gradually gets worse. The cause is not known: it is sometimes familial, and may be associated with unilateral hemihypertrophy (where people have one arm or leg bigger than the other). The dilated and baggy tubules have stagnant urine inside them where stones and infection arise. The affected part of the kidney is the medulla: it becomes swollen and honeycombed with cysts — 'medullary sponge kidney'. The radiographic appearance is typical (Fig. 4.22). If only one part of the kidney is affected it can be removed, but more often the disease is too extensive to allow this. The patients get repeated attacks of infection and ureteric colic as the little stones keep on passing down the ureter. Today, thanks to extracorporeal lithotripsy the stones can be fragmented before they give rise to serious trouble. Associated scarring from the infection often damages the distal tubule so that there is a failure of acidification and concentrating power.

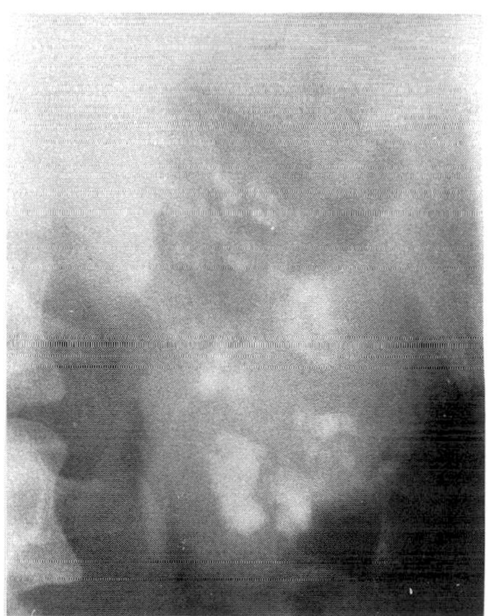

Fig. 4.22. Plain X-ray of a medullary sponge kidney: the dilated tubules are filled with innumerable small calculi.

Obstruction cysts

The metanephros may develop, but the ureter may become narrowed in fetal life. Urine is formed, and the tubules and nephrons become distended turning the kidney into a mass of cysts. When present on both sides the baby is born with *congenital multicystic kidneys* (Fig. 4.23). The fetus forms no urine, so there is no amniotic fluid, and the baby's face is squashed into a typical deformity — Potter's facies (Fig. 4.24). The condition is incompatible with life. There are usually other congenital anomalies of the cardiovascular and other systems.

A lesser form of this condition occurs when the ureter fails to develop properly on one side and the metanephros becomes *dysplastic*. Small cysts are a typical feature of these little kidneys.

A single calix is sometimes obstructed and the pyramid draining into it converted into a *caliceal cyst*. Most of these seem to be congenital, but some are acquired from late scarring (Fig. 4.25).

In pyelonephritic scarring (see p. 67) the collecting tubules are blocked and the nephrons may become grossly distended with fluid. At first this produces the typical microscopic changes of 'thyroid-like' areas as the dilated tubules are choked with protein, but later on distinct cysts

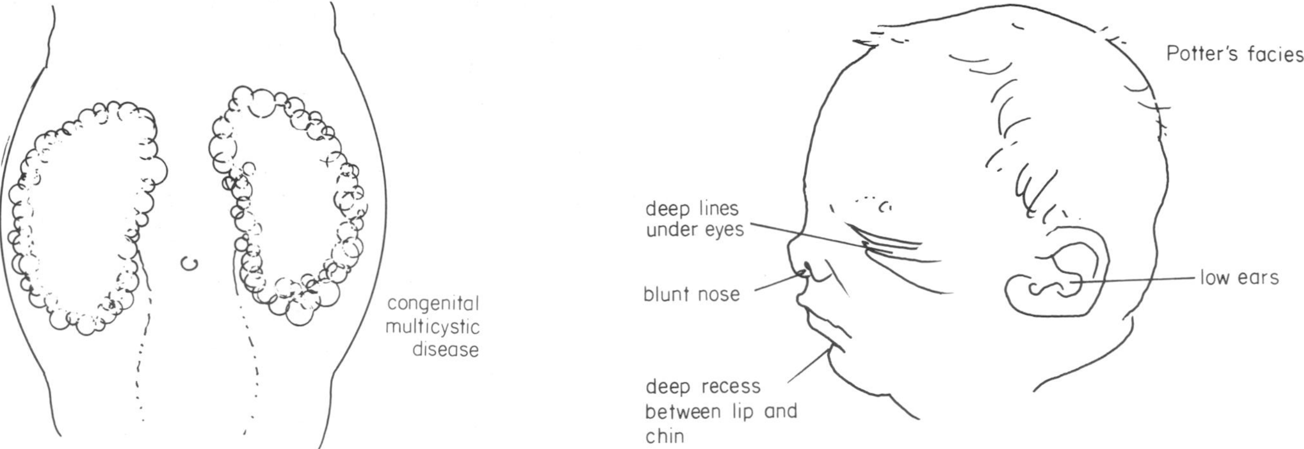

Fig. 4.23. Congenital multicystic disease. The ureters are blocked or absent. There is hydramnios and the condition is incompatible with survival.

Fig. 4.24. Potter's facies, from lack of amniotic fluid.

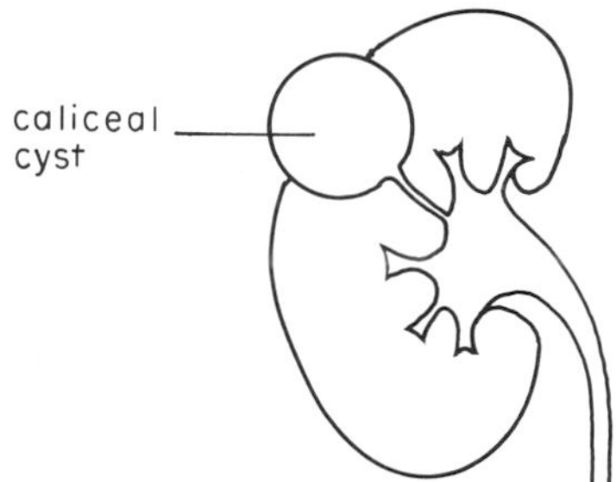

Fig. 4.25. Caliceal cyst.

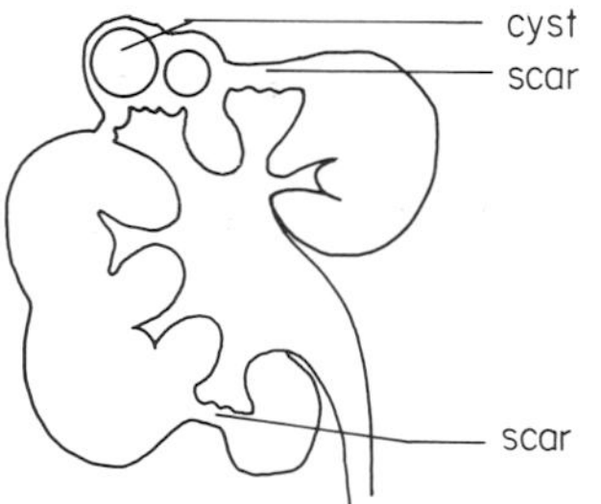

Fig. 4.26. Cysts formed as a result of obstruction to calices or collecting ducts by inflammatory scarring.

are formed (Fig. 4.26). Today these are increasingly being seen in patients with chronic renal failure who have been maintained for several years by dialysis.

Diverticula of the collecting tubules

Much more important and more common are the cysts that arise as diverticula from the collecting tubules of the kidney. One or two of these *simple cysts* (Fig. 4.27) occur in middle age in almost every kidney, and others are detected by chance in the course of the investigation of haematuria or, today, when there is some occasion to perform an abdominal ultrasound scan (Fig. 4.28). It used to be very difficult to distinguish these cysts from renal cell cancers, since both present as a 'space-occupying-mass' in the excretion urogram. Today the ultrasound scan settles the question by showing an absence of echoes from the cyst and if there is still any doubt, the fluid is aspirated and examined for malignant cells.

These simple renal cysts may cause obstruction to calices, particularly when they arise in the middle of the kidney (*parapelvic cysts*) and if they refill, as they usually do, after being aspirated, they are uncapped at an open operation (Fig. 4.29).

A bizarre exaggeration of this process is seen in *polycystic disease* which is inherited via a Mendelian dominant gene that declares itself at

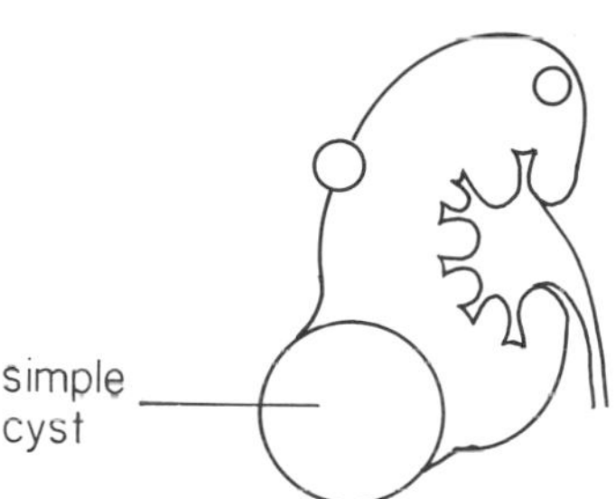

Fig. 4.27. Simple cysts—small ones are normal.

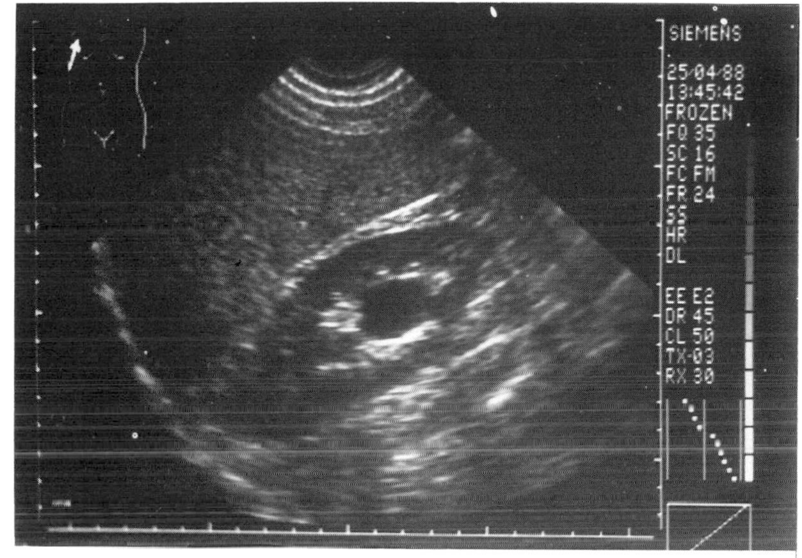

Fig. 4.28. Ultrasound of kidney showing a round cyst in the middle.

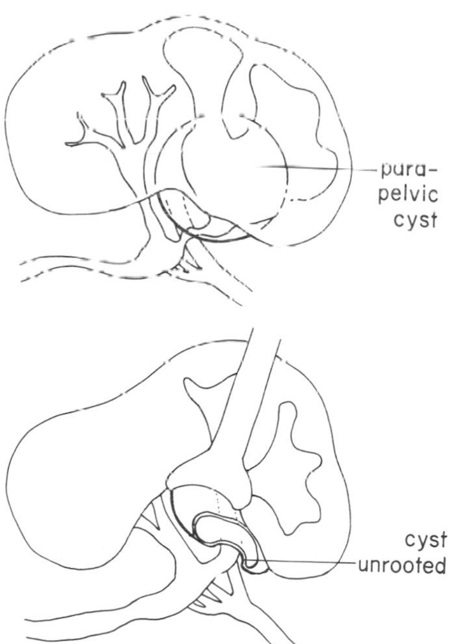

Fig. 4.29. A parapelvic cyst may cause obstruction to the neck of a calix or calices by squeezing it against a branch of the renal artery. Unroofing the cyst cures the obstruction.

different ages. It affects one or both kidneys: it may be associated with cysts in the liver and pancreas and berry aneurysms of the circle of Willis that cause subarachnoid haemorrhage. Polycystic disease usually presents in adult life when a lump is found on routine abdominal examination, or because the patient has haematuria, urinary infection, or hypertension. Occasionally the fluid inside the cyst may become infected and must be drained. Instead of there being only one or two cysts, the kidney is riddled with them (Fig. 4.30).

It is important to get polycystic disease into perspective. Although there is a slow progression of the disorder towards ultimate renal failure, the rate of progress in most patients is very slow, and they usually die of old age. Others need treatment as the years go by for their urinary infection and hypertension, and a few develop renal failure that can be controlled at first by diet, but later needs dialysis or transplantation. In former times it was the custom to aspirate these cysts at *Rovsing's operation* but this only makes the renal function worse. Very occasionally the cysts obstruct the renal pelvis or calices and then they should be unroofed.

CONGENITAL DISORDERS OF FUNCTION OF THE RENAL TUBULES

Congenital disorders of the proximal tubule result in failure of reabsorption of amino acids, glucose and phosphate. When the distal tubule is involved there may be a failure to produce acid urine, and when the collecting duct is affected there may be a failure to reabsorb water resulting in a diuresis.

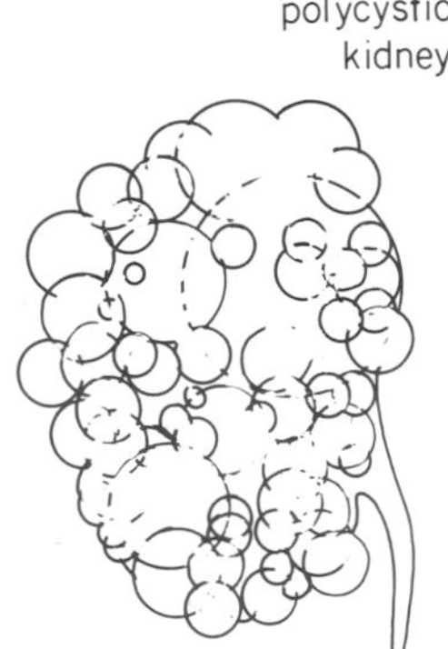

Fig. 4.30. Polycystic disease.

Proximal tubular disorders

There are many types of defect in the enzyme systems which transport the amino acids through the proximal tubule and the bowel. The most important of these is *cystinuria* (Fig. 4.31) where the transport of four amino acids is affected — cystine, ornithine, arginine and lysine ('COAL'). This is inherited as a Mendelian autosomal recessive and only about 3% of the patients are homozygous. Cystine is very poorly soluble in urine. Heterozygous patients lose about 500 mg/24 hours in their urine, and homozygous patients about 1 g so the homozygous patient is virtually bound to have urine that is supersaturated for cystine. The stones are radiodense owing to their sulphur content. Giving penicillamine binds the cystine in a soluble form (Fig. 4.31).

In *Hartnup disease* it is tryptophane that is involved. The major burden of the illness concerns not the renal tubule but the uptake of tryptophane from the bowel which results in nicotinamide deficiency and leads to pellagra and cerebellar ataxia. In *Fanconi's syndrome* there is a failure of absorption of a cluster of amino acids as well as phosphate, together with proteinuria and acidosis.

In renal glycosuria the tubules fail to reabsorb glucose and it appears in the urine even when the blood sugar is normal: it must be distinguished from diabetes but is otherwise harmless.

The tubules may fail to reabsorb phosphate from the glomerular filtrate resulting in '*vitamin D resistant rickets*'.

```
   Cysteine          Cystine        Cysteine-Penicillamine

    COOH              COOH              COOH
     |                 |                 |
  H—C—NH2          H—C—NH2           H—C—NH2
     |                 |                 |
  H—C—H            H—C—H             H—C—H
     |                 |                 |
    SH                 S                 S
- - - - - - - -        |                 |
    SH                 S                 S
     |                 |                 |
  H—C—HH2          H—C—H           H3C—C—CH3
     |                 |                 |
H3C—C—CH3          H—C—NH2           H—C—NH2
     |                 |                 |
    COOH              COOH              COOH
 Penicillamine
```

Fig. 4.31. The relationship between cystine, cysteine and penicillamine.

Distal tubular disorders

Renal tubular acidosis

When the distal tubule is unable to pump out hydrogen ions the kidney cannot form an acid urine, and instead loses potassium, phosphate, sulphate and organic acids. There is a metabolic acidosis with a low plasma bicarbonate which increases the proportion of calcium not bound to protein, and more calcium escapes in the glomerular filtrate where, because the urine is alkaline, it is precipitated in the tubules causing speckled calcification in the renal medulla — 'nephrocalcinosis'. These patients usually have normal glomerular function but the loss of calcium and phosphate may lead to osteomalacia. The diagnosis is made by the acid load test and the remedy is to give potassium bicarbonate or citrate, and perhaps additional vitamin D.

Nephrogenic diabetes insipidus

A sex-linked Mendelian recessive gene in males prevents their collecting tubules from responding to anti-diuretic hormone. The continued diuresis may lead to dehydration which may be so severe as to cause brain damage in the baby. A rather similar condition is seen in hydronephrosis, obstructive atrophy and pyelonephritic scarring.

FURTHER READING

Baert L & Steg A (1977) On the pathogenesis of simple renal cysts in the adult — a microdissection study. *Urological Research* 5, 103–8.

Crelin ES (1978) Normal and abnormal development of the ureter. *Urology* **12**, 2–7.

Gardner KD & Evan AP (1987) Cystic diseases of the kidney. In: Gonick HC (Ed) *Current Nephrology* (10). Year Book Medical Publications Inc., Chicago.

Gosling JA & Dixon JS (1985) Embryology of the urinary tract. In: Whitfield HN & Hendry WF (Eds) *Textbook of Genitourinary Surgery*. Churchill Livingstone, Edinburgh. pp. 123–31.

Graves FT (1971) *The Arterial Anatomy of the Kidney*. Wright, Bristol

Mackie GC & Stephens FD (1975) Duplex kidneys: a correlation of renal dysplasia with position of the ureteral orifice. *Journal of Urology* **114**, 274–80.

Potter EL (1973) *Normal and Abnormal Development of the Kidney*. Lloyd-Luke Medical Books, London.

Thompson BJ, Jenkins DAS, Allan PL & Winney RJ (1986) Acquired cystic disease of the kidney: an indication for renal transplantation? *British Medical Journal* **293**, 1209–10.

5 The Kidney — Trauma

PENETRATING INJURIES

Penetrating injuries of the kidney may be caused by bullet or knife wounds. Low velocity bullet and stab wounds call for abdominal exploration and conservative management of the kidney and the other viscera in the line of the missile or the knife but high velocity modern bullet injuries are a different matter: here the blast effect of the bullet inside the body devitalizes a huge sphere of tissue. There are few survivors, and a kidney found in the vicinity of such a high velocity bullet injury must be removed or there will be fatal secondary haemorrhage.

CLOSED INJURIES

Much more common in civilian practice are closed injuries of the kidney from accidents at work or in sport. The blow which damages the kidney often fractures the lower ribs and shears off some of the tips of the transverse processes of the lumbar vertebrae (Fig. 5.1). To cause such bony injuries the initial blow must be very severe, and the pain and soft tissue contusion is always considerable.

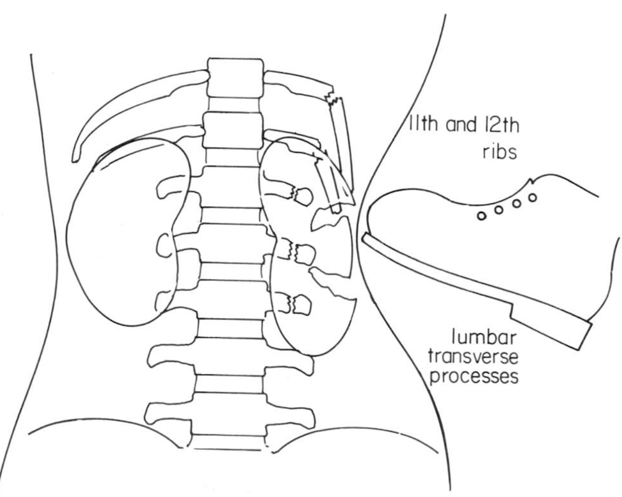

Fig. 5.1. Closed injury that damages the kidney often causes fracture of the lower ribs and lumbar transverse processes.

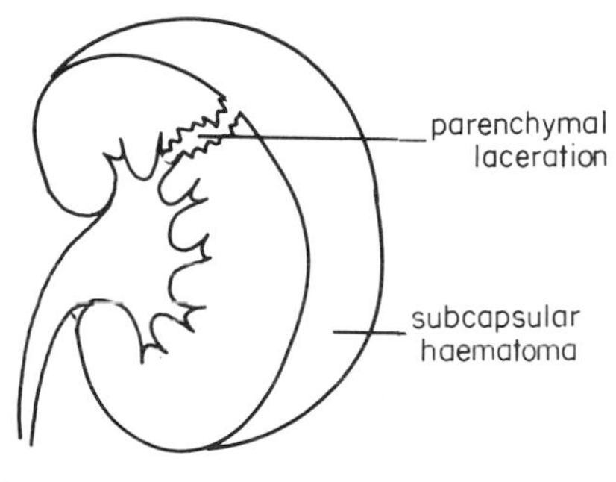

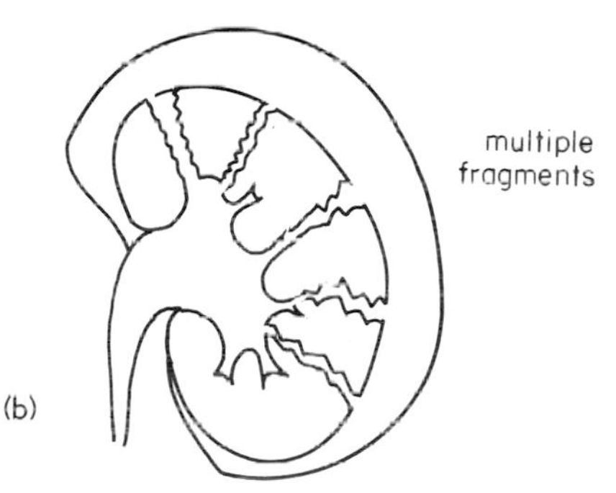

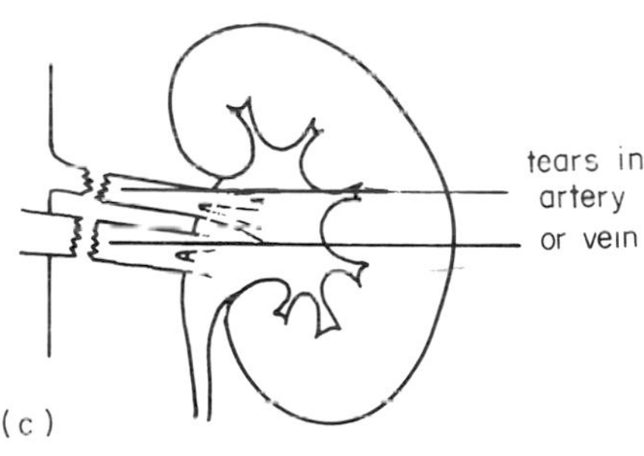

Fig. 5.2. Three grades of renal injury: (a) laceration of the parenchyma with subcapsular haematoma; (b) fragmentation of the kidney; (c) tear of the renal artery or vein or both.

There are three grades of renal injury:

1 the parenchyma is split and gives rise to haematuria and a surrounding haematoma, but is usually self-limiting, and followed by complete restoration of kidney anatomy and function after a few weeks (Fig. 5.2);

2 the kidney is split into several fragments and continues to bleed;

3 there is a tear of the main renal artery or vein.

The patient gives a history of a kick or injury to the loin. There are often other injuries, especially of the ribs (which may be important because of the risk of pneumothorax) or the spleen and liver (and the risk of internal haemorrhage). Usually the patient notices blood in the urine soon after his injury.

At first there may be no physical signs other than vague tenderness in the loin but every patient must be admitted for observation because there is no way of telling at this stage how the injury is going to develop.

On admission the patient is carefully examined with special regard to the chest and abdomen. A chest X-ray and an emergency IVU are obtained — the IVU not so much to show the type of injury, but to make sure there is a kidney on the other side. The patient is then kept under close observation, the pulse, blood pressure and abdominal girth being measured at regular intervals, and every specimen of urine saved.

Usually these patients get steadily better: the colour of the blood in the urine becomes paler and less pink. In the rare unfortunate case the pulse, blood pressure and abdominal signs suggest there is continuing internal bleeding. If these disturbing features are noticed, an emergency *renal angiogram* is obtained. This shows the exact nature of the lesion of the kidney — i.e. whether there is a single split, or total disruption. The angiogram may show that the haemorrhage is issuing from a single branch of the renal artery, which may be plugged with chopped muscle or gelfoam injected through the angiogram catheter (Fig. 5.3). If this is not possible or the patient is obviously losing blood very rapidly, a laparotomy is performed as soon as possible. The kidney is approached through a midline incision. The aorta and renal vessels are secured before Gerota's fascia is opened since this may confine the haematoma and control loss of blood by tamponade. Once the renal artery is occluded, it may be possible to control the bleeding and save at least part of the kidney.

Follow-up

There are five important complications to be watched for in the follow-up of closed renal injury (Figs 5.4, 5.5).

1 *Secondary haemorrhage.* After a tear of the renal parenchyma the clot

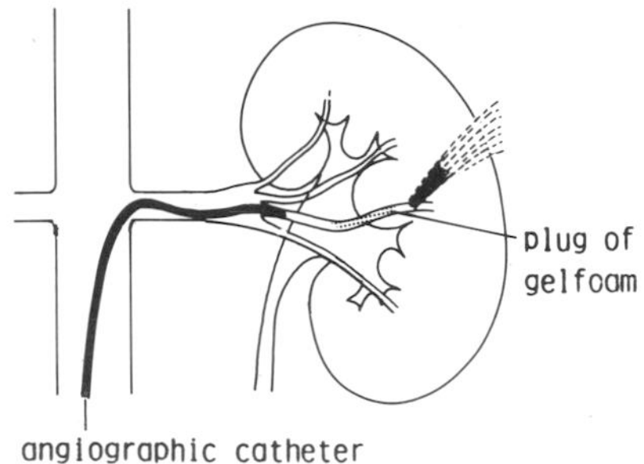

Fig. 5.3. Continuing haemorrhage from a torn segmental artery may be stopped by injecting the vessel with gelfoam or minced muscle under angiographic control.

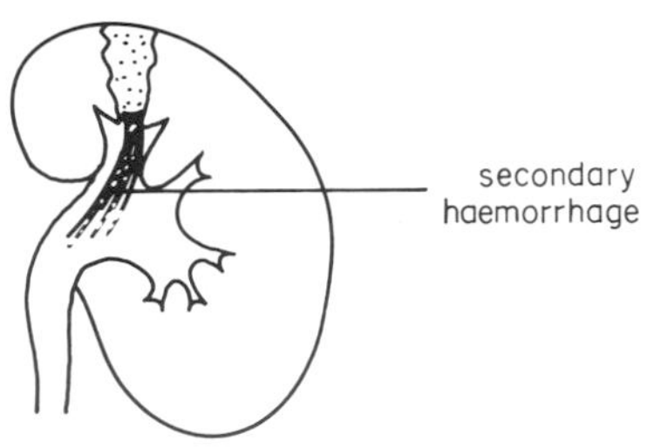

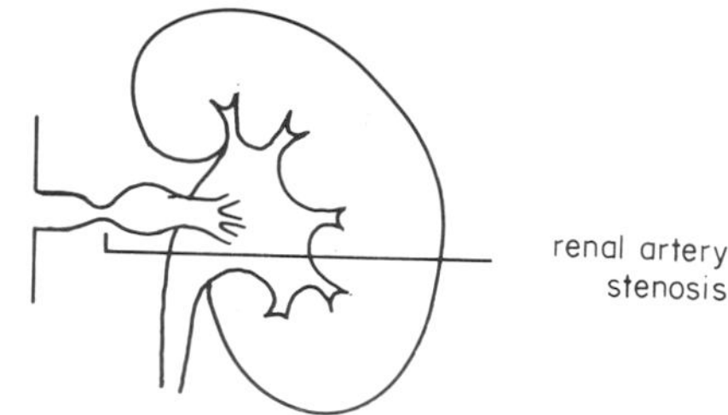

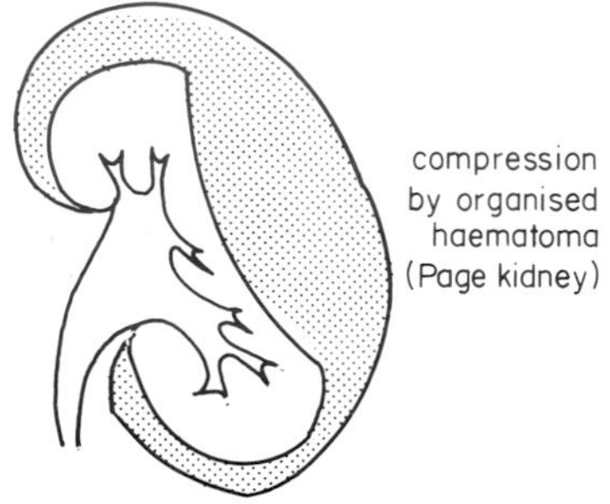

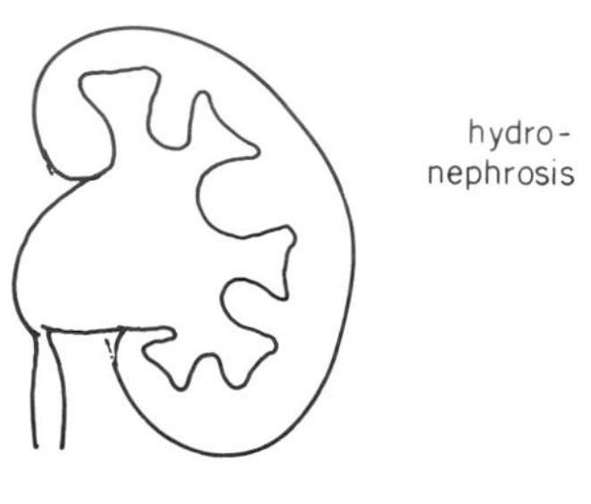

Fig. 5.4. Delayed complications of closed renal trauma—secondary haemorrhage, renal artery stenosis and compression by organized haematoma giving rise to hypertension and hydronephrosis.

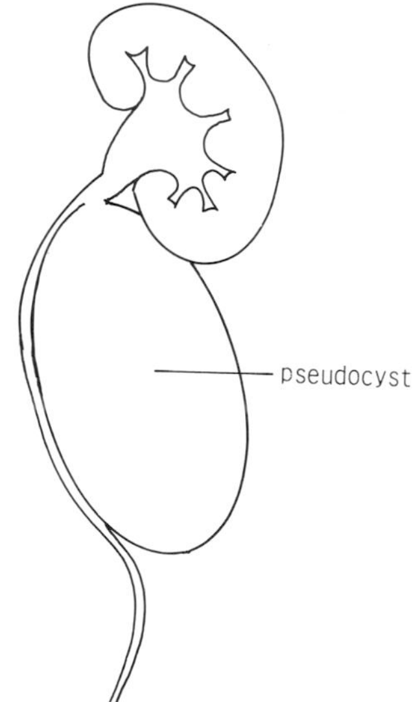

Fig. 5.5. Organization of granulation tissue around an extrarenal collection of urine urinoma—leading to a pseudocyst.

that sticks the pieces of kidney together may undergo lysis and bleeding may start again. For this reason in severe renal injuries the patient is kept in hospital for at least 10 days.

2 *Late hypertension from renal artery stenosis.* The blood pressure is measured at regular intervals during the first few months after closed renal injury. Damage to the renal artery may be succeeded by hypertension, and relieved by excising or by-passing the narrow segment of artery (see p. 115).

3 *Late hypertension from organized haematoma around the kidney — the Page kidney.* An organizing haematoma may form a thick tough rind around the kidney which compresses it and makes it ischaemic.

4 *Hydronephrosis.* There are few documented cases where a kidney known to have been normal, has developed a hydronephrosis from injury to the renal pelvis or ureter. Usually the hydronephrosis comes to light only after the injury but must have been present for a long time. A distended balloon is more likely to burst than a floppy one, and a distended hydronephrosis is more prone to trauma than a normal renal pelvis.

5 *Pseudocyst or urinoma.* This is an important but rare complication: a split in the renal pelvis allows urine to escape into the surrounding tissues where it forms a localized collection — a 'urinoma' (Fig. 5.5) which may become surrounded by a thick, sometimes partly calcified wall, which may ultimately become infected: it must be carefully dissected out if it is to be cured.

FURTHER READING

Conrad MR, Freedman M, Weiner C, Freeman C & Sanders RS (1976) Sonography of the Page kidney. *Journal of Urology* **116**, 293–6.

Page IH (1939) The production of persistent arterial hypertension by cellophane and perinephritis. *Journal of the American Medical Association* **113**, 2046–7.

Selikowitz SM (1977) Penetrating high-velocity genitourinary injuries. *Urology* **9**, 371–6.

Whitney RF & Peterson NE (1976) Penetrating renal injuries. *Urology* **7**, 7–11.

6 The Kidney — Glomerulonephritis

By tradition the diseases described in this chapter are called *glomerulonephritis* because the most distinctive features of the inflammation are found in the glomerulus, though in fact the entire nephron is always involved. These have an immunological basis and one can identify four steps:

1 damage to the glomerular basement membrane which alters its permeability and allows albumin to escape: the structural damage is minimal, and indeed, can only be detected with the electron microscope;

2 soluble complex disease — antigen + antibody forms a 'soluble complex' which damages the glomerulus in proportion to the size of the complex: it does not fix complement or excite inflammation;

3 the soluble antigen-antibody complex fixes complement, sets off the inflammatory response, and this makes the damage much worse;

4 the aftermath of inflammation, i.e. scarring.

PATHOLOGY OF GLOMERULONEPHRITIS

Anything can act as an antigen either by itself or in combination with various peptides (haptens). The list of known antigens that can cause human glomerulonephritis is very long and ranges from quite simple chemicals including many that are used in treatment such as tridione, penicillamine and butazolidine: microbes especially streptococci, staphylococci, *Treponema pallidum*, and *Plasmodium malariae* — and even the patient's own DNA, can act as the allergen in systemic lupus.

In a healthy patient with enough antibodies the immune defences of the body respond to an unwanted antigen by wrapping it in a cocoon of *insoluble complexes* which are cleared away by the reticuloendothelial system. These large complexes seldom appear in the kidney at all, and if they do they are soon got rid of. Any illness that they give rise to is brief and (usually) carries a good prognosis.

Patients may not have enough antibody to smother the antigen completely: this is when smaller *soluble complexes* are formed. The larger ones get stuck in the mesangium but the smaller ones reach the glomerulus and may penetrate the basement membrane to be trapped between the slit pores of the foot processes of the epithelial cells. A very few reach the capillary wall.

The soluble complexes may fix complement. As soon as the first of these (C1) sticks to an antigen–immunoglobulin complex it sets off a cascade of other complement factors which are immensely destructive — perforating cell membranes and causing lysis, releasing histamine from mast cells and platelets, dilating blood vessels to make them more permeable and attracting leukocytes.

CLASSIFICATION OF GLOMERULONEPHRITIS

The conventional classification of glomerulonephritis has been confused by a terminology which generally refers not to the cause or clinical features of the illness but to histological and ultramicroscopic changes seen on renal biopsy, e.g. minimal change (Fig. 6.1), focal or diffuse, mesangial or glomerular, membranous (Fig. 6.2) or proliferative (Fig. 6.3).

Whether the disease is diffuse or focal is a question of degree, reflecting the severity of the process: focal lesions being less dangerous and having a better prognosis. If complement has not been fixed, only the membrane may be affected by the accumulation of soluble complexes. When complement has been fixed and inflammation has been set off, then cells 'proliferate' in the mesangium and the glomerular tuft (Fig. 6.4), and escape into Bowman's capsule to clog up the urine space.

There are two clinical pictures. In the *nephrotic syndrome*, which is mainly seen in children, with minimal change or membranous lesions, there is loss of albumin through the damaged membrane. With the loss of albumin the plasma oncotic pressure falls and plasma water leaks,

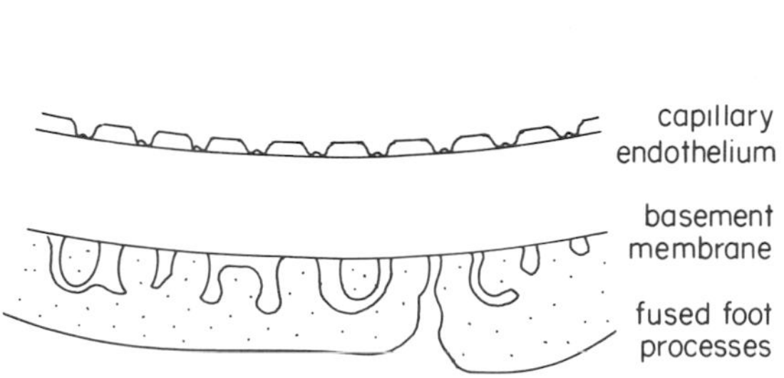

Fig. 6.1. Minimal change disease. There is an increase in the permeability of the basement membrane, probably through an alteration in its electrical charge. In response to the loss of protein, the epithelial foot processes become fused together.

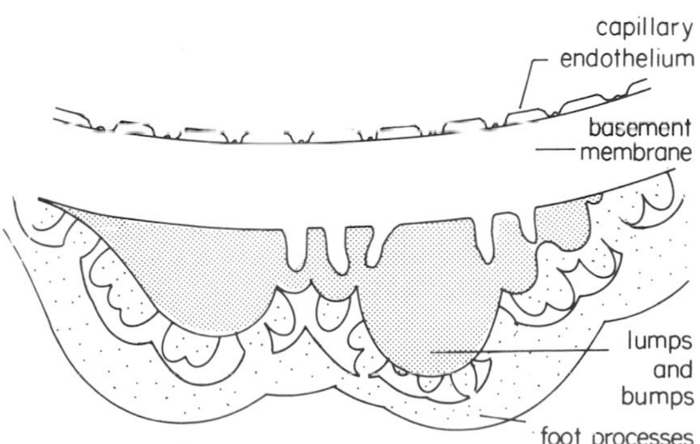

Fig. 6.2. Membranous glomerulonephritis. Lumps and bumps of soluble complex escape through the basement membrane but get trapped under the foot processes of the epithelial cells of Bowman's capsule.

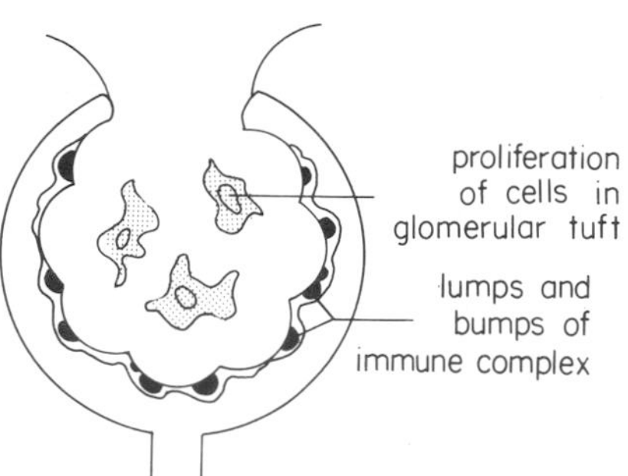

Fig. 6.3. Endocapillary proliferative glomerulonephritis. Cells in the glomerular tuft are proliferated and swollen: there are big lumps and bumps of soluble complex.

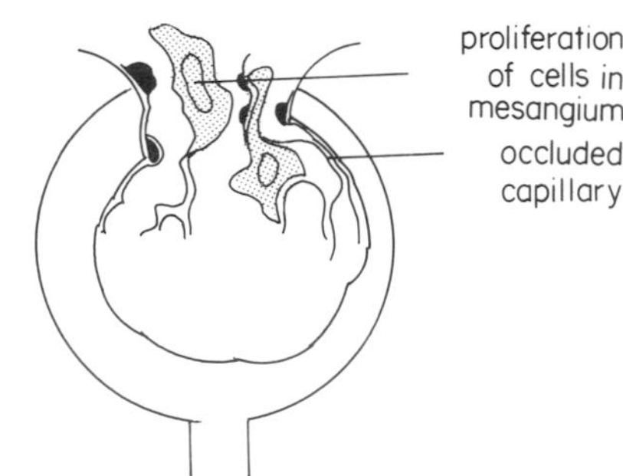

Fig. 6.4. Mesangial proliferative glomerulonephritis. Proliferation of cells mainly in the mesangium, perhaps because the complexes are so large that they are held up here.

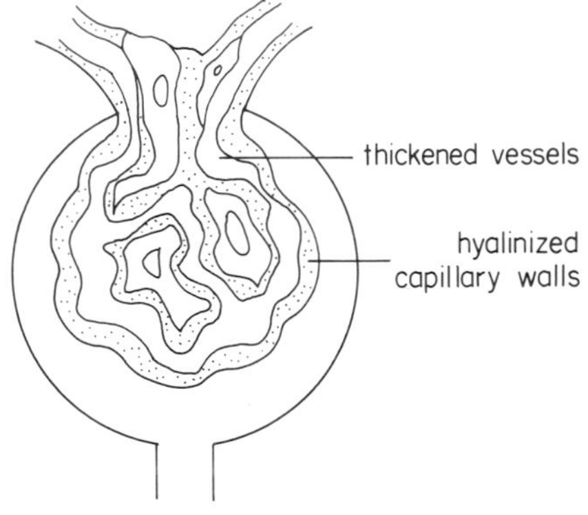

Fig. 6.5. Mesangiocapillary glomerulonephritis. More sinister changes occur—thickened vessels and hyalinized capillaries.

causing widespread oedema. Along with albumin there is also a leak of cholesterol which the tubules reabsorb, causing hypercholesterolaemia, and streaking the oedematous kidneys with lipid. Usually there is spontaneous recovery, and the condition may be reversed by steroids.

In the *nephritic syndrome* there is usually a more rapid onset of the disease. Destruction resulting from complement fixation leads to larger breaches in the filter, with loss of protein, red and white cells which appear in the urine as granular casts. Hypertension is often severe. There may be oliguria or anuria. The outlook depends to some extent on the pattern of the damage in the kidney, and renal biopsy may be useful in predicting the outcome. Where proliferation of cells is mainly in the mesangium or the glomerular tuft (Fig. 6.5) the changes are often reversible. Where both lots of vessels are involved and collections of cells are seen proliferating in the space of Bowman's capsule (Fig. 6.6), the outlook is bad. It is worst of all when the kidneys reach the end stage, where the glomeruli become replaced by little spheres of hyaline debris and there is scarring between and around the tubules.

You will undoubtedly come across several of the more important syndromes within this group of diseases.

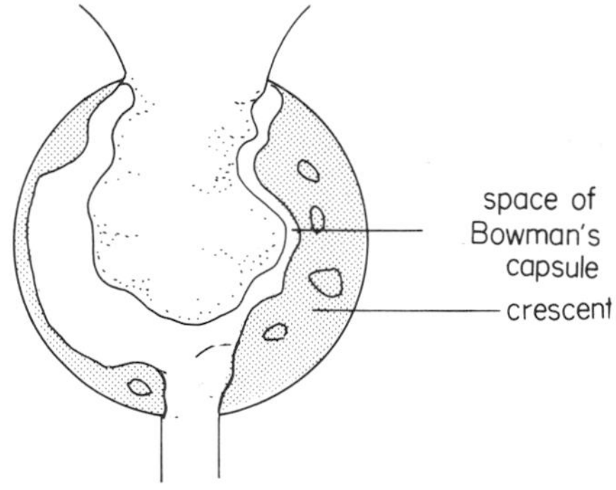

Fig. 6.6. Extracapillary proliferative glomerulonephritis. Bowman's capsule is beginning to fill up with 'crescents.'

Goodpasture's syndrome

It seems that the glomerular basement membrane has elements in common with the basement membrane of the pulmonary alveoli. In Goodpasture's syndrome after a pulmonary infection, antigenic material is released to which antibodies form which attack the basement membrane, fix complement, and set off a rapid and irreversible nephritic syndrome. Characteristically there is a vivid combination of haemoptysis, haematuria and renal failure.

Henoch-Schönlein nephritis

A sudden onset of abdominal and joint pains in a child is accompanied by purpura and sometimes by the nephritic syndrome. The outlook is usually good. The glomeruli show only mesangial changes but if crescents are seen in Bowman's space the outlook is less favourable.

Polyarteritis nodosa

Necrotizing inflammation in the walls of arteries all over the body includes changes in the arcuate arteries of the kidney and glomeruli: tufts are entirely replaced by fibrinoid necrosis. Others show severe extracapillary proliferation of cells in Bowman's space. The outlook is very bad.

Lupus nephritis

The antigen is the patient's own DNA. Soluble complexes in the glomeruli may give rise to the whole range of changes, but fortunately are usually limited to the membrane and cause the nephrotic syndrome.

Alport's syndrome

There are abnormalities in the basement membrane with proteinuria, and eventually crescents. It is inherited as an autosomal dominant, appears in boys before puberty, and is accompanied by deafness, ocular abnormalities and polyneuropathy.

Diabetic renal disease

This is not a glomerulonephritis and immunological mechanisms are not involved, but it presents with the nephrotic syndrome, and is characterized by the presence of an eosinophilic matrix in the mesangium and the glomerulus, with thickening of the afferent and efferent arterioles and the basement membrane.

Amyloidosis

Amyloid may be deposited in both primary and secondary amyloidosis between the basement membrane and the mesangium, going on to form eosinophilic deposits which make the tufts less and less cellular, and fill up the space of Bowman's capsule. The tubules are also involved, and the whole picture may be made suddenly worse by thrombosis of the renal vein.

Myelomatosis

In multiple myeloma there is an excessive production of immunoglobulins. In about half the patients light-chain immunoglobulins are found which appear in the urine as a protein which coagulates as the urine is warmed to 45–55°C and then dissolves again as the temperature is increased (Bence-Jones protein).

FURTHER READING

Cameron JS (1985) Glomerulonephritis. In: Marsh FP (Ed) *Postgraduate Nephrology*. Heinemann Medical Books, London. pp. 237–96.

Haverty T, Kelly CJ & Neilson EG (1987) Immune-mediated renal disease. In: Gonick HC (Ed) *Current Nephrology* (10). Year Book Publications Inc., Chicago. pp. 1–36.

Little PJ, Sloper JS & de Wardener HE (1967) A syndrome of loin pain and haematuria associated with disease of peripheral renal arteries. *Quarterly Journal of Medicine* **36**, 253–9.

Risdon RA & Turner DR (1980) *Atlas of Renal Pathology*. MTP Press, Lancaster.

Shuki WH, Massry SG (Eds) (1984) Therapy of renal diseases and related disorders. Martinus Nijhoff Publishing, Dordrecht.

Thompson IM (1987) The evaluation of microscopic haematuria: a population-based study. *Journal of Urology* **138**, 1189–90.

7 The Kidney and Urinary Infection

ACUTE URINARY INFECTION

Ascending

Bacteria in the urethra can reach the bladder whence reflux may carry them to the kidney if the ureteric valve is deficient. If, in addition, there are compound renal papillae, then infected urine may be forced into the renal pyramid where it will set up inflammation.

Haematogenous

Bacteria may also reach the kidney through the bloodstream. Here multiple small miliary abscesses may be found throughout the kidney. They are usually dealt with by the defence mechanisms but are often seen post-mortem in patients who have suffered an episode of bacteraemia before death. In experimental animals injected organisms are dealt with and the kidneys heal up unless there is some localized damage in the kidney. It is the same in man: a kidney that has previously been scarred from whatever cause, is more susceptible to clinical infection from a haematogenous source.

Ascending infection is usually from an organism that has originated in the patient's own intestinal flora, e.g. *Escherichia coli, Klebsiella, Streptococcus faecalis, Proteus mirabilis.* A patient given broad-spectrum antibiotics or who has had to sit around in hospital for any length of time, may have more dangerous organisms because the intestine is likely to have been colonized by resistant micro-organisms from the hospital environment. This is one of the chief reasons why urologists are reluctant to use prophylactic antibiotics. In patients with relapses of urinary tract infection the new organism may not be of the same strain as on the previous occasion.

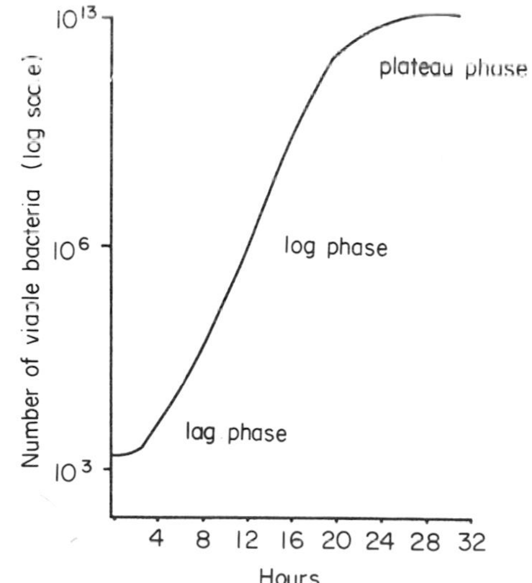

Fig. 7.1. Growth of micro-organisms in the urine.

FACTORS PREDISPOSING TO URINARY INFECTION

Stagnant urine

Urine is a good culture medium for many organisms (Fig. 7.1), allowing them to multiply very rapidly at normal body temperature once they

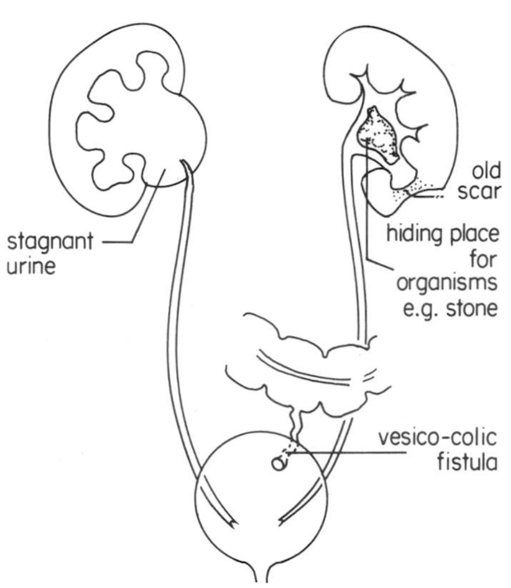

Fig. 7.2. Some of the common causes of persistent or relapsing urinary infection.

enter a pool of urine that is not regularly and completely emptied (Fig. 7.2). Such stagnant pools are seen under four circumstances as follows:

1 *Infrequent voiding.* Some women are in the habit of emptying their bladders only once or twice a day. Dividing every 15 minutes, an inoculum of only 10 organisms can, within 6 hours, have multiplied to 8 million. One of the chief weapons in the therapy of urinary infection is to encourage frequent emptying of the bladder so that organisms are never given time to multiply.

2 *Mechanical obstruction to the urinary tract.* This results in incomplete emptying of the bladder, ureters or kidneys. Overcoming this obstruction forms a large part of routine urological surgery. There may be hydronephrosis from obstruction at the pelviureteric junction, dilatation of the ureter from obstruction from a stone, obstruction to the outflow of the bladder by the prostate or a urethral stricture, or because the bladder does not empty because its detrusor is defectively innervated.

3 *Undrained pockets of urine.* Diverticula occur in the bladder and in the kidney, and similar pockets may be seen elsewhere in the urinary tract.

4 *Dilated or refluxing ureters.* There are a number of conditions in which the ureters are dilated: sometimes this is due to an obstruction at the lower end: sometimes the ureterovesical valve is deficient and the urine reaches the kidney by vesicoureteric reflux. The effect is to produce a pool of urine that is pushed up and down from the bladder but never empties out completely. One of the most important causes of urinary infection and renal damage in childhood is due to congenital vesicoureteric reflux and reflux nephropathy (see below).

Hiding places for micro-organisms

The most common hiding place for organisms is a stone: they are often crumbly and porous and between the collections of crystals there is room for organisms to lurk. A stone may shelter billions of bacteria year after year, protecting them from antibiotics which cannot diffuse into the very centre of the stone.

Other important causes of persistent infection are foreign bodies or dead tissue, e.g. a carcinoma whose surface has undergone necrosis, a non-absorbable suture or a fragment of broken-off catheter.

Fistulae

Diverticular disease, Crohn's disease or cancer may give rise to an abscess which bursts into the bladder and allows micro-organisms to enter from the intestine (Fig. 7.3).

Lowered resistance to infection

Many patients will tell you that their symptoms of urinary infection begin a few days after an influenza-like illness. It is seldom possible to detect a virus in urine, and it is not certain that a virus infection precedes a bacterial one, or whether it merely lowers the host resistance. No less important are other causes of lowered host resistance, e.g. diabetes mellitus, immunosuppression for transplantation and chemotherapy for cancer.

Infection is also more apt to attack tissues that have already been damaged, e.g. old tuberculosis in the urinary tract which has left calcified scars, and previous damage from interstitial nephritis due to causes other than infection.

THE END RESULT OF URINARY INFECTION IN THE KIDNEY

Infection in the kidney, like infection anywhere else in the body, is followed by one of four processes (Fig. 7.4) — resolution, suppuration, scarring and granuloma.

The commonest end result is *resolution*. Most patients with common

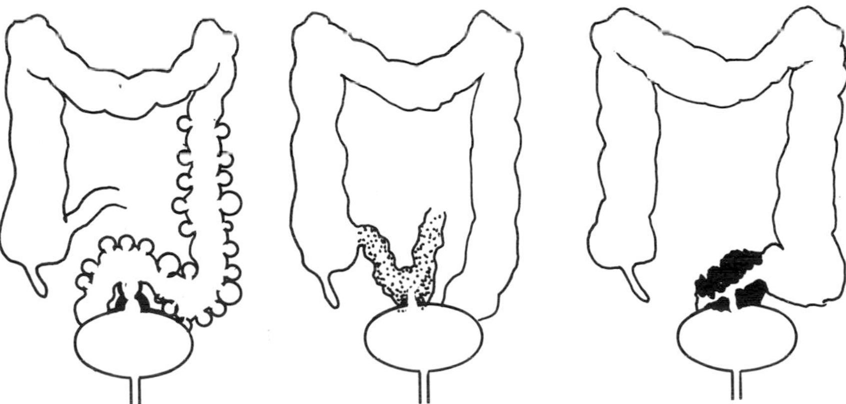

Fig. 7.3. Infection can be caused by an abnormal communication (fistula) between bowel and bladder due to diverticular disease, Crohn's regional ileitis, or carcinoma of the sigmoid colon.

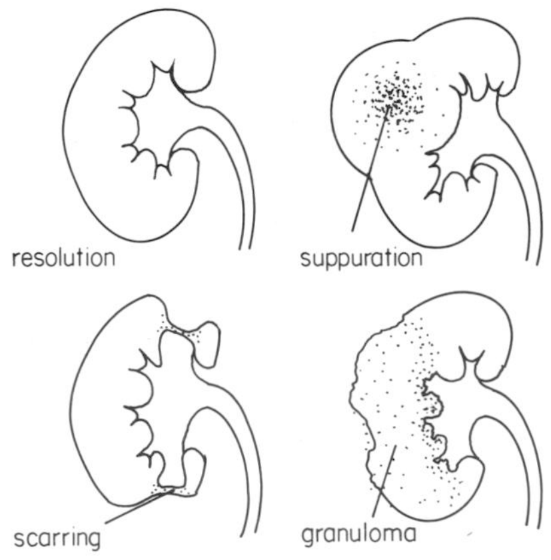

Fig. 7.4. The four possible results of infection in the kidney—resolution, suppuration, scarring or chronic granuloma formation.

bacterial infection in the bladder or kidney end up with an absolutely normal bladder and an undamaged kidney.

Suppuration is common in kidneys where there is already obstruction. At its worst this takes the form of a pyonephrosis, and the entire kidney is converted into a bag of pus. Minor forms of this occur when the calices are obstructed and infected, and form pyocalices. In these instances high pressure upstream of the obstruction forces infected urine into the renal parenchyma and even when the obstruction is relieved, there is always some loss of renal function and scarring.

Suppuration is also a rare consequence of haematogenous infection where it gives rise to renal parenchymal abscess and carbuncle (see below p. 72).

Scarring in the kidney is a very important and common sequel of urinary infection, and is almost entirely restricted to those cases where there has been a combination of infection and obstruction. But almost identical scarring may be produced by a number of other causes without any infection, the whole group being sometimes referred to as 'interstitial nephritis'.

Granulomas occur in kidneys infected by any of the organisms that are known elsewhere in the body to cause chronic inflammation so, as one might expect, granulomatous changes are seen in tuberculosis and brucellosis. There are also a group of granulomas in the urinary tract which follow infection with what might seem to be quite innocuous *E. coli* etc. Among these are malakoplakia and xanthogranuloma.

RENAL SCARRING, REFLUX NEPHROPATHY, INTERSTITIAL NEPHRITIS

Reflux nephropathy

Many children are born with defective valves where the ureters enter the bladder, often associated with duplex ureter or ureterocele. In most of these children the valve matures and becomes competent at about puberty. Sometimes reflux of urine up the ureter is associated with the presence of compound renal papillae. When the urine squirts up the ureter it is forced up through the tip of the papilla into the collecting tubules, rupturing their walls and injecting urine into the renal parenchyma. Uninfected urine probably causes little harm, but infected urine causes havoc: it sets up acute inflammation, and this is invariably followed by scarring — the typical deeply pitted scars of 'reflux nephropathy'.

As the child grows and the kidneys grow too, so the unaffected parts of

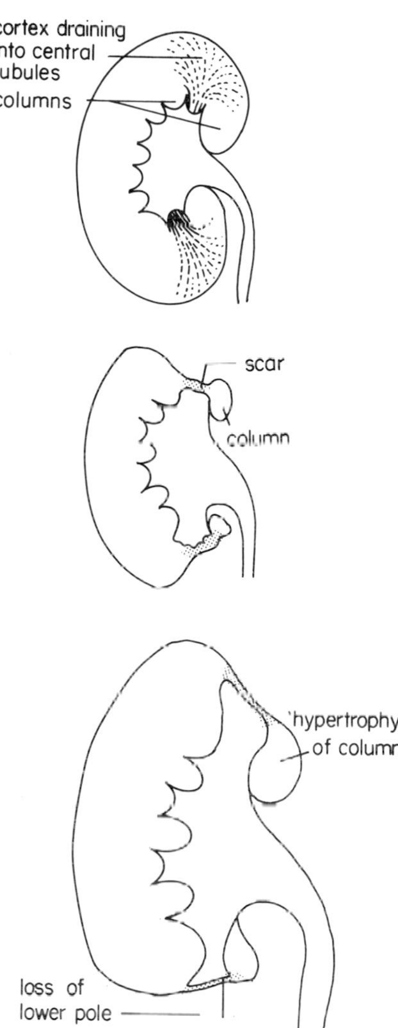

Fig. 7.5. Compound papillae that allow reflux to occur into the interstitium are usually found at the upper and lower poles. When these undergo scarring, the rest of the undamaged kidney continues to grow but the adult kidney continues to show the site of the scarring (below).

the kidney enlarge while the pitted scars become even deeper and more pronounced (Fig. 7.5). The deformed compound papillae are usually found at the upper and lower poles of the kidney so it is here that the brunt of the scarring in reflux nephropathy is to be found.

The diagnosis is made (see p. 20) by a micturating cystogram. If the reflux is not severe, and if the urine can be kept sterile by suitable medication, it is safe to wait for the valve to mature. If the reflux is very gross, and it is impossible to keep the urine sterile with daily medication, or if the child keeps getting break-through infection, then most paediatric urologists will perform an operation to prevent the reflux — ureteroneo-vesicostomy.

There are several methods of doing this: they all in essence make a new long tunnel for the ureter under the mucosa. One of the most simple and effective techniques is that of Cohen. The ureter is dissected out of its tunnel in the wall of the bladder: a new tunnel is made for it to the opposite side of the trigone through which the ureter is drawn and sewn to the bladder mucosa (Fig. 7.6).

In recent years it is claimed that equally good results follow the injection of a small blob of Teflon or collagen paste under the mucosa of the ureteric orifice to convert it into a kind of crescent (Fig. 7.7).

Interstitial nephritis from non-infective causes

Papillary necrosis

Many conditions cause death of the renal papilla, either partial or complete: it may occur in the extreme examples of suppuration which are seen in infection combined with obstruction, but it is also seen in

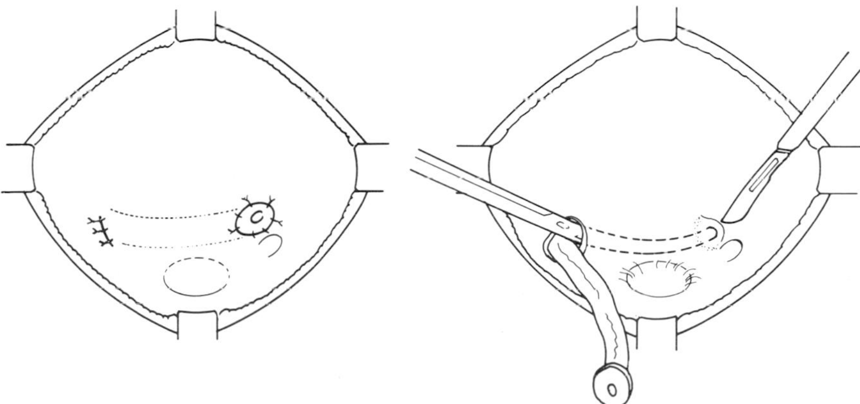

Fig. 7.6. Reimplantation of the ureter for reflux using Cohen's method.

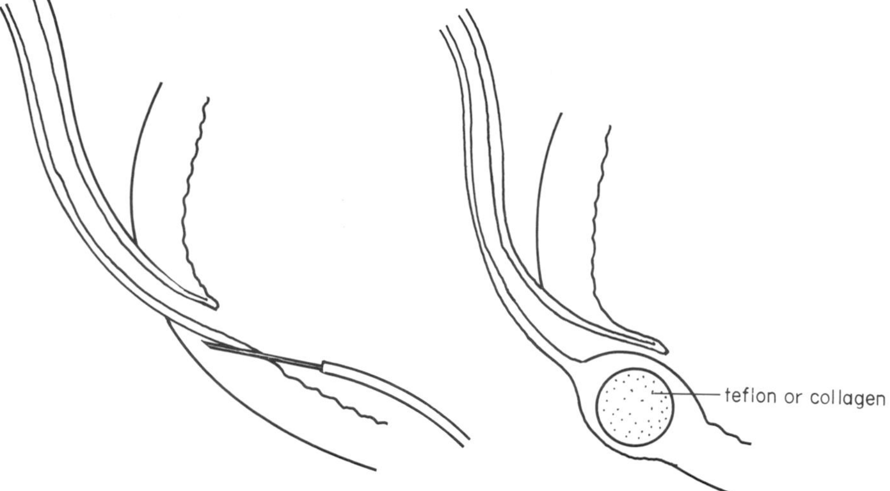

Fig. 7.7. A tiny blob of Teflon or collagen paste is injected below the mucosa of the floor of the ureteric orifice. This prevents reflux—STING—Submucosal Teflon Injection.

analgesic abuse, sickle-cell disease and Balkan nephropathy. The effect can be patchy: sometimes it seems that only one kidney is affected, and only two or three of the papillae, on other occasions it seems as though all the papillae have sloughed.

When the papilla dies, there is always some blockage of the overlying collecting tubules and scarring in the cortex. Sometimes a pyelogram will show a papilla that is not completely detached, with a line of demarcation forming around its base. Later on the detached papilla may become stuck in the ureter and give rise to ureteric colic like a stone, and sometimes a dead papilla lingers in the renal pelvis and acts as a nidus for the further growth of a stone.

Analgesic abuse

There was once a charlatan who persuaded the entire population of Husqvarna to take a certain phenacitin-containing powder to protect it from influenza and all other evils. Twenty years later Dr Hjorten's powder had produced an epidemic of scarred kidneys. Although there is no infection, the scarring is very similar to that of reflux nephropathy. Sometimes the papillae slough as well.

Balkan nephropathy

This occurs in isolated villages in the Balkans. It is thought that it may be due to a toxin produced by a fungus which attacks grain stored in damp barns. As with analgesic nephropathy, the scarring may be in the renal parenchyma with or without sloughing of the papilla. A late sequel of both can be multifocal cancer arising in the urothelium of the renal pelvis and calices.

Gout and nephrocalcinosis

The sharp needles of uric acid are deposited in and around the tubules where they provoke scarring. Something very similar may follow nephrocalcinosis of whatever cause.

COMPLICATIONS OF URINARY TRACT INFECTION

Acute renal failure

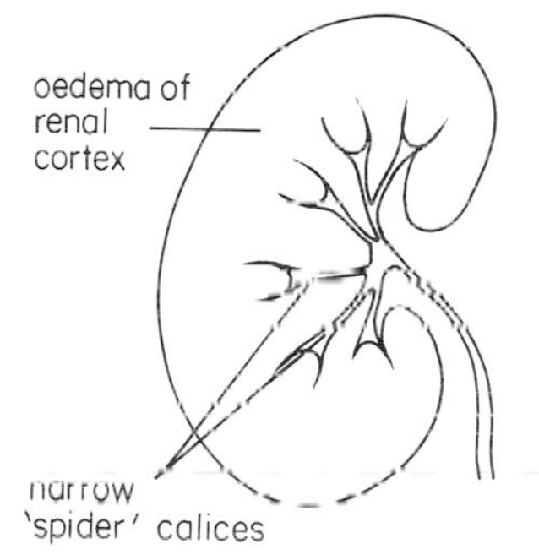

Fig. 7.8. Urography in acute infection—oedema makes the calices long and thin. Impaired filtration may (temporarily) give a very poor picture.

Whether the infection is haematogenous or comes up the ureter, its immediate effect upon the parenchyma is like inflammation elsewhere — *rubor, calor, dolor* and *laesio functionis*. The rubor and calor cannot be seen unless there is occasion to explore the kidney (when it is red, swollen and incredibly vascular): small wonder that the patient has pain and tenderness over the kidney. A urogram at this stage shows a swollen renal outline, and oedema masks the edge of the psoas muscle. The swelling of the renal parenchyma makes the necks of the calices seem narrow and drawn-out (Fig. 7.8).

These changes need not be uniform: depending on the cause, they can be limited to only one or two pyramids of the kidney, and if a DMSA scan is performed, since the isotope is taken up by the tubules, it may show large silent areas. On occasion, when the entire kidney is inflamed, it may stop working. The DMSA scan is blank, and an IVP will show no trace of excretion of the contrast medium. Nevertheless, there may be complete recovery. It is most important to bear this in mind when receiving a report which states that there is 'no function' in the kidney.

Septicaemia

The most serious of all the complications of urinary tract infection is septicaemia. Never forget how huge is the blood supply to the kidney or how thin are the membranes that line the collecting tubules or how narrow the interval which separates urine from the surrounding veins and lymphatics of the kidney. Whenever the pressure is increased inside the kidney for whatever cause, if there are micro-organisms in the urine they will be injected directly into the veins and lymphatics that issue from it straight into the vena cava and the cisterna chyli. The organisms in the urinary tract are usually Gram-negative bacilli which harbour potent 'lipid-A' endotoxin. This stimulates the hypothalamus to cause fever: it releases kinins which cause vasodilatation, increase capillary permeability and depress the function of the cardiac muscle (Fig. 7.9). Gram-negative septicaemia may occur after any urological operation without warning. It is notoriously common when there are both obstruction and an infected urine.

In the first phase of septicaemia the peripheral circulation is dilated, the patient may have a rigor, fever and a bounding pulse: his face and limbs may be flushed and warm. Within half an hour the picture has changed dramatically: the blood pressure falls to an unrecordable level; the limbs become cold from vasoconstriction; the patient looks as if he has had a myocardial infarct.

The first thing is to suspect the diagnosis: the next is to make sure. Get a needle into a vein (not always easy) and send blood for culture.

A massive dose of the most appropriate antibiotic is now given intravenously but the question is: which one? It may be obvious from preoperative cultures of the urine which organisms are already in the urinary tract, but often the urine has until now been sterile. The microbiologists in the hospital laboratory will know which is the most probable cause of septicaemia and will advise as to the choice of antibiotic.

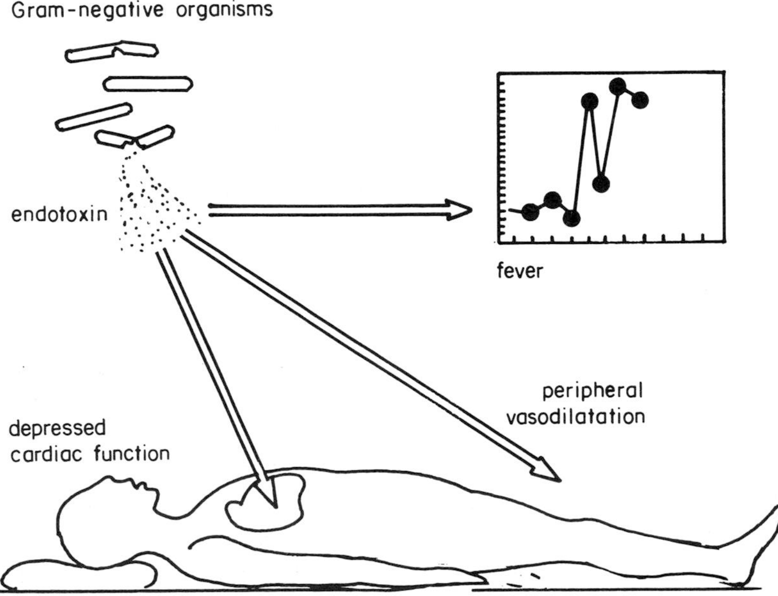

Fig. 7.9. Gram-negative septicaemia.

Remembering that there are two pathological processes that may be contributing to the state of shock — a massive dilatation of the circulatory space and a possible depression of myocardial activity — it is necessary to refill the circulatory volume and at the same time monitor the cardiac output. If possible get help from the team in the Intensive Therapy Unit.

Through the same needle an intravenous infusion is started with saline: later give a plasma-expander. As soon as possible get a central venous cannula in position to monitor the pressure in the right heart. Give enough plasma-expander until the central venous pressure returns to normal. This replacement may need 5 or 10 litres of fluid, and unless the central pressure is carefully watched there is a risk of overloading the heart.

In most patients improvement is seen within an hour and within two the peripheral vessels have recovered their tone. Now the lost fluid begins to return to the circulation and there is a danger of precipitating heart failure. Usually natural diuresis gets rid of the surplus fluid, but it may be necessary to perform venesection to keep the patient out of heart failure.

As soon as the patient has been resuscitated it is necessary to consider very carefully the underlying urological problem: any localized pocket of infected urine under pressure must be drained, e.g. by percutaneous nephrostomy, emptying the bladder or draining an abscess.

Stones

Stones may form within a few weeks of an episode of infection: sometimes it is obvious that they have formed around sloughed renal papillae, but more often it is not possible to identify a missing papilla and it seems that the stone has formed around bacterial debris in the urinary tract (Fig. 7.10). Stones are most common in patients with a urea-splitting infection, e.g. *Proteus mirabilis*.

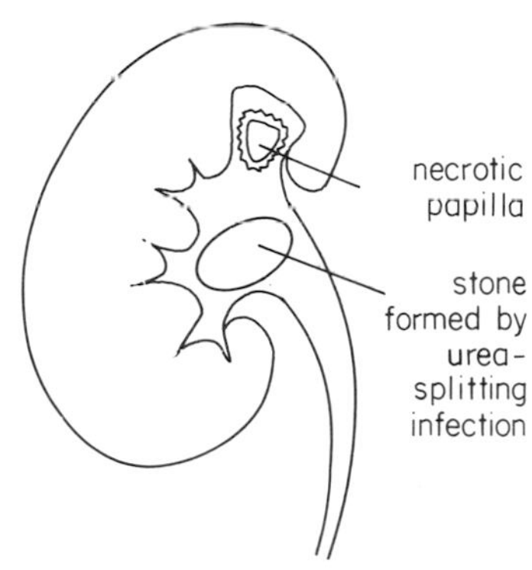

Fig. 7.10. Stone may form *de novo* in the renal pelvis from urea-splitting organisms, or by being precipitated on a dead papilla.

Suppuration

Haematogenous infection of the renal parenchyma beginning as a series of little abscesses may later coalesce and form a large inflammatory lump in the parenchyma of the kidney followed by an abscess. In the days before antibiotics bacteraemia from a staphylococcal boil would lead to a *renal carbuncle* (Fig. 7.11). Today the same lesion is seen in people ill for other reasons, e.g. diabetes, drug addicts who inject themselves with infected equipment, and those with impaired immune defences. When the infection is confined to the parenchyma there is no pus in the urine.

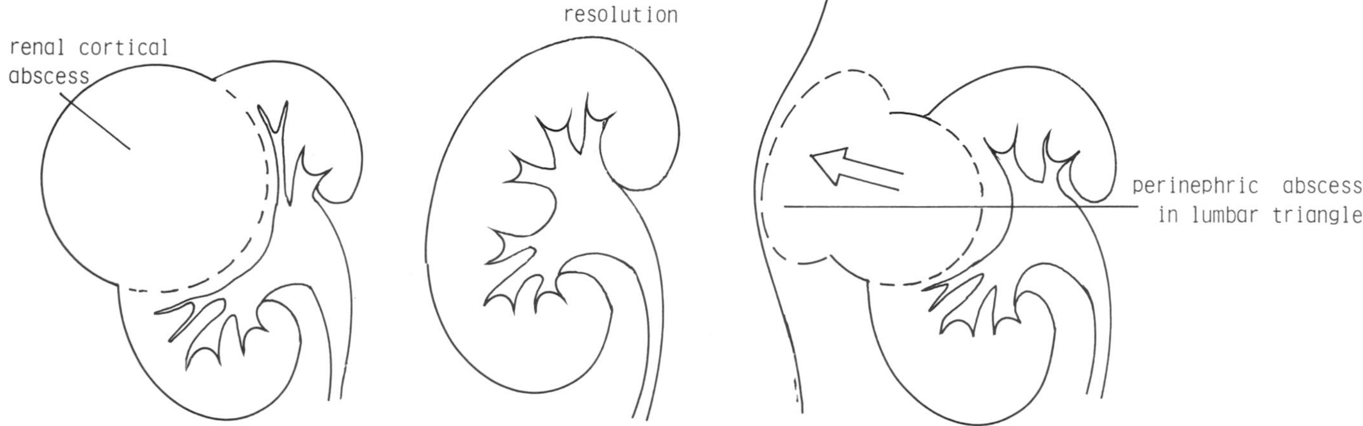

Fig. 7.11. Suppuration in the cortex forms an abscess (renal carbuncle) which usually resolves with treatment, but may rupture into the perinephric fat and even point in the lumbar triangle.

The kidney is swollen and tender. The X-rays show a soft tissue mass: ultrasound shows echoes suggestive of a neoplasm rather than a cyst. One needs a high index of suspicion to make the right diagnosis. It may be necessary to aspirate pus from the abscess in order to confirm the diagnosis and get bacteriological sensitivities for chemotherapy.

An abscess in the parenchyma often forms a perinephric abscess which will point in the lumbar triangle of Petit and call for drainage.

Granuloma

Xanthogranuloma

This is a rare change seen in association with a stone in the kidney. Histiocytes become laden with lipid, so yellow in colour that they resemble a carcinoma of the kidney. The inflammation spreads into the tissues around the kidney (Fig. 7.12). Amongst the stiff adherent yellow tissue are many small abscesses: some invade the liver or burrow under the fascia of the psoas muscle to form a honeycomb of sinuses that can even invade the colon to form a nephrocolic fistula. The patient loses weight and deteriorates. There is a lump: the radiological features are those of any other solid space-occupying tumour and it is difficult to distinguish the mass from a renal parenchymal cancer. The stone should alert one to the possibility of xanthogranuloma. Even at operation the mass may look like a tumour, but it is important to remove it since it will not respond to conservative measures and one must be almost as radical as if it were a cancer.

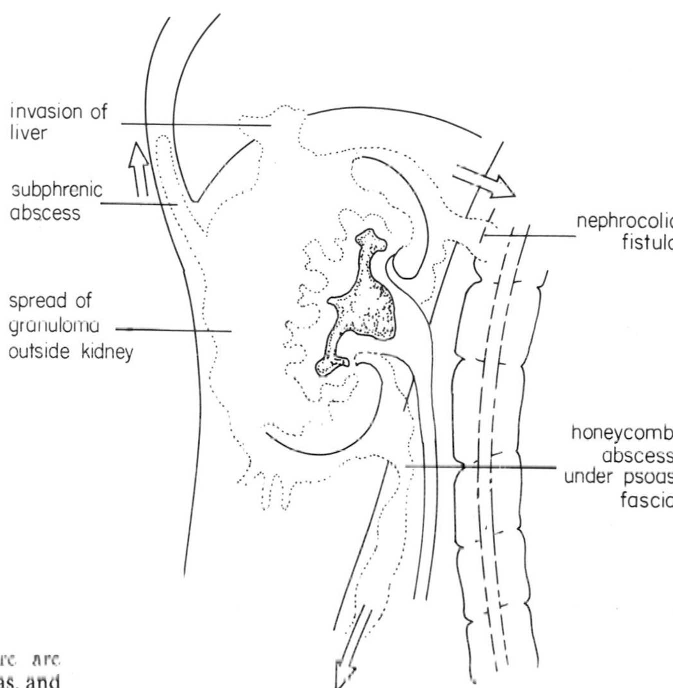

Fig. 7.12. Chronic granulomas usually occur where there are neglected stones. They track all round, burrow under the psoas, and cause fistulae into the bowel.

Malakoplakia

This is a similar granuloma which occurs in the kidney, bladder, ureter and testis. There are multiple abscesses, dense fibrosis, and in the bladder and ureter, heaped up brown plaques that may bleed and cause obstruction. The specific feature which makes the diagnosis is to find Michaelis–Guttman bodies (peculiar calcified spherules) in and around the chronic inflammatory cells. Only an inflammation, this is as bad as xanthogranuloma: unless removed, it persists, invades and kills the patient.

TUBERCULOSIS

Tuberculosis was once a common and important urological entity. Today in the West it has almost disappeared: not so elsewhere in the world. The offending organism is usually the human variety of *Mycobacterium tuberculosis*: in Britain usually Phage type B, but in patients from overseas more often Phage type I. Only 2 to 3% of patients with pulmonary tuberculosis develop genitourinary tuberculosis which reaches the kidney via the bloodstream. In the early cases there is a small focus in a renal papilla (Fig. 7.13): at this stage the patient notices

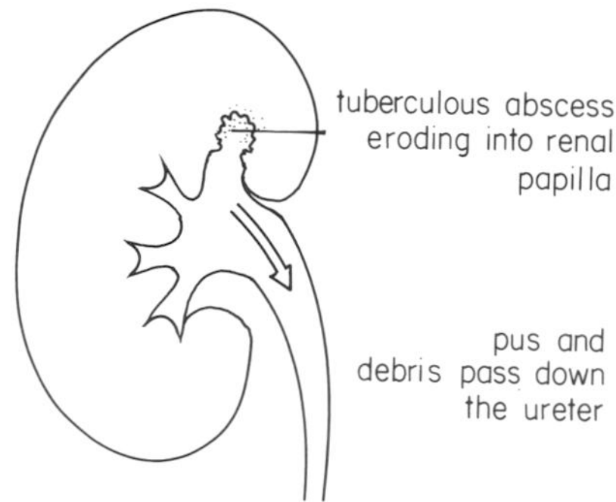

Fig. 7.13. The early lesion in tuberculosis is a small abscess that erodes a renal papilla.

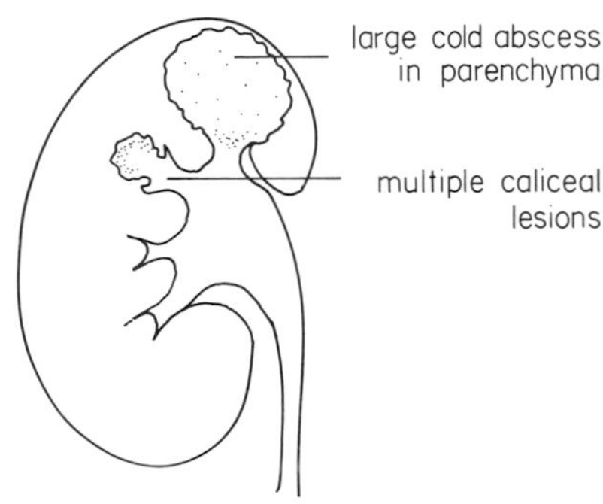

Fig. 7.14. In later stages, large, cold abscesses destroy the entire pyramid and more and more papillae are affected.

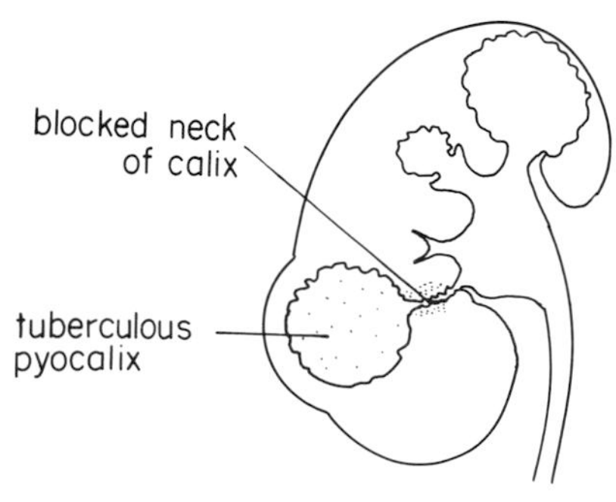

Fig. 7.15. Granulation tissue obstructs some caliceal necks, giving pyocalices upstream of them.

frequency of urination and perhaps haematuria. The excretion urogram shows a barely-detectable irregularity in a renal papilla which is very easy to miss.

Later the tuberculoma in the papilla enlarges and grows out to the cortex to form an abscess which may be calcified (Fig. 7.14). Still later, granuloma narrows the necks of the calices and they fill up with calcified debris (Fig. 7.15). Ultimately the entire kidney may be converted into a bag of more or less calcified tuberculous caseation tissue (Fig. 7.16). This gives a striking appearance in the plain abdominal radiograph: it used to be called the 'cement kidney'.

Spread to the ureter and bladder

Although in the beginning the infection is in the kidney, soon there is active tuberculous granulation tissue in the ureter and bladder. In the ureter inflammation makes the ureter thicker and shorter so that the ureteric orifice is pulled up to give a typical appearance on cystoscopy of a 'golf-hole' ureter (Fig. 7.17). With anti-tuberculous therapy the active granulomas in the wall of the ureter heal with fibrosis and cause a stricture (Fig. 7.18). In the bladder the early phase of tuberculosis may cause oedema looking like a tumour on cystoscopy. Tiny tubercles (as one might expect) are never seen. Biopsy of the oedematous mass or the red bladder seen at this stage may show acid–fast bacilli and characteristic tubercles. As the disease progresses and the granulomas heal under treatment the muscle of the bladder is infiltrated with fibrous tissue which contracts so that the volume of the bladder is diminished and the patient gets severe frequency of micturition.

Diagnosis

Early diagnosis calls for a highly suspicious mind: every patient with pus in the urine not explained by associated bacterial infection must have tuberculosis excluded by examination of three early morning specimens of urine for acid-fast bacilli in the deposit with the Ziehl–Neelsen stain, and culture using the Loewenstein–Jensen medium — a culture medium which contains an agent which inhibits growth of other bacteria and fungi during the 6 weeks that it may take for the tubercle bacilli to appear on the slope. A negative result is declared at 6 weeks: in fact, the microbiologists can often discover tubercle bacilli within 2 weeks. In cases of doubt at least six specimens of urine should be sent for examination. Inoculation of guinea-pigs has been given up — it was too risky for the laboratory staff.

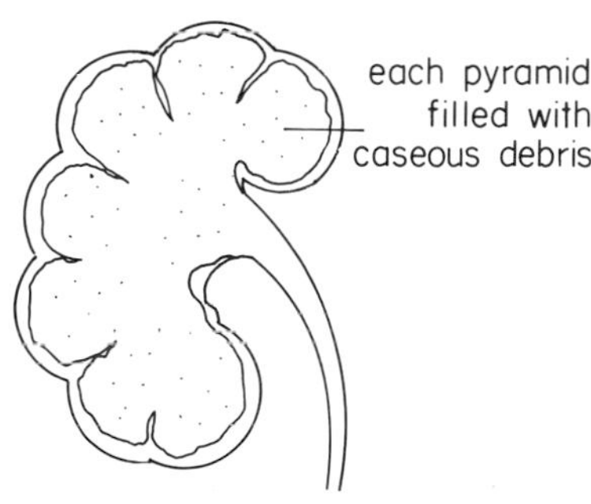

Fig. 7.16. Eventually the kidney is converted into a calcified bag of caseous debris—the cement kidney.

Urography

In early cases the IVU might show an eroded papilla: later there would be traces of calcification and larger hollow areas in the cortex with perhaps some narrowing of calices and ureter. Later large parts of the kidney — several complete pyramids — might be replaced by calcified caseating tissue. Little stones are common on previously damaged tissue. In Africa one should be wary — calcification seems to be uncommon in tuberculosis and doctors trained in the West can be badly mistaken.

Cystoscopy

Cystoscopy may show uniform inflammation of the mucosa of the bladder, occasionally a shallow ulcer, sometimes the deformed golf-hole ureter, and rarely a papilloma-like area of oedema. There is no room for

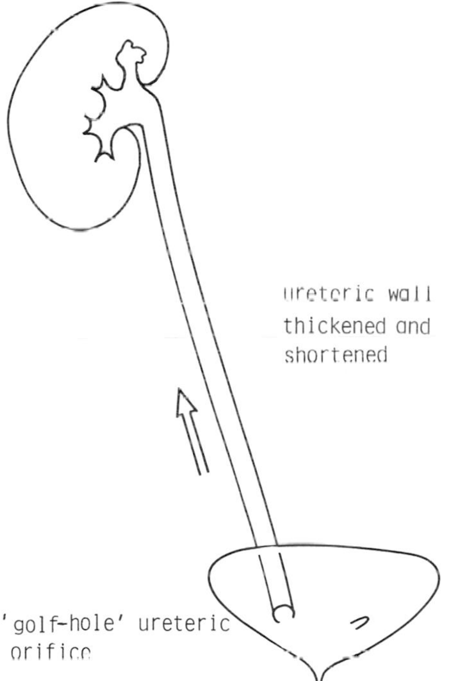

Fig. 7.17. The ureter in tuberculosis is oedematous and shortened, pulling out the ureteric orifice.

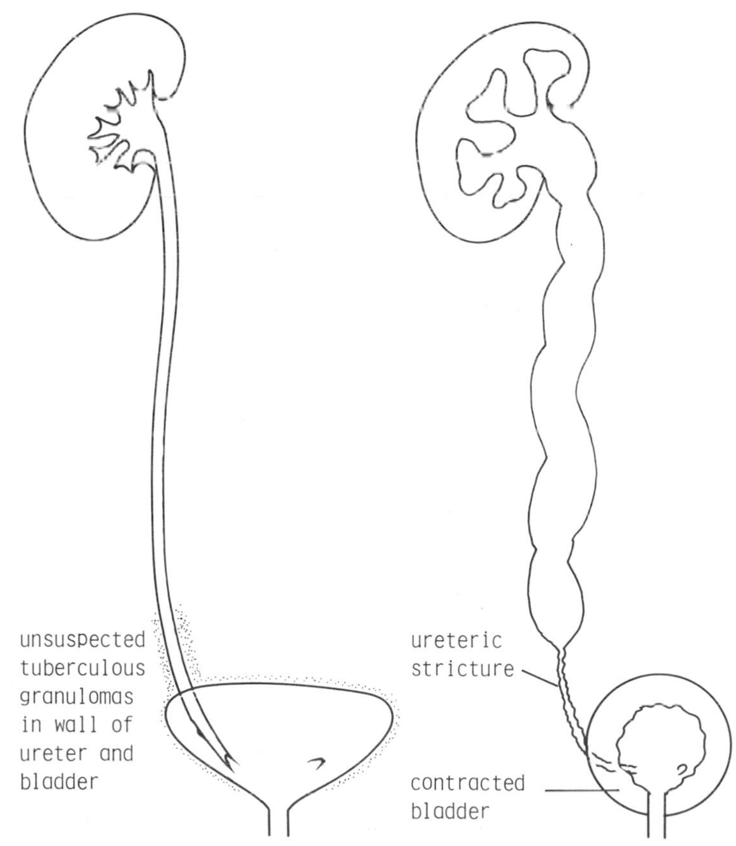

Fig. 7.18. Unsuspected tuberculous granulation tissue in the wall of the ureter will undergo fibrosis and shrinkage with treatment and so gives rise to obstruction. Similar scarring makes the bladder shrink down.

guesswork. Biopsy will give the diagnosis. Irrigation of a catheter passed up the suspected ureter will provide urine rich in pus cells that may reveal the tubercle bacilli on staining and culture.

Management

One must never forget the whole patient: many will have active tuberculosis elsewhere. Their families and their workmates must be checked up. The disease is notifiable, and you can be sued if you do not inform the authorities.

The urologist is well-advised to consult his colleagues who see many cases of tuberculosis, and with their concurrence, treatment may be started off with rifampicin 450 mg, INAH 300 mg and ethambutol 800 mg daily for the first 3 months: after this, treatment is continued with rifampicin and INAH (in the same dose) for a further 3 to 6 months. If the organism is resistant to the first-line drugs, others may be needed.

In the early case with a small lesion in one or more renal papillae one expects to see complete resolution of the disease with, at worst, a fleck of calcification to mark the place where the tuberculous granuloma had been active. But you never know whether there are silent but still active tuberculous granulomas in the wall of the ureter or bladder.

With treatment these heal up very rapidly and unless you are on your guard you may miss the formation of a stricture in the ureter before it has caused needless atrophy of the kidney upstream. The rule today is that the IVU should be repeated within 3 weeks of beginning treatment. If the ureter is seen to be narrowed at this early stage one may try steroids to prevent oedema (but they do not usually work) and it is necessary to operate to bypass the obstruction. When the narrowing is at the pelviureteric junction a modification of a pyeloplasty (see p. 142) is performed. When the narrowing is at the junction of ureter with bladder the ureter is reimplanted (see p. 139). When it is the entire wall of bladder that has shrunk with fibrosis then it can be enlarged by the operation of caecocystoplasty (Fig. 7.19).

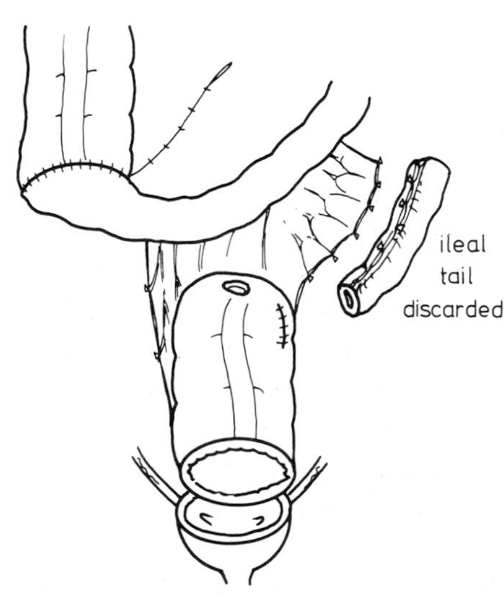

Fig. 7.19. Caecocystoplasy enlarges the capacity of the contracted tuberculous bladder.

Even today we still see patients who only come up when the kidney is entirely destroyed. For them the right treatment (after preliminary chemotherapy) is removal of the kidney. It used to be necessary to take the ureter as well, in case tuberculosis came back. Today modern chemotherapy is so efficient that there is no need to remove the ureter.

Genital tuberculosis involving the prostate, seminal vesicles, *vasa deferentia*, epididymes and sometimes testes in males — and Fallopian tubes and uterus in females, may be seen alongside urinary tuberculosis. They do not necessarily coincide.

BRUCELLOSIS

Although this is rare it is worth remembering that *Brucella* may lead to a granuloma in the kidney which is almost indistinguishable from tuberculosis. It occurs in communities where brucellosis is still rife in cattle. It occurs in testis and kidney.

HYDATID DISEASE

Hydatid disease is very rare in the West. It is caused by the tapeworm *Echinococcus granulosus*. Pet dogs have been fed uncooked sheep offal containing the worm: the worms breed in the dogs. Their ova are shed in the dogs faeces which dry but survive on the dogs fur. Children fondle the dogs, and forget to wash their hands. They ingest the ova. The worms invade the gut and form cysts in the viscera — usually the liver but sometimes the kidney. The cysts are multilocular: their walls are sometimes calcified. They resemble tumours on ultrasound, CT scanning and angiography. Only experience and a high index of suspicion is likely to give the right diagnosis. There is a complement fixation test which confirms the diagnosis.

The cysts are filled with dilute formalin or hypertonic saline to kill the little tapeworms inside them, then they are aspirated, and then removed by operation. If unkilled tapeworms are spilt they will engender a whole new population of cysts in the surrounding tissues — an outcome which is usually fatal.

CHYLURIA AND FILARIASIS

In the population of the Far East a fistula may form between the perirenal lymphatics and the renal pelvis. Lymphangiography depicts the communication between the two systems. There is a continual loss of fat, absorbed from food into the lymphatics, into the urine. The urine laden with fat (mixed with blood) presents an appearance like anchovy sauce. Sometimes the patient becomes so starved that treatment is necessary. More often it is better to do nothing. Some of these patients can be proven to have been infested with the microfilaria worm *Wuchereria bancrofti* — but they are the exception. Usually no such cause can be found. If the patient is so ill that something must be done, a lymphangiogram is performed to delineate the communication between lymphatic system and renal pelvis. The kidney is explored, all its surrounding tissue is meticulously dissected away and all the lymphatic connections very carefully ligated.

FURTHER READING

Arneil GC (1985) Urinary tract infection in children. *British Medical Journal* **290**, 1925–6.

Birmingham Reflux Study Group (1987) Prospective trial of operative versus non-operative treatment of severe vesicoureteric reflux in children: five years' observation. *British Medical Journal* **295**, 237–41.

Bonal J, Caralps A, Lauzurica R, Serra A, Romero R & Inaraja L (1987) Cyst infection in acquired renal cystic disease. *British Medical Journal* **295**, 25.

Gow JG & Barbosa S (1984) Genitourinary tuberculosis. A study of 1117 cases over a period of 34 years. *British Journal of Urology* **56**, 449–55.

Haddad FS (1987) Re primary retroperitoneal pelvic echinococcal cyst. (Letter.) *Journal of Urology* **137**, 1248.

Ibrahim AIA, Awad R, Shetty SD, Saad M & Bilal NE (1988) Genitourinary complications of brucellosis. *British Journal of Urology* **61**, 294–8.

Marsh FP (1985) Infection of the urinary tract, In: Marsh FP (Ed) *Postgraduate Nephrology*. Heinemann Medical Books, London. pp. 296–324.

Monsour M, Asmy AF & MacKenzie JR (1987) Renal scarring secondary to vesicoureteric reflux. Clinical assessment and new grading. *British Journal of Urology* **60**, 320–4.

O'Donnell B & Puri B (1984) Treatment of vesicoureteric reflux by endoscopic injection of Teflon. *British Medical Journal* **289**, 7–9.

Ozen HA & Whitaker RH (1987) Does the severity of presentation in children with vesicoureteric reflux relate to the severity of the disease or the need for operation? *British Journal of Urology* **60**, 110–2.

Smellie JM, Ransley PG, Normand ICS, Prescod N & Edwards D (1985) Development of new renal scars: a collaborative study. *British Medical Journal* **290**, 1957–60.

Weinberg AC & Boyd SD (1988) Short-course chemotherapy and role of surgery in adult and pediatric genitourinary tuberculosis. *Urology* **31**, 95–102.

8 Urinary Calculi

Surgery traces its origins to the ancient operation of cutting for the stone which by the time of Hippocrates was well recognized as a procedure that should be left to those who were specially trained to do it — advice which deserves to be repeated today. In the ancient world, without postmortem dissection or X-rays, 'stone' meant stone in the urinary bladder. It was centuries before it was realized that most stones originated in the kidney.

Epidemiological studies show that the incidence of stones varies greatly in different populations, and that in the West there has been a stepwise increase in the incidence of calculi in the kidney and ureter, year by year, interrupted only by the two world wars. The inference is that the incidence of stones reflects affluence and overfeeding, particularly with refined sugar and protein. Stones are not rare: nearly 20% of doctors are likely to have at least one attack of ureteric colic, and in other professions where dehydration is even more severe, the incidence may be higher.

STRUCTURE OF A STONE

Stones do not consist only of crystalline material like stones on the road. They have an organic scaffold surrounded by crystals like the iron reinforcement of ferroconcrete or the glass fibre in fibre-glass supporting a 'fill' of crystalline material (Fig. 8.1). In most stones the crystalline 'fill' is arranged in rings. These look like the growth rings of a tree, but they do not mark episodes of precipitation of calculus or episodes of infection: similar growth rings can be produced artificially when crystals are deposited in media containing organic matrix-forming material. We may know more about the 'fill' than we do about the matrix but the matrix may be just as important.

STONE FORMATION

Salt added to water continues to dissolve until a point is reached when no more will dissolve: this is the *saturation concentration* and every schoolchild knows that it can be measured by the solubility product of the concentration of the ions making up the salt (Fig. 8.2). However, under the conditions found in biological fluids there may be a supersaturated solution which does not precipitate crystals — the *metastable* region —

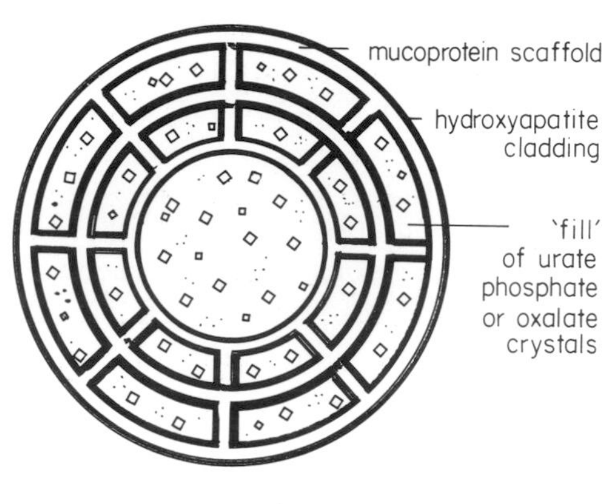

Fig. 8.1. Diagrammatic representation of the structure of a stone.

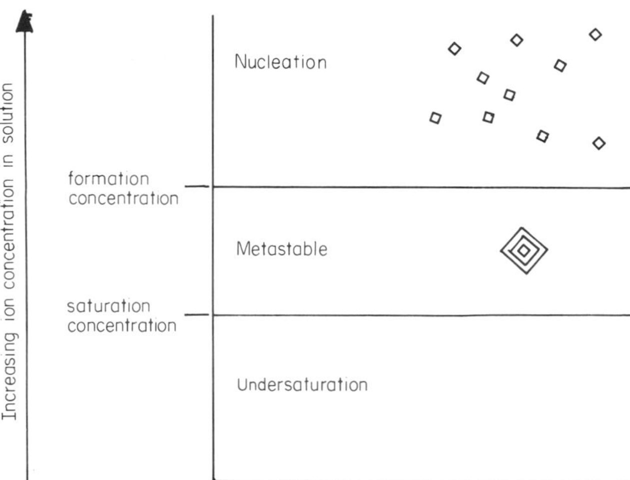

Fig. 8.2. Effects of increasing ion concentration in a solution such as urine.

unless the solution is left undisturbed for a considerable time, or is provided with a nucleus on which stones can form. Above the metastable region is a concentration at which crystals precipitate, i.e. make their own nuclei — this is the range of *nucleation*. For practical purposes human urine is *metastable* with respect to the principal ingredients of stones — calcium and oxalate.

Many factors influence this metastable range: temperature, the presence or absence of colloids and the turbulence and rate of flow of the fluid, but the concentration of the solute remains of chief importance. It will be influenced by an excess of the solute in the urine or anything that makes the urine more concentrated.

Equally important is the presence of something that acts as a nucleus, and in the urinary tract many things will do this: dead papillae; dying fronds of cancer; foreign bodies such as a non-absorbable suture, a fragment of a burst catheter balloon, or an existing fragment of stone are ideal nuclei for the formation of a new calculus (Fig. 8.3).

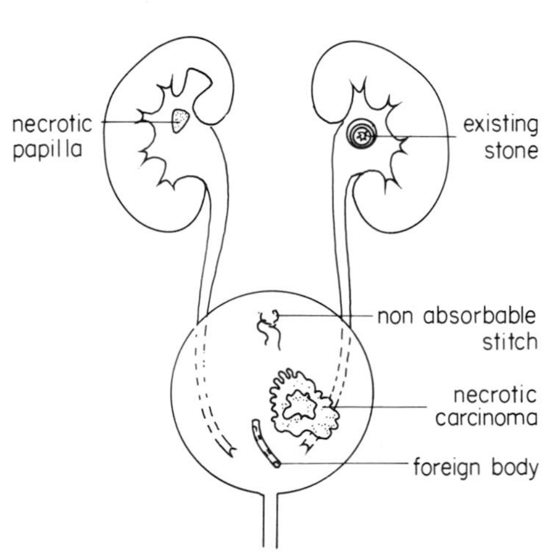

Fig. 8.3. Common conditions that act as nuclei for stone formation.

Many crystalline substances have a greatly different solubility in urine of different pH: magnesium ammonium phosphate is insoluble in an alkaline urine such as that provided by *Proteus mirabilis* which converts urea to ammonia; urate is insoluble in an acid urine but may be completely dissolved by keeping the urine alkaline by suitable medication.

All crystals like rest and quiet if they are to grow to any size and they tend to form wherever there is stagnant urine as in a ureterocele, a caliceal diverticulum, hydronephrosis or chronically obstructed bladder.

SUPERSATURATION STONES

The purest example of the simple supersaturation stone is *cystine*: there is an inherited defect in the transport of cystine, ornithine, arginine and lysine both in the renal tubule and in the gut. Cystine is almost insoluble in urine. A patient who is homozygous for cystinuria may be passing almost 1 g/24 hours and is certain to form stones. If heterozygous the quantity of cystine is halved and stone formation less common. By giving cystinuric patients a very high fluid intake, stones may be prevented or even dissolved. Cystine is more soluble in an alkaline urine. Giving penicillamine breaks the bond between the two molecules of cysteine to form a soluble penicillamine-cysteine compound (Fig. 8.4).

Another good example of a supersaturation stone is *uric acid*. Urate is soluble in alkaline urine with a pH > 6.8 but may precipitate in acid urine, especially when concentrated as in the tropics. Sometimes there is a congenital error in tubular function when patients have difficulty in forming an alkaline urine and form urate stones unless they take additional alkali. Others may pass large amounts of uric acid in the urine because of gout or the catabolism of protein (as in chemotherapy of carcinoma). In these patients one may block the formation of uric acid by giving allopurinol which inhibits xanthine oxidase.

Classical *calcium oxalate* or *calcium phosphate* stones are found when the urinary calcium concentration is excessive as in hyperparathyroidism, inactivity, metastases and other bone-destroying conditions. In these patients the ion in excess is calcium, but it is just as dangerous to have an excess of oxalate in the urine.

An excess of *oxalate* may occur in the rare congenital disease hyperoxaluria which leads to the formation of little calculi in the

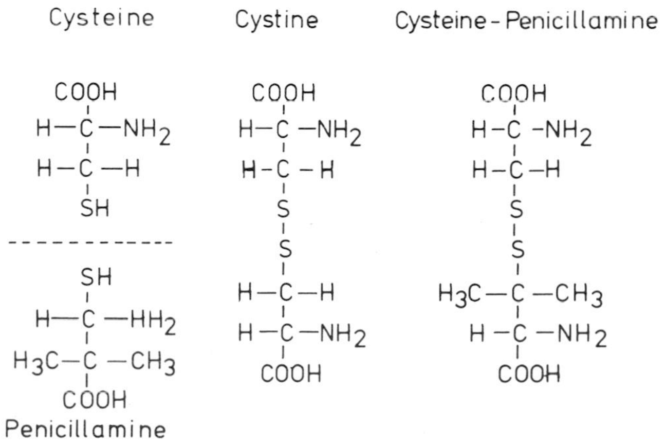

Cysteine
COOH
H—C—NH2
H—C—H
SH
- - - - - - - - - - - -
SH
H—C—HH2
H3C—C—CH3
COOH
Penicillamine

Cystine
COOH
H—C—NH2
H—C—H
S
S
H—C—H
H—C—NH2
COOH

Cysteine-Penicillamine
COOH
H—C—NH2
H—C—H
S
S
H3C—C—CH3
H—C—NH2
COOH

Fig. 8.4. Penicillamine forms a soluble compound with cysteine.

collecting tubules of the kidneys. Many of these cases respond to treatment with large doses of pyridoxine. Hyperoxaluria may also occur in disorders such as Crohn's disease, of the last few feet of the ileum — or its surgical removal, because bile acids are normally absorbed in this part of the bowel and if they are no longer absorbed, they are not available to be recycled in the liver to be excreted in the bile (Fig. 8.5). Fat in the diet cannot be emulsified and absorbed: it remains in the bowel where it forms insoluble soaps with dietary calcium. This in turn leaves a relative excess of dietary oxalate which is absorbed and finds its way into the urine. This hyperoxaluria may be avoided by refraining from food containing oxalate (chocolate, tea, coffee, spinach and rhubarb) and by giving cholestyramine which binds oxalate in the lumen of the bowel.

Idiopathic hypercalciuria, i.e. an excess of calcium in the urine (> 350 mg/24 hours in males; > 300 mg/24 hours in females), is often thought to be a cause of calculi. It is doubtful if this is significant in females, but in a small group of males who keep on passing stones this may be important. Three kinds of idiopathic hypercalciuria are recognized: *renal* — where there is decreased renal tubular reabsorption of calcium; *resorptive* — where calcium salts are reabsorbed from bone; *absorptive* — where too much calcium is absorbed from the bowel. Treatment is a matter for debate: one may try to limit the quantity of calcium and oxalate in the diet (by refraining from milk products that are rich in calcium and the chocolate and fruit referred to above); one may try to prevent resorption by giving cellulose phosphate etc. to precipitate calcium salts in the bowel; or one may give magnesium and other compounds in the hope that they will keep calcium particles in suspension in the urine and prevent them sticking together. Few of these measures have any effect.

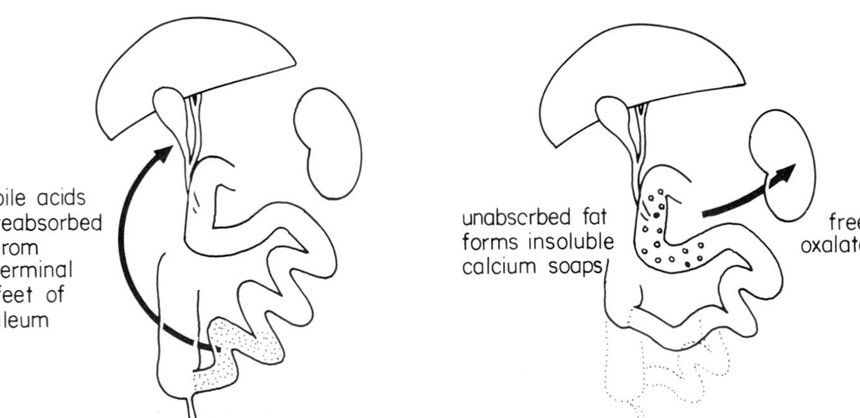

Fig. 8.5. Hyperoxaluria after disease or surgical removal of the last feet of the ileum.

Hyperparathyroidism

The most important type of supersaturation stone is seen in hyperparathyroidism. The parathyroid gland secretes a hormone which encourages osteoclasts to dissolve the bony skeleton and release calcium into the blood. Normally the secretion of the parathyroid is regulated by the level of ionized calcium in the blood. Most of the calcium in the blood is bound to protein: only a small fraction exists in solution and of this only a small part is ionized. In blood the product [Ca $\times$ P] is kept constant: if [Ca] is increased [PO_4] must fall, and vice versa. There are three types of hyperparathyroidism.

Primary hyperparathyroidism

For no clear reason the parathyroid glands start to secrete more parathormone than is needed (Fig. 8.6). More calcium salts are leached out of the skeleton and added to the blood to raise the level of plasma [Ca]. In turn the plasma [PO_4] falls: the superfluous calcium is filtered into the urine and may precipitate in the renal tubules as a form of *nephrocalcinosis*. More often stones form downstream in the renal calices or pelvis.

The diagnosis may be made by finding an elevated plasma [Ca] in the course of a routine check-up of a seemingly healthy patient, or the standard investigation that is performed for every patient with a calculus. Today it is very rare to find the gross changes of *osteitis fibrosa cystica*, where massive collections of osteoclasts have eroded cystic areas in the bones — especially the jaws.

The finding of an elevated plasma [Ca] is always checked, and if confirmed, the plasma parathormone is measured by radioimmunoassay.

Secondary hyperparathyroidism

Among the metabolic products that cannot be excreted by the ailing kidney in renal failure is phosphate. As the plasma [PO_4] rises so the plasma [Ca] must fall. The plasma [Ca] may be precipitated in soft tissues (*heterotopic calcification*) or replaced in the bones. The parathyroids respond to the lowered plasma [Ca] by secreting more parathormone for which they hypertrophy. This secondary hyperparathyroidism is seen in patients on regular dialysis for renal failure. It may be controlled by giving large doses of vitamin D to encourage the absorption of calcium from the bowel (Fig. 8.7).

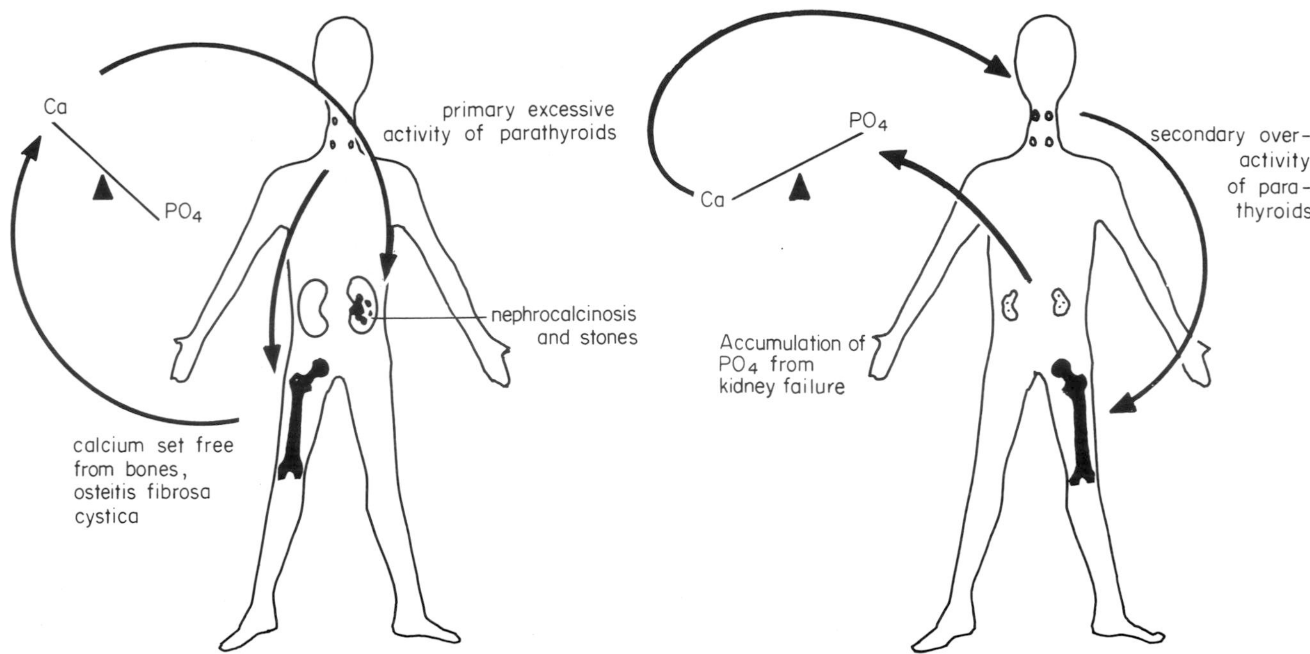

Fig. 8.6. Scheme of the sequence of events in primary hyperparathyroidism.

Fig. 8.7. Events in secondary hyperparathyroidism begin with the accumulation of phosphates along with other waste products as a result of renal insufficiency.

Tertiary hyperparathyroidism

There comes a time when the overactive parathroid glands seem not to know when to stop: they keep on growing and putting out far more parathormone than is needed to keep the plasma [Ca] constant. The bones become eroded while the excessive calcium is laid down in the soft tissues. This can no longer be controlled by giving vitamin D and the parathyroid glands must be removed.

Parathyroidectomy

There are four parathyroid glands each the size of a pea. They lie behind and buried in the lateral lobes of the thyroid gland along the course of the superior and inferior thyroid arteries (Fig. 8.8). Primary hyperparathyroidism may be caused by an adenoma in one gland, or hyperplasia of all four. In former days it was often very difficult to find these little glands, and when one was found, it was necessary to make sure (by means of a frozen section) that the little lump was a parathyroid rather than one of the little nodules which are so common in the thyroid. Today it is

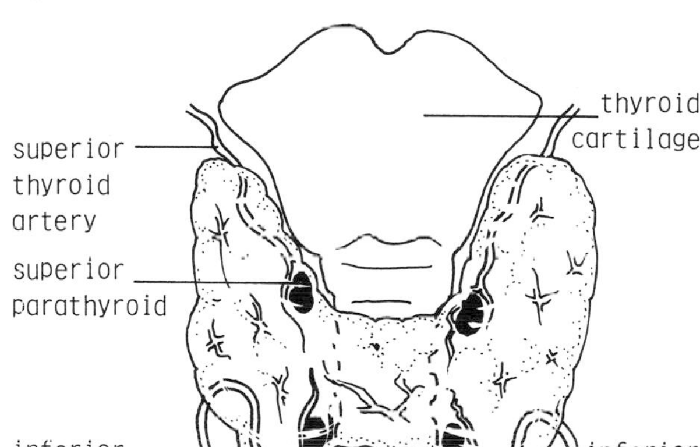

Fig. 8.8. Situation of the four parathyroid glands behind the thyroid, in close relationship to the thyroid arteries.

possible to localize the parathyroid nodules before operation by means of subtraction radioisotope scans but frozen section verification of each nodule is still necessary. Occasionally a 'missing' parathyroid is found in the mediastinum.

HOW STONES FORM IN THE KIDNEY

In the kidneys of patients with recurrent calcium stones, tiny spherical concretions are found in the collecting ducts of the papillae: they are made of calcium phosphate and a mucoprotein. These are *Carr's concretions*. Later these little spherules gather under the epithelium of the tip of a papilla where they form little shining plaques easily seen with a nephroscope at operation. These are *Randall's plaques* and some of them fall off into the collecting system to act as a nucleus for further stone formation (Fig. 8.9).

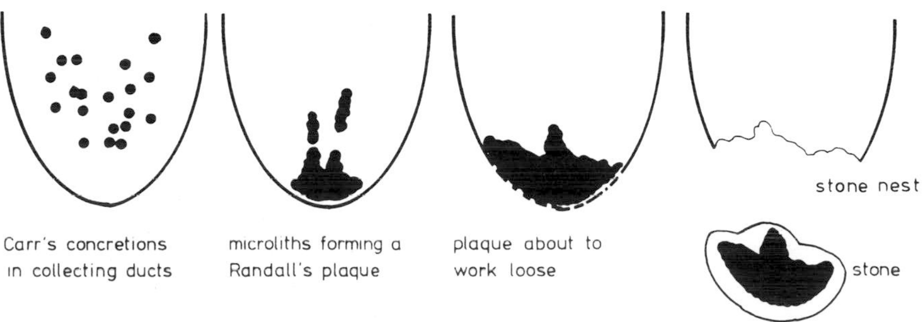

Fig. 8.9. How most stones begin in the renal papilla.

A more massive nucleus for stone formation is formed when an entire renal papilla dies off and is shed into the collecting system. *Papillary necrosis* is seen in many conditions (see p. 67). Whatever its cause, stone forms on the dead tissue. In some little stones a careful section through a stone may reveal the ghost of the original papilla in its centre.

INVESTIGATION OF A CALCULUS

There are always two distinct questions to be answered:

1 Exactly where is the stone, and is it likely to do any harm?

2 What is the cause of the stone, and can it be prevented?

To answer the first, a plain X-ray supplemented by an IVU will show where the stone is situated, and whether or not it is likely to get stuck in the collecting system and give rise to obstruction.

To answer the second, it is necessary to consider all the likely causes of stone formation: e.g. is the urine infected with a urea-splitting organism?; is there any underlying foreign body giving rise to the stone?; is there a pool of stagnant urine?; is there an elevated plasma or urinary [Ca]?

MANAGEMENT OF A STONE

If a stone is too large to pass down the urinary tract, and in general, the ureter will not let through stones larger than 5 mm in diameter, then it should be got rid of. If a stone is stuck, and there is obstruction upstream of the stone, it must be removed to prevent obstructive uropathy (see p. 66). If the urine is infected, the infection will not be controlled so long as a stone is present to act as a hiding-place for micro-organisms, and infection with any organisms that turn urea into ammnoia will cause the stone to grow.

Sometimes it is necessary to relieve the obstruction and control infection before it is safe to remove the stone: a percutaneous nephrostomy will relieve pressure in the renal pelvis, and antibiotics will control the immediate and systemic effects of infection. But when these urgent measures have been taken, the stone must be removed.

METHODS OF REMOVING STONES

In the last few years methods for removing stones have been so wonderfully improved that open surgical operations have become quite rare. The new techniques use radically new principles.

Extracorporeal lithotripsy

This uses the principle of the depth-charge: a shock wave travelling through water. There are several different machines but all generate a series of shock waves, and focus them on the stone. The shock waves travel through water and then through the tissues of the body (which are mostly made of water). When they reach the stone they break it up and the succession of shock waves is continued until the stone has been broken up into fragments that are small enough to pass down the urinary tract.

These machines differ in the way the shock waves are generated, how the stone is localized, and how the waves are focused on the stone.

The original system (Dornier) used a huge spark-plug to emit the shock wave. The spark-plug was placed at the first focus of an ellipsoidal mirror (Fig. 8.10). When the spark went off, one shock wave struck the patient directly, followed by another which was reflected from the mirror, and was concentrated at the second focus of the ellipse where the stone was localized, using two sets of X-ray equipment. The patient was placed in a water-bath while this was done. The double force of the two shock waves was painful — especially when it might take 1000 shocks to break a stone up — and so, as a rule patients required epidural or general anaesthesia.

Other systems (EDAP, Wolf) generated the shock wave from a set of tiny ceramic piezoelectric generators mounted on a spherical basin (Fig. 8.11). Every schoolboy remembers how he could irritate his schoolmaster by making the chalk squeak on the blackboard — applying

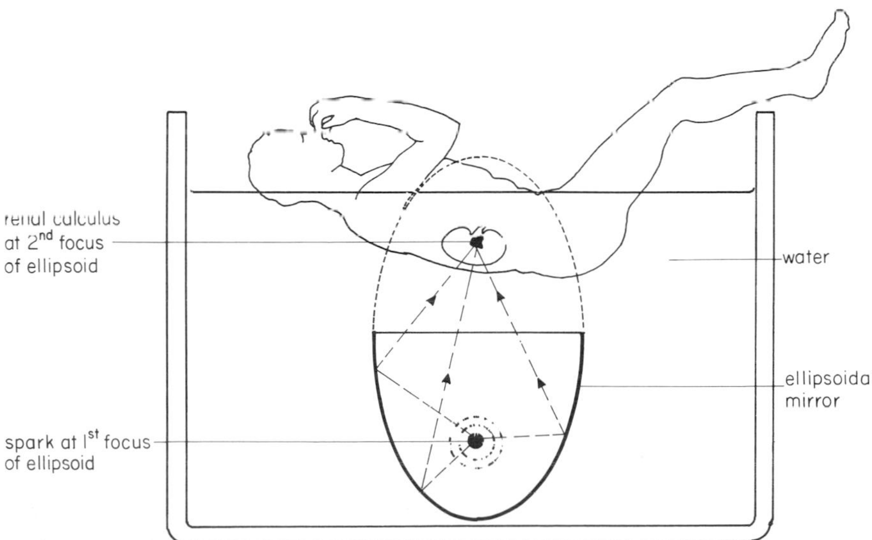

Fig. 8.10. Dornier shock wave system of fragmenting stones within the renal pelvis. A powerful spark is discharged at the first focus of an ellipsoidal mirror. The shock waves pass through the water-bath to concentrate at the second focus of the ellipse, where the stone is carefully sited using cross-beams of X-rays.

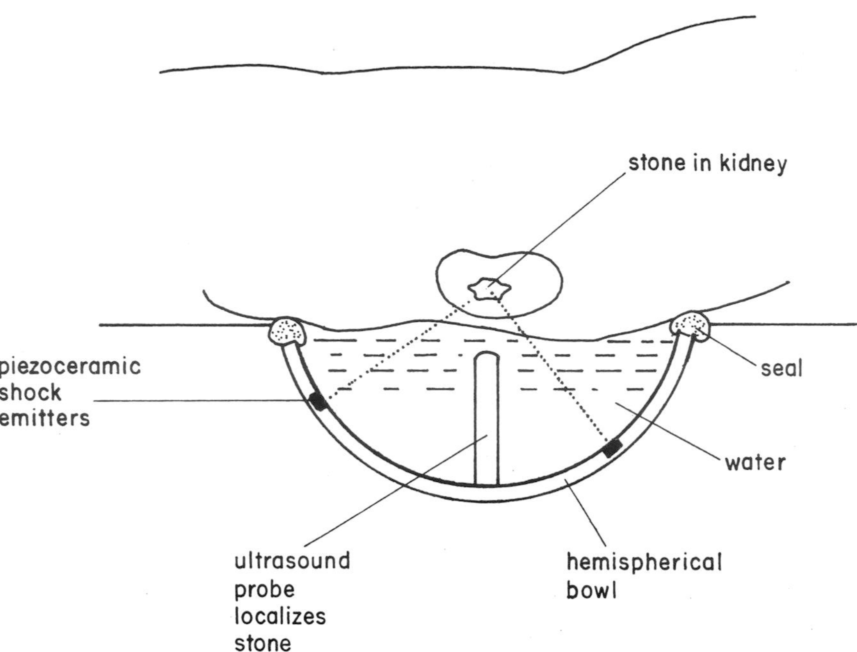

Fig. 8.11. Piezoceramic shock emitters mounted in a spherical basin focussed on the stone.

force to a crystalline structure to emit sound waves. The same principle is used for lithotripsy, except the force is an electrical current rather than the schoolboy's fingers and the sound waves are focused on the centre of the sphere. The system is aimed by ultrasound rather than X-rays.

Percutaneous nephrolithotomy (PCNL)

When a guide-wire is introduced through a needle into a renal calix or pelvis, the track can be enlarged with appropriate dilators until a sheath about 8 mm in diameter can be introduced (Fig. 8.12). Through the sheath various instruments can be passed: a nephroscope allows a stone to be seen; small forceps allow small stones to be seized and extracted; and instruments can be passed to break the stone into smaller fragments which can then be extracted. There is no end to the ingenuity of these instruments. To break the stone up one may use a strong forceps, a little rock-drill which oscillates at ultrasonic speed, a concentric electrode which emits a tremendous spark to shatter the stone, and a Q-switched laser which does much the same thing (Fig. 8.13).

When stones are broken up in the kidney, the pieces must be passed. If they are small, and the flow of urine is copious, they are washed out of the ureter. If they are larger, they can get jammed in the ureter, forming a typical *steinstrasse* or log-jam of stone fragments at the lower end of the ureter (Fig. 8.14).

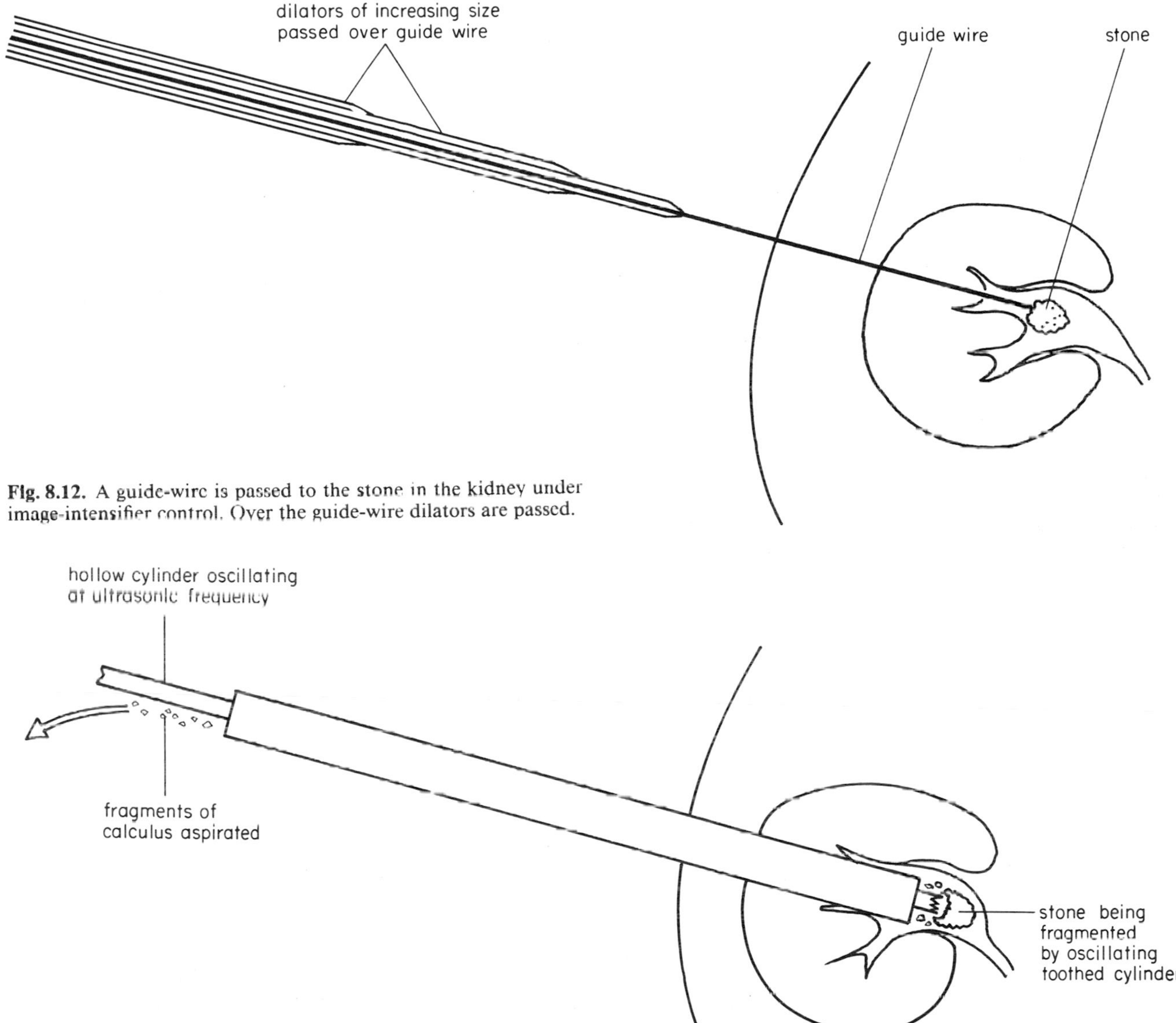

Fig. 8.12. A guide-wire is passed to the stone in the kidney under image-intensifier control. Over the guide-wire dilators are passed.

Fig. 8.13. The stone is fragmented by the oscillating toothed cylinder passed down the nephroscope tube.

Ureteroscopy

To help remove tiny bits of stone jammed in the lower end of the ureter one may pass a *ureteroscope* (see p. 91). Through this, small forceps or baskets can be passed to extract bits of stone that have got stuck (Fig. 8.15).

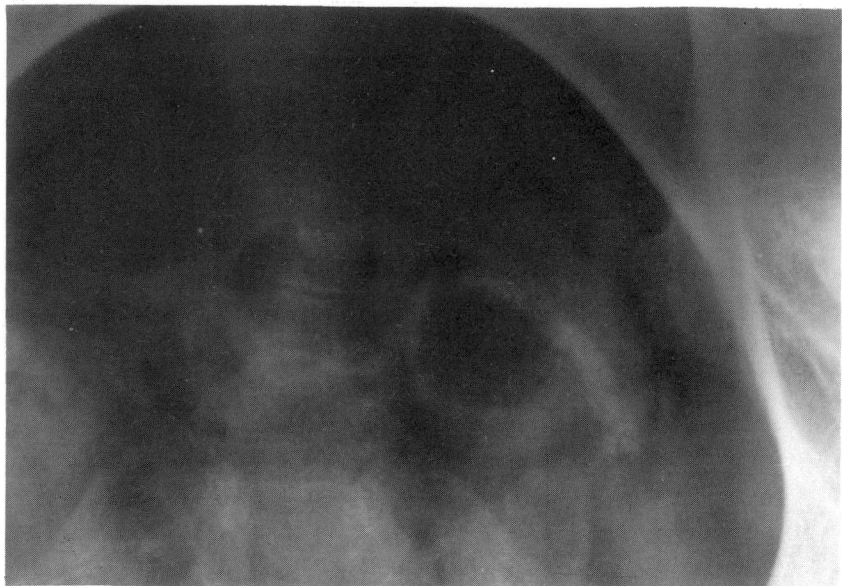

Fig. 8.14. 'Steinstrasse' — collection of stone fragments in the lower end of the right ureter after successful electrohydraulic lithotripsy of a renal calculus. They passed spontaneously within 48 hours.

Double J splints

More useful is the *double-J* splint. This is passed up the ureter through a cystoscope over a guide-wire (Fig. 8.16). It can be left in the ureter for 3 to 4 months at a time. The presence of this foreign body in the ureter has the effect of causing it to dilate with the result that bits of stone which might otherwise have got stuck in the ureter, pass easily down to the bladder.

Classical open operations for stones

When all else fails, the stone can be removed by an open operation. How the stone is approached, and exactly how it is removed depends upon its *position.*

Stone in a calix

In this location a stone is always quite small. At first it has a pyramidal shape: later it may grow and bulge out through the neck of the calix. Small ones are common and cause no trouble. Very exceptionally they cause pain, probably from intermittent obstruction (Fig. 8.17). At other times there are recurrent urinary infections which never clear up because the offending organisms hide from antibiotics in the porous crevices of the stone. When such a stone is jammed in a caliceal neck it may give rise to a pyocalix upstream of the stone. When a patient has persistent pain, infection, or demonstrable pyocalix the stone has to be removed. In other patients small caliceal stones are usually kept under review (Fig. 8.18) but in some patients — e.g. aircrew — it may be wise to get rid of them by means of ESWL as a preventative measure.

In the days before ESWL was available these stones were quite difficult to remove by an open surgical operation unless there was an obviously dilated calix. After exposing the kidney through a 12th rib tip incision and mobilizing it, the renal artery was isolated to make sure that bleeding could be prevented, and then an incision was made into the parenchyma over the stone. Alternatively the calix was approached by the Gil–Vernet technique (see below).

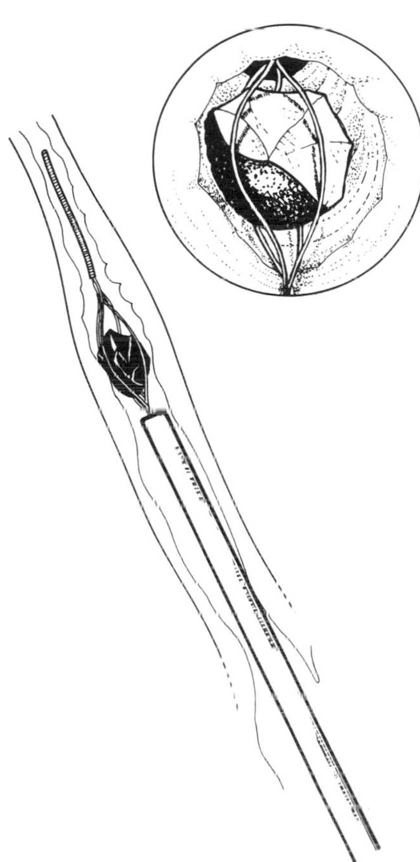

Fig. 8.15. Small fragments of stone that get jammed in the ureter can be safely extracted under vision by means of a forceps or basket introduced through the ureteroscope which makes it possible to see that the wall of the ureter is not being torn.

Stone in the renal pelvis

Often a stone which begins in a calix will slip into the renal pelvis but cannot get out down the ureter. It acts as a nucleus for further stone formation, and gradually increases in size (Fig. 8.19). A pelvic stone less

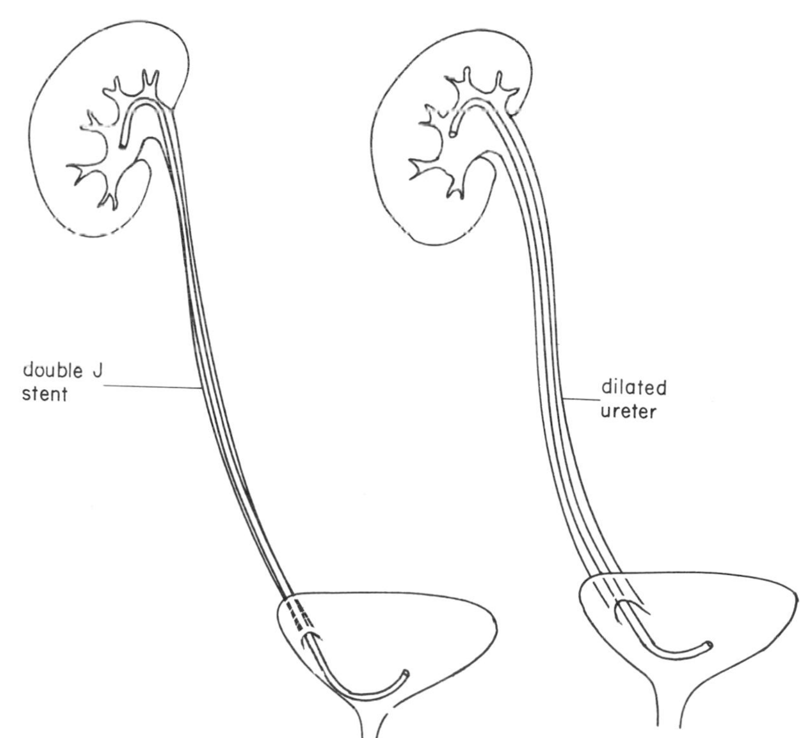

Fig. 8.16. A double-J stent in the ureter causes it to dilate.

than 5 mm in diameter may go down the ureter, but any that are larger than this should be removed before they get stuck in the pelviureteric junction or upper ureter. These stones may not give rise to any pain unless they become jammed in the ureter when there is pain in the loin,

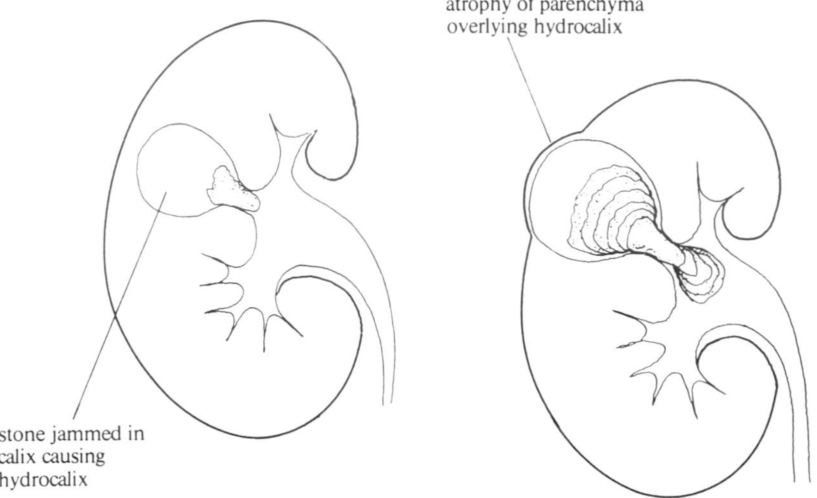

Fig. 8.17. Stone in a calix.

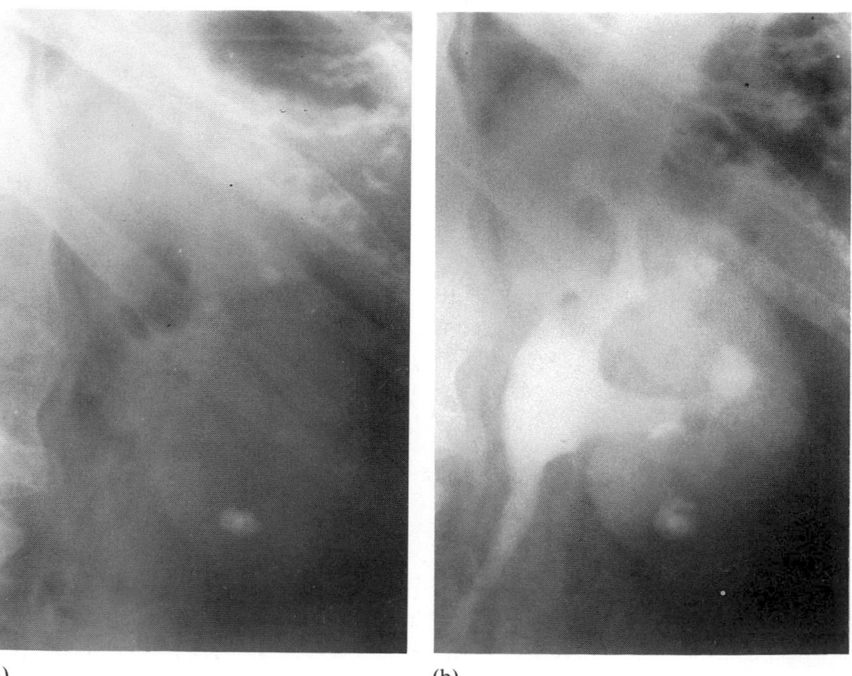

Fig. 8.18. (a) Small stones lying in calices (b) causing negligible obstruction. These are very common, seldom cause symptoms and probably do not need to be treated.

groin or vulva. They may cause increasing irritability of the bladder and the patient may have frequency and discomfort on voiding — symptoms that are difficult to explain. Haematuria is common in these patients, but even when a stone has been found, the patient must still be cystoscoped to rule out a tumour of the bladder.

The treatment of these stones today is by ESWL using any of the machines described above. When the stone is more than 2 cm in diameter, and a large amount of pulverized stone must be passed down the ureter, a double-J stent is often passed up the ureter before ESWL to cause it to dilate and help the little fragments pass down.

In some instances the shock wave cannot reach the stone because a rib — or sometimes the iliac crest — is in the way. Sometimes too, the stone is so large that the amount of debris that will have to be passed down the ureter will inevitably mean prolonged obstruction and pain. For these cases *percutaneous nephrolithotomy* is used (see p. 88). The main body of the stone is broken up and extracted through the sheath: a nephrostomy is left in the pelvis to help fragments to escape, and the rest of the stone is broken up with ESWL. When ESWL or PCNL is not available — or when they are, for some unusual reason, contraindicated, the kidney is approached through the 12th rib tip incision and mobilized

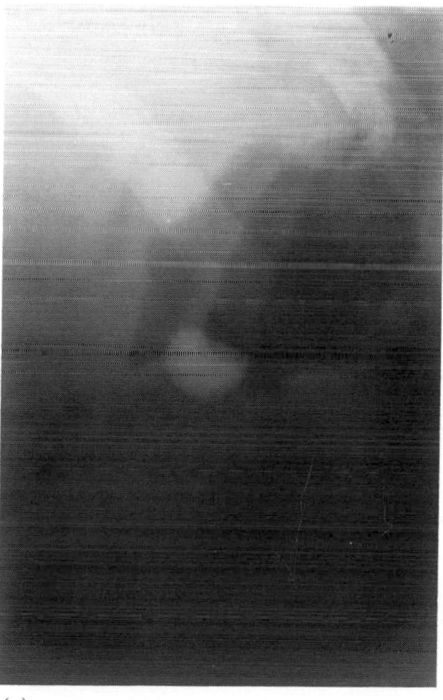

(a)

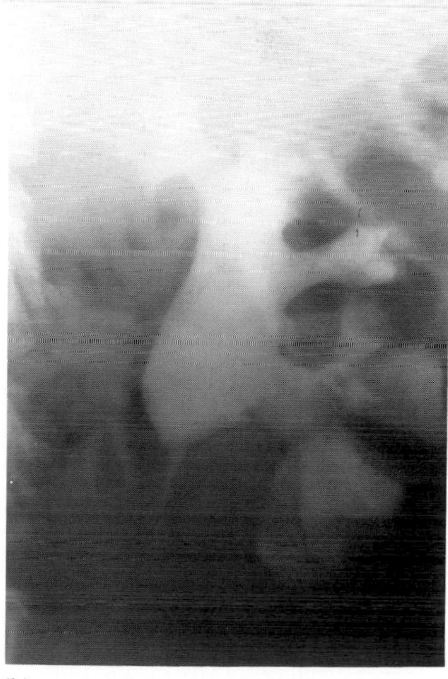

(b)

Fig. 8.19. (a) When a stone in the renal pelvis gets too large to go down the ureter it causes obstruction (b) and must be got rid of.

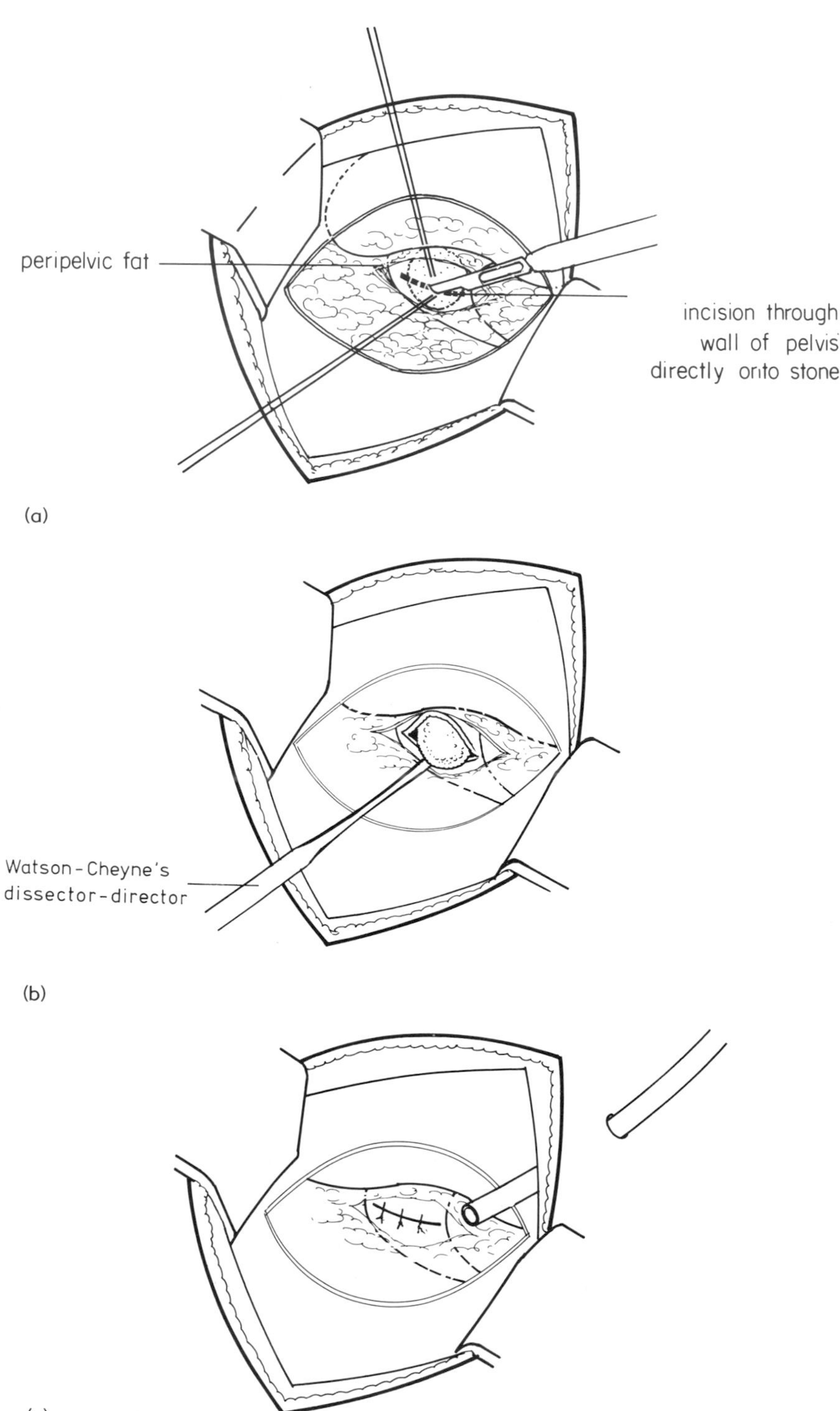

Fig. 8.20. Pyelolithotomy: through a short loin incision (a) the renal pelvis is opened between stay sutures and (b) the stone lifted out and (c) the pelvis closed.

sufficiently far as to permit access to the renal pelvis. This is incised between two stay sutures (Fig. 8.20), the stone is removed, and the pelvis is closed. The wound is closed with drainage.

Staghorn calculi

Here the stone has progressively enlarged until it fills not only the pelvis but also the calices, producing a large branched 'coralliform' or 'staghorn' calculus (Fig. 8.21). Most of them are seen in patients with urinary infection with *Proteus mirabilis* and are composed of mixed magnesium ammonium phosphate, but any type of stone can end up by forming a staghorn calculus.

These stones are so bulky that to remove them requires great skill and care in selecting the best combination of PCNL for the main body of the stone, leaving the outlying fragments to be broken up by ESWL.

Before ESWL or PCNL techniques were available these stones were removed by the Gil-Vernet operation of the *extended pyelolithotomy*. The kidney was approached through a 12th rib bed incision (Fig. 8.22) and fully mobilized. Its artery was isolated so that it could be taped (to prevent loss of blood), and the plane of cleavage between the renal pelvis and the parenchyma was opened up. This is a bloodless plane, and it allows the parenchyma of the kidney to be lifted away from the renal

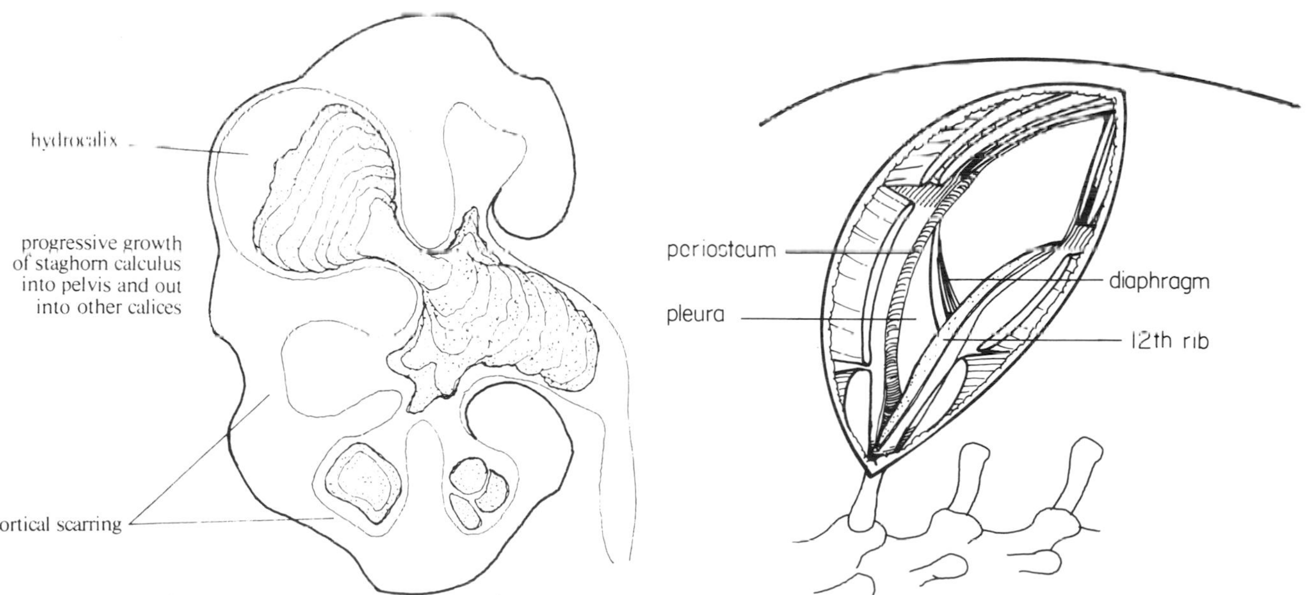

Fig. 8.21. Formation of a typical staghorn calculus.

Fig. 8.22. 12th rib-red incision.

pelvis and the necks of the calices. An incision is now made from the upper calix to the lower one (Fig. 8.23) and the main body of the stone is removed (Fig. 8.24). Often there are outlying mushroom-shaped fragments, and to get these out it is necessary to incise the parenchyma — *nephrolithotomy* (Fig. 8.25). This is apt to bleed, and while the outlying fragments are being removed the renal artery is occluded. Removing all the outlying fragments can take a considerable time, and to protect the kidney from ischaemic damage various methods were devised to cool the kidney — of these the simplest and most effective was to pack it in sterile ice-slush and irrigate it with ice-cold saline.

Stone in the ureter

Little dogs make the most noise, and stones in the ureter often cause pain in inverse proportion to their size. The pain comes on suddenly. It can be excruciating. Women who have experienced a difficult childbirth as well as a ureteric calculus would rather have another baby than another stone. The pain comes on in waves: it makes the patient roll and twist in the attempt to get relief. The accompanying disturbance of intestinal transport makes them vomit. There is gaseous distension of the small and large bowel, constipation, or sometimes diarrhoea. Experienced surgeons may be deceived into a diagnosis of intestinal obstruction when these bowel symptoms are particularly severe. There may be tenderness over the kidney or the loin (Fig. 8.26). The urine may show haematuria on testing, and microscopy soon after the colic nearly always reveals a few red cells.

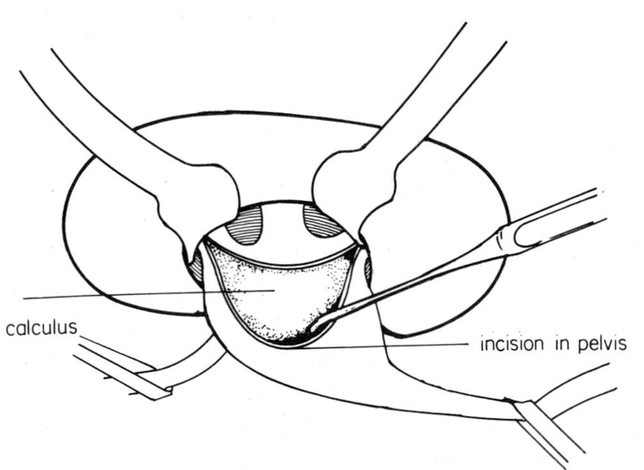

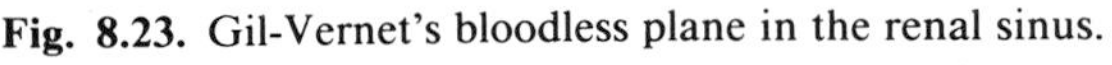
Fig. 8.23. Gil-Vernet's bloodless plane in the renal sinus.

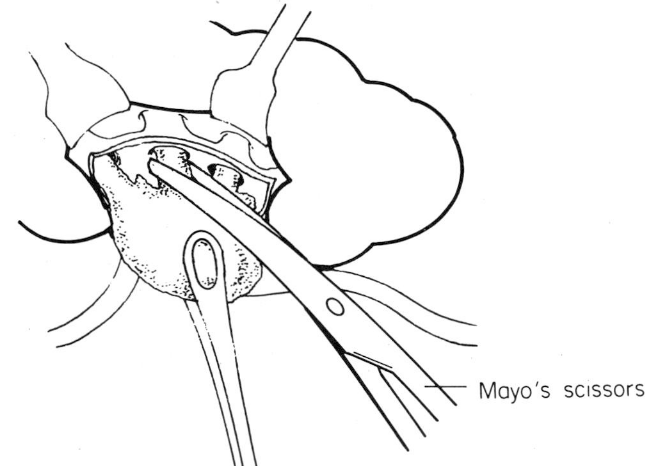

Fig. 8.24. Breaking off the 'mushroom' extensions of a staghorn stone.

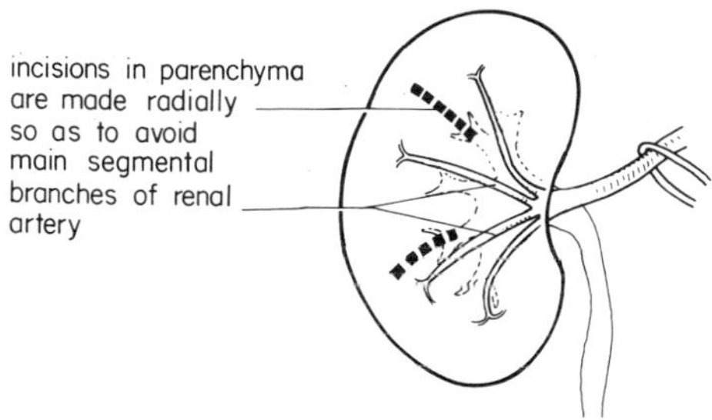

Fig. 8.25. Radial incisions in the renal parenchyma avoid the segmental arteries of the kidney.

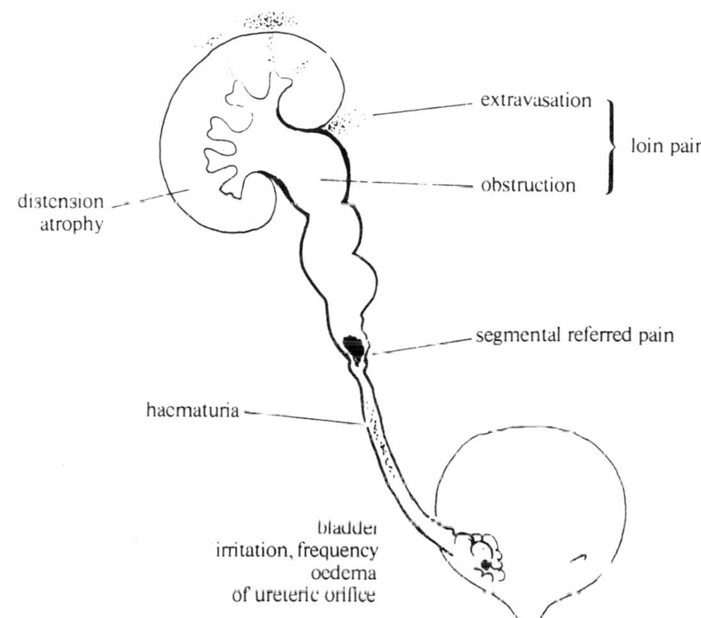

Fig. 8.26. Clinical features of a stone in the ureter.

Stones less than 5 mm in diameter usually pass down the ureter. They may have difficulty in doing so, and the patient may suffer several bouts of pain, but so long as these stones make steady progress and so long as there is no atrophy of the kidney upstream of the stone, it is safe to defer surgery. Infection changes all this: when obstruction is accompanied by infection there is a risk of septicaemia and the kidney may suffer inflammatory damage.

Stone in the bladder

Many calculi reach the bladder having safely passed down the ureter, and most are passed in the urine without being noticed. If there is obstruction to the outflow from the bladder the stones cannot get out, so they are seen nowadays in the West almost exclusively in elderly men with prostatic obstruction. In women, stones are rare in the bladder except when they form on some foreign material such as a stitch or a fragment of catheter.

The symptoms are usually those of outflow obstruction without pain or haematuria (Fig. 8.27). A few will still give the classical history of pain referred to the tip of the penis, worse on taking exercise, relieved by lying down, the result of the altered position of the stone giving most discomfort when it sits on the trigone.

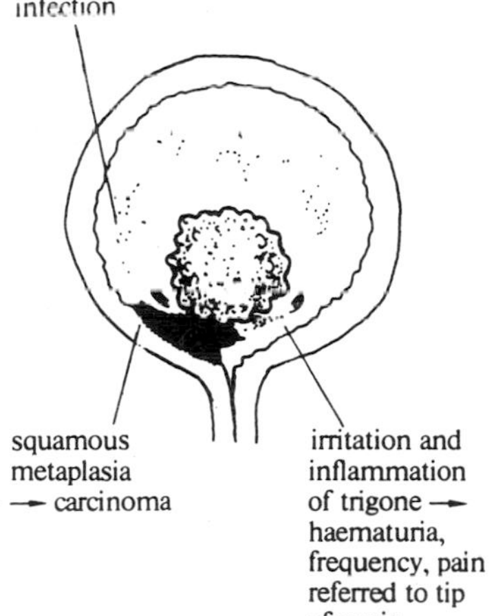

Fig. 8.27. Clinical features of a stone in the bladder.

Management of a stone in the bladder. Most stones are removed via the urethra. Small stones are seen through a resectoscope sheath, broken up with forceps, and evacuated with an Ellik evacuator. Larger ones are better crushed with the classical *lithotrite* (Fig. 8.28) — an instrument that has remained unchanged in design for a century: with it the stone is crushed to powder and then evacuated. Modern devices — the *ultrasonic lithotriptor* (Fig. 8.29) and the *electrohydraulic lithotriptor* pulverize the stone with an oscillating toothed cylinder or a series of sparks, and are used by surgeons who are unfamiliar with the classical instrument. As a last resort, the bladder is opened suprapubically and the stone extracted — *lithotomy*. In most cases it is also necessary to treat the underlying cause of the outflow obstruction, e.g. the enlarged prostate or the urethral stricture.

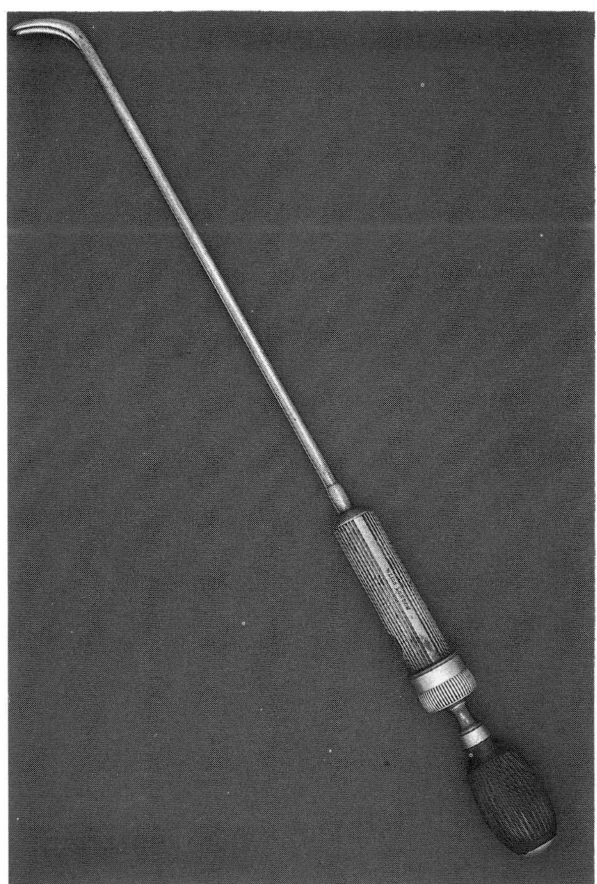

Fig. 8.28. The classical lithotrite. This one, still in use at St Peter's Hospital for Stone, was made for Sir Peter Freyer in 1886.

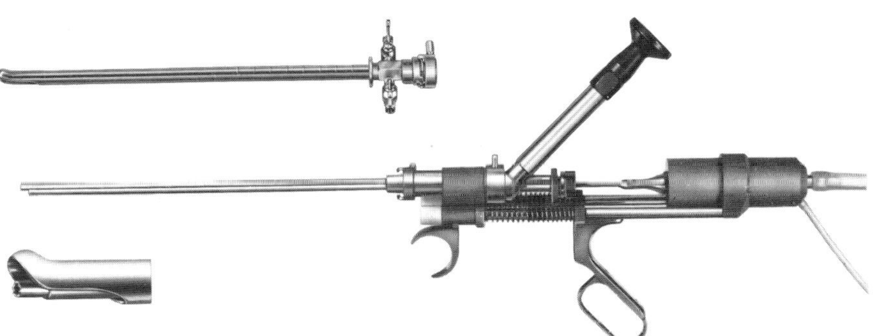

Fig. 8.29. Storz ultrasonic lithotriptor (courtesy Messrs Rimmer Bros, UK Agents for Karl Storz A.G.).

FURTHER READING

Amplatz K & Lange PH (1986) *Atlas of Endourology*. Wolfe and Year Book Publications, Chicago & London.

Blandy JP (1986) *Operative Urology*. 2nd Ed. Blackwell Scientific Publications, Oxford. pp. 40–61.

Coptcoat MJ, Webb DR, Kellet MJ, Fletcher MS, McNicholas TA, Dickinson IK, Whitfield HN & Wickham JEA (1986) The complications of extracorporeal shockwave lithotripsy; management and prevention. *British Journal of Urology* **58**, 578–80.

Dickinson IK, Fletcher MS, Bailey MJ, Coptcoat MJ, McNicholas TA, Kellett MJ, Whitfield HN & Wickham JEA (1986) Combination of percutaneous surgery and extracorporeal shockwave lithotripsy for the treatment of large renal calculi. *British Journal of Urology* **58**, 581–4.

Gravenstein JS & Peter K (Eds) (1988) *Extracorporeal Shock-Wave Lithotripsy for Renal Stone Disease*. Butterworths, Boston.

Jamieson MJ (1985) Hypercalcaemia. *British Medical Journal* **290**, 378–82.

Marickar YMF & Rose GA (1985) Relationship of stone growth and urinary biochemistry in long-term follow-up of stone patients with idiopathic hypercalciuria. *British Journal of Urology* **57**, 613–7.

Ryall RL, Darroch JN & Marshall VR (1984) The evaluation of risk factors in male stone-formers attending a general hospital out-patient clinic. *British Journal of Urology* **56**, 116–21.

9 Neoplasms of the Kidney

Tumours arise either from the parenchyma or the urothelium that lines the renal pelvis. There are two main types of parenchymal tumours, one in children, the other in adults.

EMBRYOMA — WILMS' TUMOUR

This tumour was described by Rance in 1814 long before Wilms (1899) was born (such is the injustice of eponymous fame). It accounts for 10% of all childhood malignancies and occurs in 1:13 000 children. Odd genetic associations link Wilms' tumour with congenital aniridia, hemihypertrophy, exomphalos and macroglossia. In some family trees there is an excess of children with Wilms' tumour or multicystic disease, and adults with renal cell (Grawitz) carcinoma and neurofibromatosis. Few of these tumours occur after the age of six although rare examples are seen in adults.

An important sub-group occurs in the first few months of life which behaves almost as if it were benign — this is the *mesoblastic nephroma* (Fig. 9.1), and it is made up of diffuse mesenchymal proliferation between islands of healthy-looking kidney tissue, whereas in the usual *embryoma* there is no such clear distinction between the healthy and the malignant parts.

About one in ten Wilms' tumours are bilateral. They show almost every tissue that can arise from mesoderm — bone, cartilage, smooth and striated muscle — but the most malignant parts usually resemble rhabdomyosarcoma. They spread by direct invasion into the psoas, bowel and adjacent tissues. In addition they may be carried in the bloodstream to the lungs. They erode the renal pelvis relatively late, so that haematuria is a late feature and carries a bad prognosis.

Clinical features

A big lump in a wasted child (Fig. 9.2) is the classical presentation, but these tumours may cause pain. Haematuria, found in one in three, is a late feature. Other features — hypertension, fever, and a raised red cell or white cell count — may at first mislead the doctor.

The main differential diagnosis is from a *neuroblastoma*. Today the

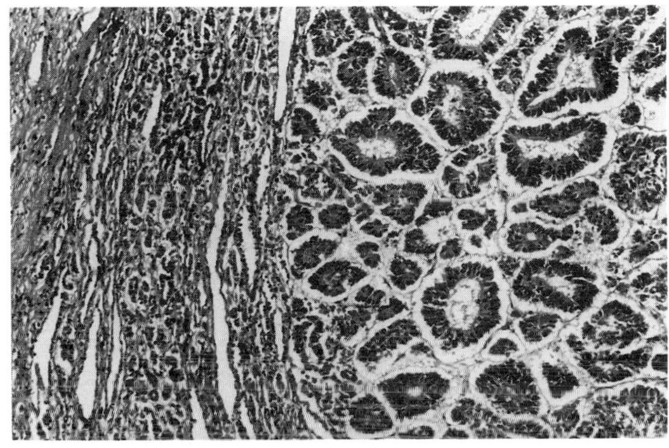

(a)

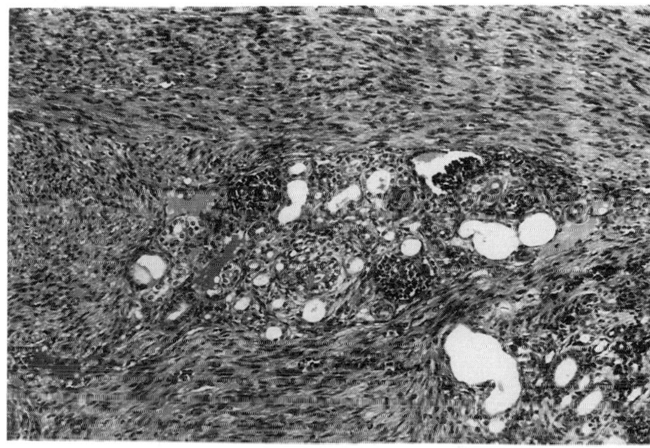

(b)

Fig. 9.1. (a) Wilms' tumour of kidney (b) Mesoblastic nephroma of kidney. (Courtesy of Dr Jo Martin. The London Hospital Institute of Pathology).

most useful investigation is ultrasound, but it may need urography, and sometimes it is helpful to inject the contrast medium into the vena cava to provide a cavogram at the same time. Speckled calcification is more often seen in a neuroblastoma than a Wilms' tumour, and a neuroblastoma usually shifts the kidney to one side or downwards rather than distorting the pyelogram. In practice, CT scanning gives the most information in these children, but may require heavy sedation. Angiography is indicated in bilateral tumours to define the presence of a tumour on the other side and to plan treatment, e.g. by partial nephrectomy.

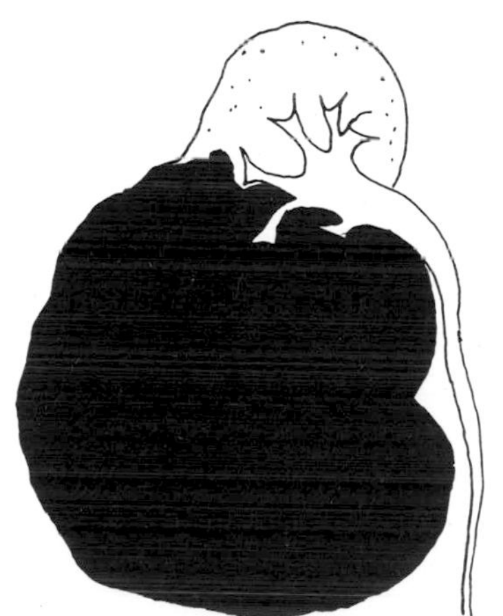

Fig. 9.2. Embryoma of the kidney (Wilms').

Staging of Wilms' tumour (Fig. 9.3)

Stage I. Tumour completely excised, no tumour rupture.
Stage II. Tumour extending outside kidney but completely excised, vessels invaded, local spillage of tumour.
Stage III. Tumour incompletely excised at operation, lymph nodes involved, tumour spilt into peritoneum.
Stage IV. Distant metastases.
Stage V. Bilateral renal tumours from the beginning.

Management

The outlook for the child with a Wilms' tumour has been completely transformed by chemotherapy which today allows a cure in > 80% — a figure which is only achieved by making sure that every child with this unusual tumour is offered the most up-to-date team management by

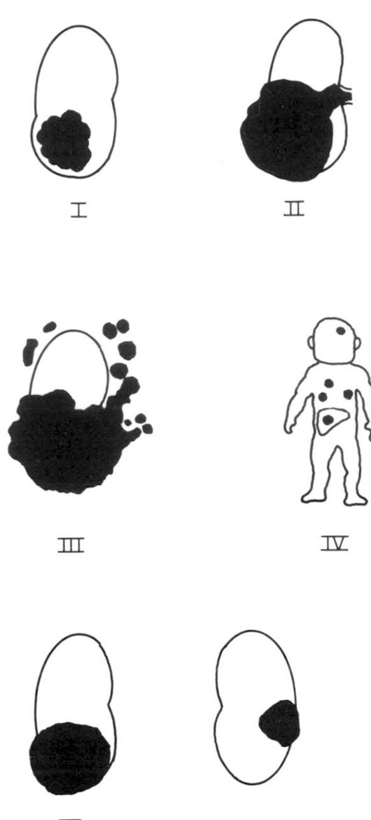

Fig. 9.3. Staging of embryoma (Wilms' tumour). Stage I. Tumour limited to kidney; capsule intact; completely excised. Stage II. Tumour beyond kidney but completely excised; or local extension; infiltration of vessels; biopsy or tumour spilt. Stage III. Residual local tumour; lymph nodes; spill into peritoneum; incomplete excision. Stage IV. Distant metastases to lung, liver, bone, brain etc. Stage V. Bilateral renal tumour at time of diagnosis.

surgeon and oncologist in a centre that is actively participating in trials of the latest protocols of treatment. It is as important to make sure the child is referred to such a centre as it is to make the diagnosis in the first instance: it is not a task for the occasional surgeon in a small hospital.

Treatment begins with a 5 day course of *actinomycin D* followed by laparotomy at which the renal vessels are ligated before the kidney is handled. A full exploration of the abdomen is carried out, and the other kidney meticulously inspected. After the kidney has been removed — and its removal must be radical, taking, when necessary, part of the psoas and other adjacent organs — a course of *vincristine* is given, and in some trials, *adriamycin* is given as well.

Radiotherapy

Radiotherapy is unnecessary in Stage I tumours: it is always given in Stage III, and whether or not it is needed in Stage II is still the subject of prospective carefully-controlled trials.

GRAWITZ TUMOUR, RENAL CELL CARCINOMA, HYPERNEPHROMA

Grawitz has no better title to his eponym than Wilms to his, nevertheless Grawitz is a convenient shorthand for this tumour (Fig. 9.4). It is rare before puberty, more common in males than females, and typically a cancer of old people. There is an undue incidence of Grawitz tumours in certain families and it may be associated with the von Hippel–Lindau syndrome (cerebellar and retinal angiomas together with cysts in the liver and pancreas). It may perhaps be associated with cadmium pollution, oestrogen ingestion, and in one form is being seen as a kind of epidemic in people with renal failure on chronic dialysis.

Pathology

Many healthy adults have tiny areas in their kidneys which resemble this tumour but by convention are not called adenocarcinomas until they are at least 3 cm in diameter — well within the size that can be detected by ultrasound or angiography. The distinction is not absolute, rare cases are described where there have been widespread metastases from primary tumours < 2 cm in diameter. Macroscopically these tumours, which are thought to arise from the renal tubule, are bright yellow in colour, but blotchy from extravasated blood and necrosis (Fig. 9.5).

Microscopically three grades are recognized: G1 has large orderly

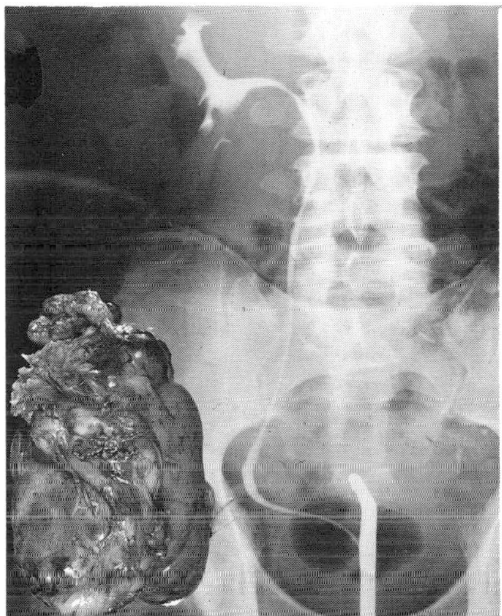

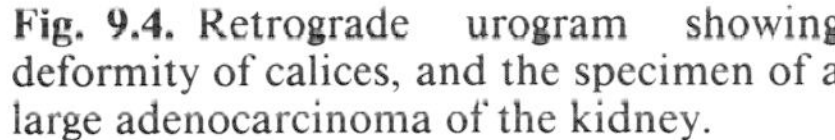

Fig. 9.4. Retrograde urogram showing deformity of calices, and the specimen of a large adenocarcinoma of the kidney.

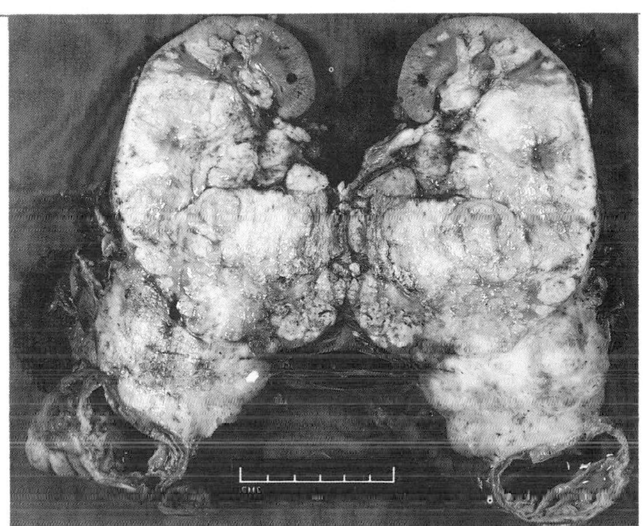

Fig. 9.5. Macroscopic appearance of a large carcinoma of the kidney which extended outside the kidney and invaded the colon.

clear cells stuffed with lipid, G3 shows sheets of anaplastic cells and G2 is somewhere in between (Fig. 9.6). There is one variety which deserves notice since it is almost always benign — *oncocytoma*: here the cells are well differentiated and eosinophilic (Fig. 9.7).

Clinical features

Haematuria, pain and a lump are the three cardinal features of a Grawitz tumour (Fig. 9.8). Haematuria is a relatively late feature, meaning that the cancer has eroded into the collecting system, but it occurs in about 40% of the cases seen today. Pain is common, difficult to describe or localize: there may be a lump in the abdomen. Today these tumours are more and more often detected in the course of abdominal ultrasound performed for some other indication, or as an incidental finding when contrast is injected for some other condition, e.g. coronary angiography.

One most interesting group of patients present with loss of weight, illness, tiredness, unexplained fever and sweating. They have a raised sedimentation rate, polycythaemia, or a raised white cell count. Others have hypercalcaemia from the secretion by the tumour of a substance similar to parathormone: still others have clubbing and pulmonary osteodystrophy. Many a tumour is only detected on biopsy of a distant metastasis. It is worth remembering that the histological picture of a

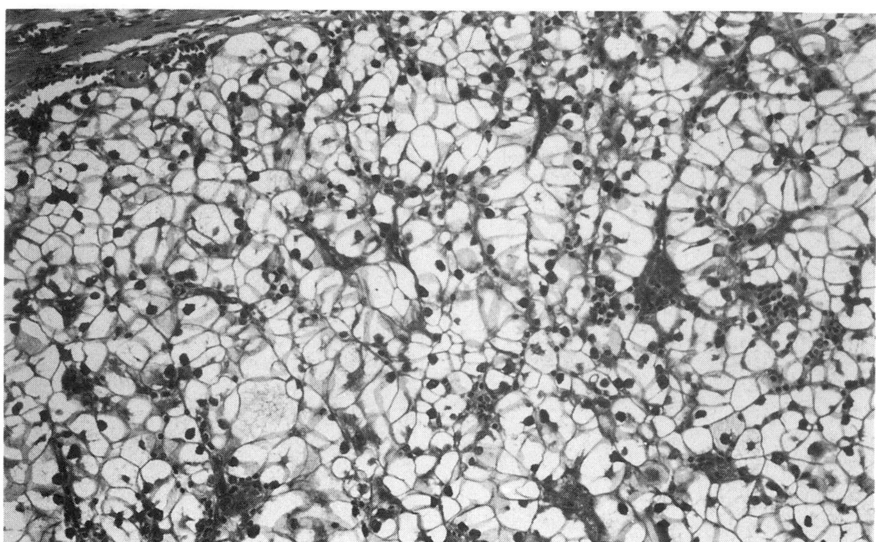

Fig. 9.6. Grawitz carcinoma of the kidney: a moderately differentiated (G2) carcinoma showing large clear cells stuffed with lipid. (Courtesy of Dr Jo Martin. The London Hospital Institute of Pathology.)

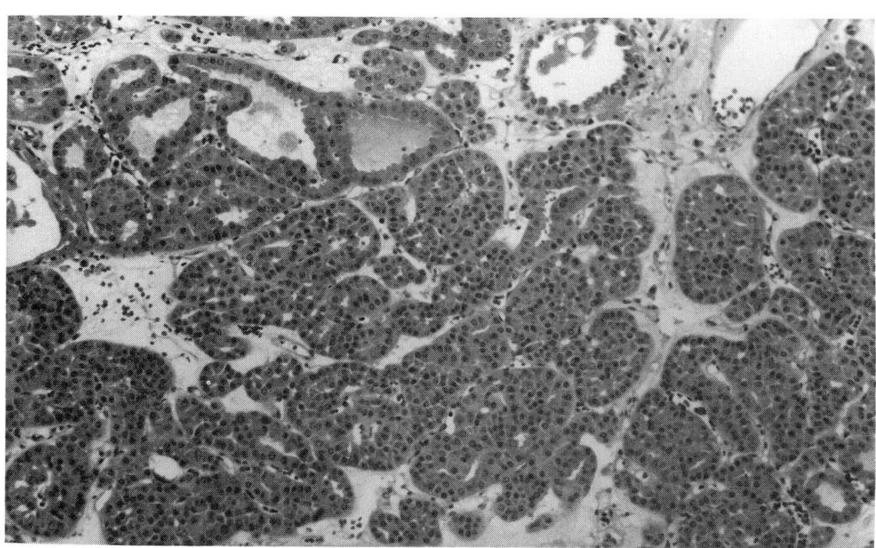

Fig. 9.7. Oncocytoma of kidney: these cells are brightly eosinophilic. (Courtesy of Dr Jo Martin. The London Hospital Institute of Pathology.)

Grawitz tumour is usually so characteristic that the pathologist who reports that a metastasis has arisen from a primary in the kidney is usually right, however improbable this may seem.

Investigations

An *excretion urogram* will show a soft tissue mass which distorts the adjacent collecting system (Fig. 9.9). The next step is an *ultrasound* scan

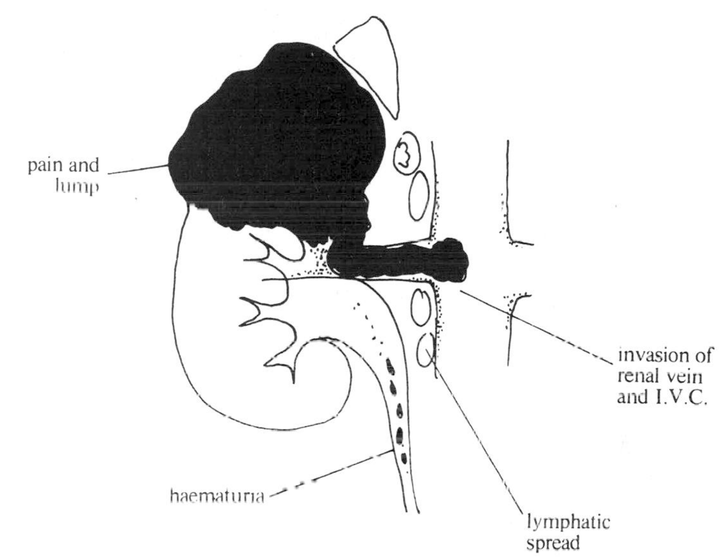

Fig. 9.8. Adenocarcinoma of the kidney.

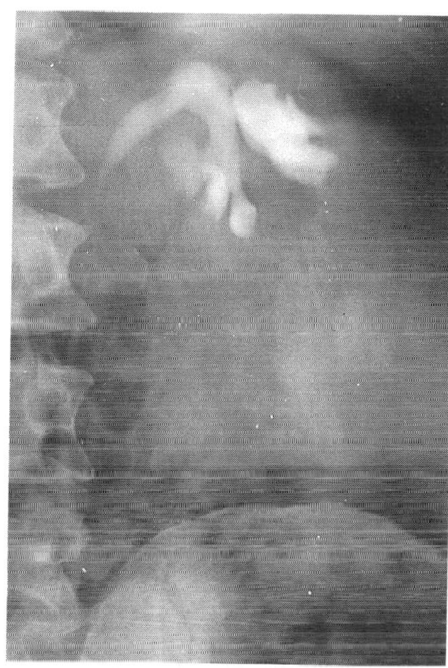

Fig. 9.9. IVU showing the left renal pelvis and calices grossly distorted by a huge soft tissue mass arising from the lower pole.

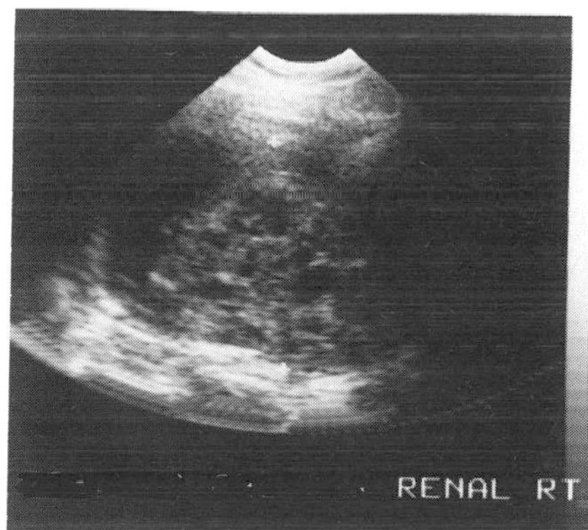

Fig. 9.10. Ultrasound scan of right kidney showing a mass full of echoes in the middle of the kidney.

which will show whether there are echoes in the mass or not (Fig. 9.10): if there are no echoes, the swelling is a cyst and the diagnosis may be confirmed by aspiration of its fluid. Turbid or blood stained fluid suggests a carcinoma. Echoes within the mass may be due to a multilocular cyst, hydatid disease, fibrin or pus inside a cyst — but are more likely to be due to cancer.

In practice, few additional investigations are needed, but in very large tumours, before embarking on nephrectomy, it is sometimes of practical value to the surgeon to know whether the inferior vena cava is invaded or not: as a rule the suspicion of vena caval involvement is raised by the ultrasound scan. It can be confirmed by superior and inferior cavography. Angiography was formerly a standard investigation but today seldom adds any useful additional information.

Treatment

Through a generous abdominal incision (Fig. 9.11), which may be vertical, transverse or thoracoabdominal (when the upper pole is involved), the colon and duodenum are reflected from the front of the kidney (Fig. 9.12). The renal artery is ligated and divided (Fig. 9.13) (to cut off most of the blood going to the kidney). The renal vein is then divided, and finally the entire mass of kidney together with all the

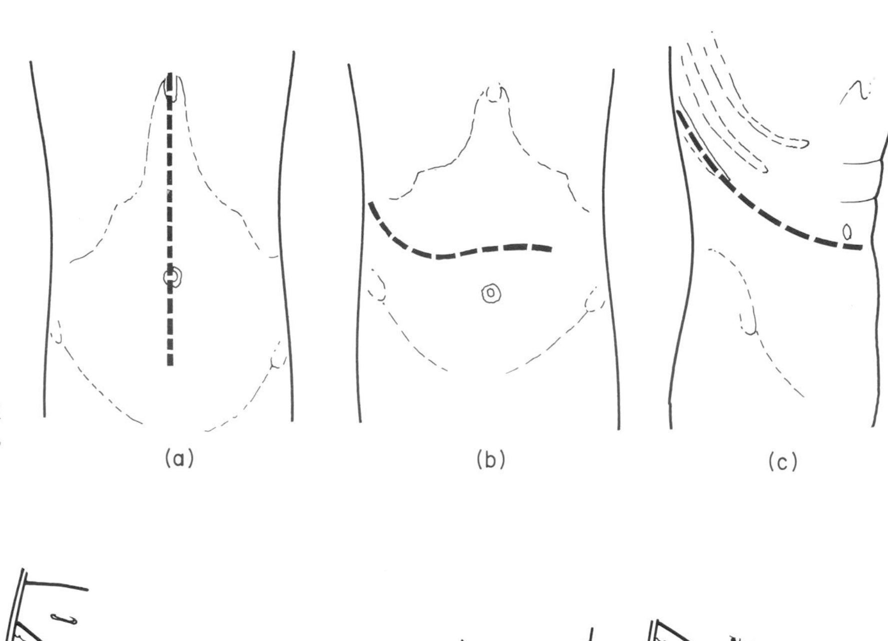

Fig. 9.11. Choice of incisions for removal of a carcinoma of the kidney. (a) Midline, (b) transverse, (c) thoracoabdominal.

Fig. 9.12. Transabdominal nephrectomy.

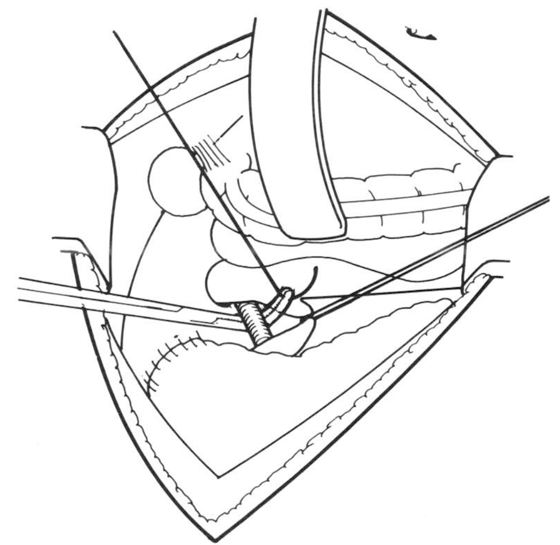

Fig. 9.13. Ligature of the right renal artery.

surrounding fat and fascia, and all the lymph nodes alongside the aorta (on the left) and the inferior vena cava (on the right) are removed *en bloc*. If the inferior vena cava is invaded, it is taped above and below the renal vein, the lumbar veins are all divided, and the opposite renal vein occluded (Fig. 9.14). Then the vena cava is opened and the lump or tumour removed *en bloc* with the specimen. The vena cava is closed with a vascular suture. When a mass of tumour has been discovered by the

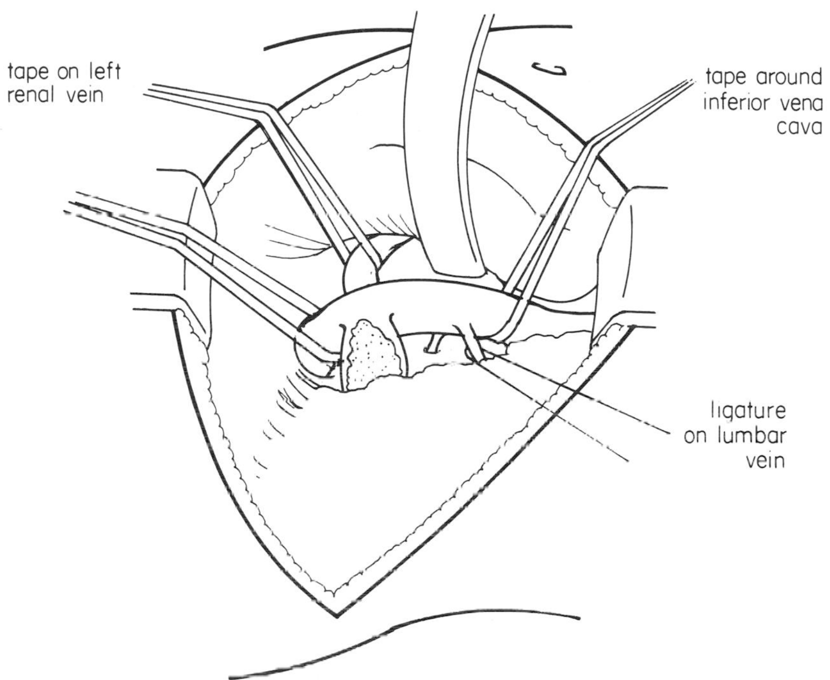

Fig. 9.14. Removing a malignant thrombus from the vena cava.

pre-operative cavogram to extend up inside the vena cava, the chest is opened and preparations made for cardiac bypass in order to allow the malignant thrombus to be removed from the right atrium.

Adjuvant treatment and prognosis

If the tumour is confined to the kidney there is a > 80% 5 year survival: unfavourable features are invasion of the surrounding lymph nodes, fat, and inferior vena cava. Even when there are metastases some of these patients do well when the primary tumour is removed, and in up to 8% of cases the metastases can be shown to disappear during the first few months after nephrectomy — though most of them return elsewhere later on. This suggests that the system of immune surveillance is particularly effective in renal parenchymal cancer, and that if only one could find the right stimulus, this natural defence could be helped. To this end there are many studies in progress with BCG, interferon and interleukin and the early results seem promising.

Hormonal therapy was formerly in vogue: it was based on observations in the golden hamster whose renal tumours responded to progestogen treatment. Controlled trials have long since shown that this does not work in man.

Rare tumours that imitate renal cell carcinoma

Oncocytoma has already been mentioned: it is said to have a characteristic 'cartwheel' angiogram, but this is of little value today when angiography is so seldom indicated, and in any event, oncocytoma is probably not as benign as was once thought. *Benign multilocular cysts* occur which exactly mimic all the radiological, CT, and ultrasonic features of the cystic form of a Grawitz tumour. *Angiomyolipoma* is a benign tumour which is often — but not always — seen in patients with tuberose sclerosis: it is most often seen on the right. Its fat gives it a striking and unmistakable appearance in the CT scan. It is usually benign and only needs to be explored when the diagnosis is uncertain (not all tumours in patients with tuberose sclerosis are benign) or because of haemorrhage into the mass.

UROTHELIAL TUMOURS OF THE RENAL PELVIS

The upper tract is lined with urothelium identical with that lining the bladder. Most of the tumours that arise from it are *urothelial* or *transitional cell* carcinomas, but just as the urothelium of the bladder can undergo squamous or adenomatous metaplasia, so too in the renal pelvis and ureter there may be *squamous carcinoma* and *adenocarcinoma* — though these are very unusual.

Urothelial cancer in the renal pelvis is seen in association with bladder tumours, especially in people with very active bladders that keep producing crop after crop of multiple tumours, probably because there is some carcinogenic agent in the urine. Multiple urothelial carcinoma is particularly common in the renal pelvis as a long-term sequel of Balkan nephropathy and analgesic abuse (see p. 68).

Pathology

Urothelial tumours are classified exactly as for tumours of the bladder — Grades 1, 2 and 3 (where G1 is well differentiated and G3 highly malignant). Squamous cancers may be seen in patients with very long-standing stones in the kidney, and adenocarcinoma is a rare sequel of prolonged infection. All these tumours spread directly through the thin muscular wall of the renal pelvis into the surrounding fat or the renal parenchyma. They metastasize usually via the lymph nodes rather than the renal veins.

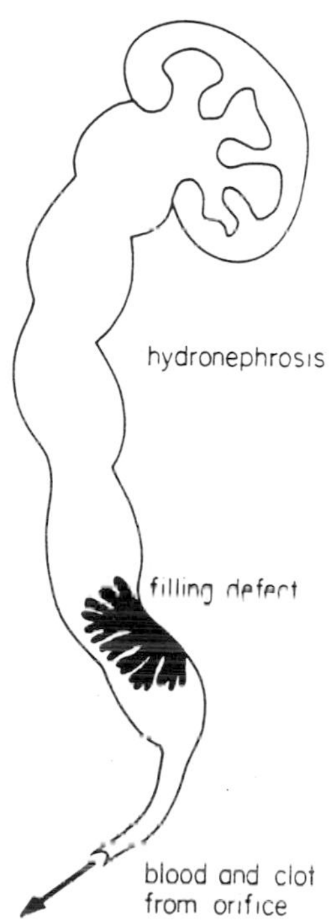

Fig. 9.15. Clinical features of carcinoma of the ureter.

Clinical features

Haematuria is the most important feature of these tumours, and pain a late one (Fig. 9.15). An IVU will show a filling defect in the pyelogram, often difficult to detect when the tumour is small. Malignant cells are usually present in the urine.

Investigations

To confirm the diagnosis a retrograde urogram will provide a more clear picture of the upper tract, especially when the outline of a calix is not very clear. At this investigation a *brush* (Fig. 9.16) may be passed up the ureter to get tissue from the tumour for histological examination and *ureteroscopy* may permit a biopsy to be taken under direct vision (Fig. 9.17).

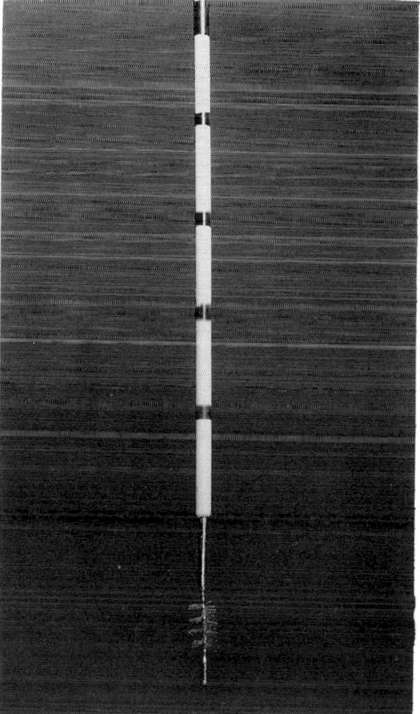

Fig. 9.16. Brush passed via ureteric catheter to obtain tissue from a ureteric or renal pelvic tumour.

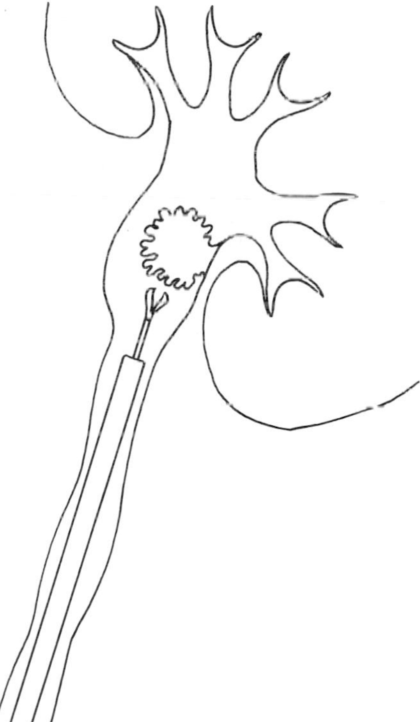

Fig. 9.17. Through the ureteroscope a biopsy forceps may give a histological sample from the tumour.

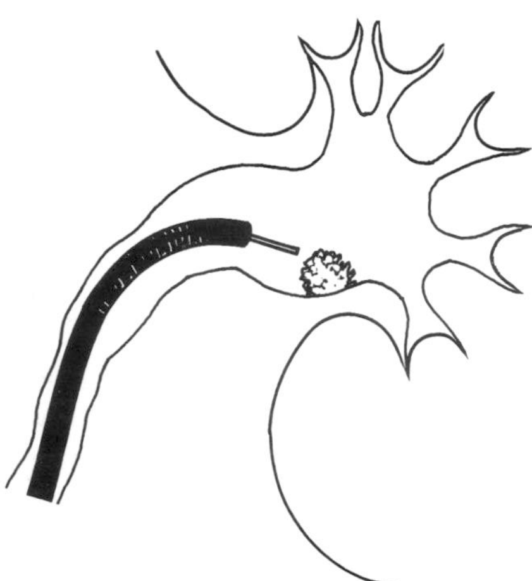

Fig. 9.18. Through the flexible ureteroscope the quartz fibre from the Neodymium YAG laser may be used to destroy a renal pelvic tumour.

Treatment

In small, single, G1 tumours, local treatment may be performed. The renal pelvis may be approached through the ureteroscope, and after a biopsy has been obtained, the tumour may be destroyed using the *Neodymium-YAG laser*, whose thin quartz fibre can be passed up the ureteroscope (Fig. 9.18). If this is not feasible, the kidney may be approached through the usual 12th rib-tip incision, the renal pelvis may be opened, and a local excision of the tumour performed (Fig. 9.19).

In multiple G1 tumours this approach is insufficient because recurrence further down the ureter is almost inevitable, and it is usual to perform a complete *nephroureterectomy.* The kidney and ureter are removed *en bloc* (Fig. 9.20). If there are multiple tumours along the ureter it is necessary to open the bladder and remove an ellipse of its wall where the ureter enters it, to prevent the recurrence of tumour in the stump of intramural ureter (Fig. 9.21).

Few G3 tumours are detected at a stage before they have invaded the renal parenchyma, and their prognosis is so poor that in many centres a course of preoperative radiotherapy is given as a routine before proceeding to nephroureterectomy. In other centres chemotherapy using *methotrexate, vincristine, adriamycin* and *cis-platinum* is given prior to surgery.

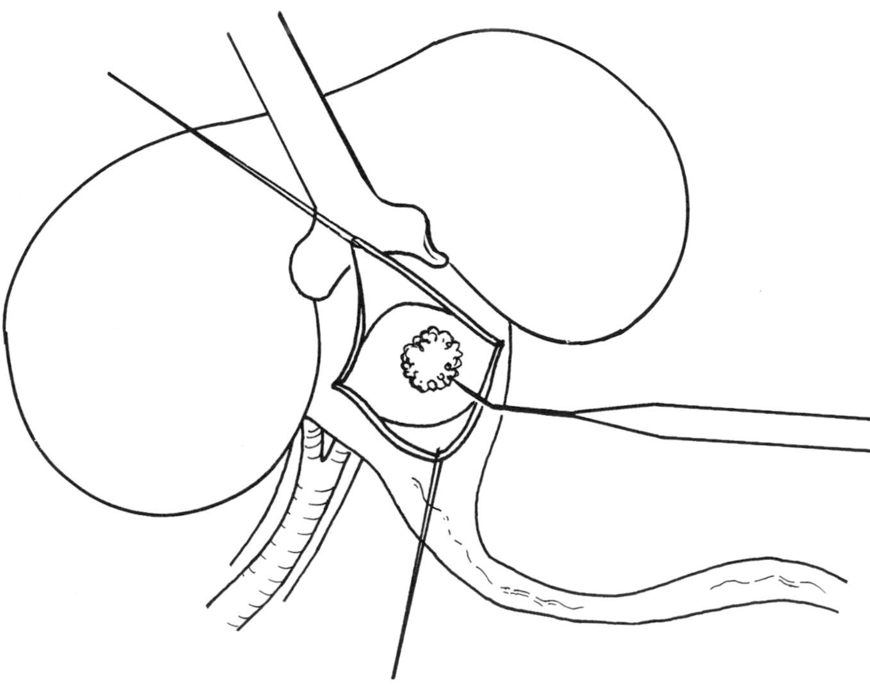

Fig. 9.19. Local excision of a G1 (well-differentiated) renal pelvic tumour. The renal pelvis is exposed through gil-Vernet's approach and opened between stay sutures: the tumour is excised with its pedicle using the diathermy needle.

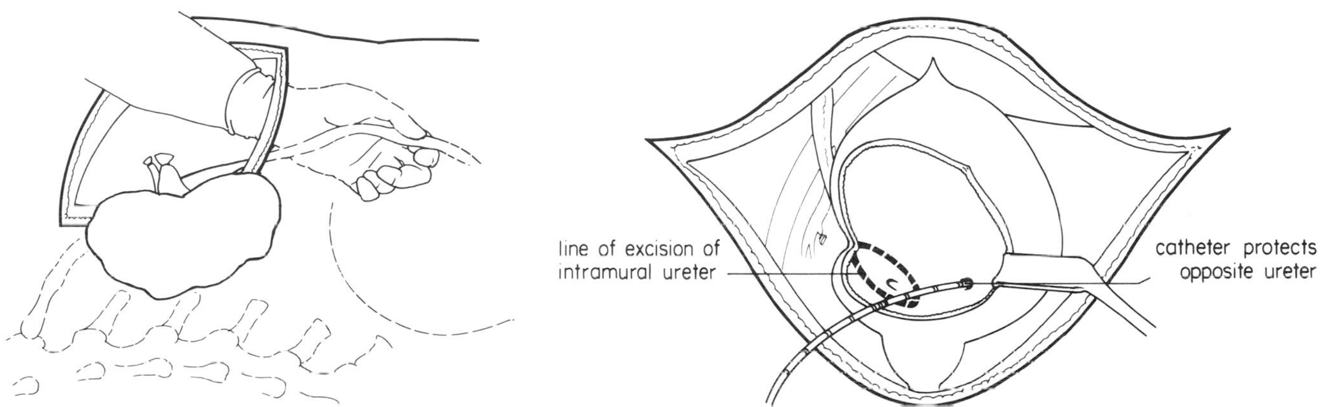

Fig. 9.20. Nephroureterectomy for tumour of renal pelvis or ureter: the kidney and its surrounding fat are removed through an upper abdominal or loin incision.

Fig. 9.21. The lower end of the ureter is removed together with a cuff of healthy bladder through a separate Pfannenstiel incision.

FURTHER READING

Ahuja S, Loffler W, Wegener O-H & Ernst H (1986) Tuberose sclerosis with angiomyolipoma and metastasized hypernephroma. *Urology* **28**, 413–9.

Bartsch G (1984) Renal carcinoma. *World Journal of Urology* **2**, 1–165.

Blute ML, Malek RS & Segura JW (1988) Angiomyolipoma: clinical metamorphosis and concepts for management. *Journal of Urology* **139**, 20–4.

Hardy BE (1988) Wilms' tumor. In: Skinner DG & Lieskovsky G (Eds) *Diagnosis and Management of Genitourinary Cancer.* WB Saunders, Philadelphia. pp. 362–71.

Kirchner FK, Braren V, Smith C, Wilson JP, Foster IH, Hollifield JW & Rhamy RK (1976) Renal cell carcinoma discovered incidentally by arteriography during evaluation for hypertension. *Journal of Urology* **115**, 643–5.

Pritchett TR, Lieskovsky G & Skinner DG (Eds) (1988) Clinical manifestations and treatment of renal parenchymal tumors. In: Skinner DG and Lieskovsky G (Eds) *Diagnosis and Management of Genitourinary Cancer.* WB Saunders, Philadelphia. pp. 337–61.

Richie JP (1988) Carcinoma of the renal pelvis and ureter. In: Skinner DG & Lieskovsky G (Eds) *Diagnosis and Management of Genitourinary Cancer.* WB Saunders, Philadelphia. pp. 323–36.

Steffens J & Nagel R (1988) Tumours of the renal pelvis and ureter. Observations in 170 patients. *British Journal of Urology* **61**, 277–83.

Woodhouse CRJ, Kellett MJ & Bloom HJG (1986) Percutaneous renal surgery and local radiotherapy in the management of renal pelvic transitional cell carcinoma. *British Journal of Urology* **58**, 245–9.

Ziegelbaum M, Novick AC, Streem SB, Montie JE, Pontes JE & Straffon RA (1987) Conservative surgery for transitional cell carcinoma of the renal pelvis. *Journal of Urology* **138**, 1146–9.

10 Vascular Disorders of the Kidney and Hypertension

INFARCTION

Since the renal arteries are end-arteries (Fig. 10.1), if one of them is blocked, the territory it supplies will die. Infarcts occur from mural thrombi after cardiac infarction and operations on the heart. These patients may have pain, sometimes haematuria, and in subsequent urograms one can follow the atrophy of a segment of the kidney. If the whole main renal artery is blocked the entire renal parenchyma undergoes atrophy but, typically, the renal pelvis and the collecting system is unaffected, so that a retrograde urogram will show a surprisingly normal renal pelvis without any overlying parenchyma.

Venous thrombosis

In contrast, the veins of the kidney intercommunicate freely, so that even when there is a complete thrombosis of the main renal vein there is some alternative pathway for the blood to leave the kidney and recovery is usually complete (Fig. 10.2). Clinically the condition may occur in debilitated dehydrated children, ill from some other disorder, who have pain and swelling in the loin, with profuse haematuria. At this stage a

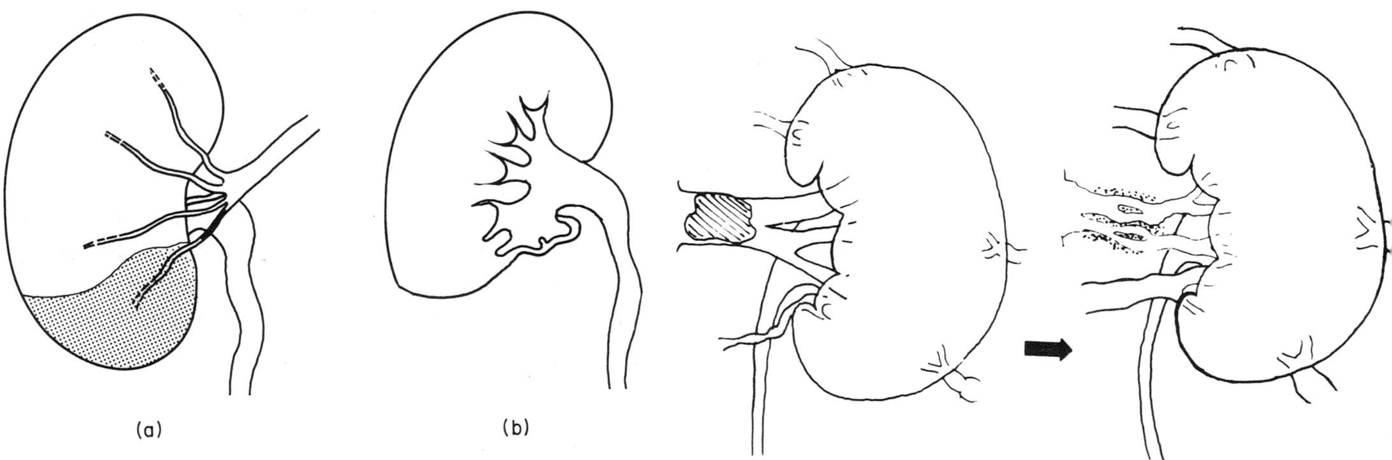

Fig. 10.1. (a) An embolus blocking the inferior segmental artery of the kidney leads to (b) infarction of the lower pole.

Fig. 10.2. Venous obstruction.

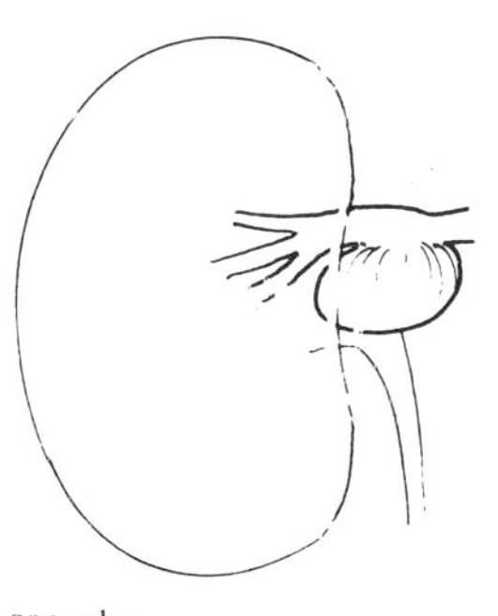

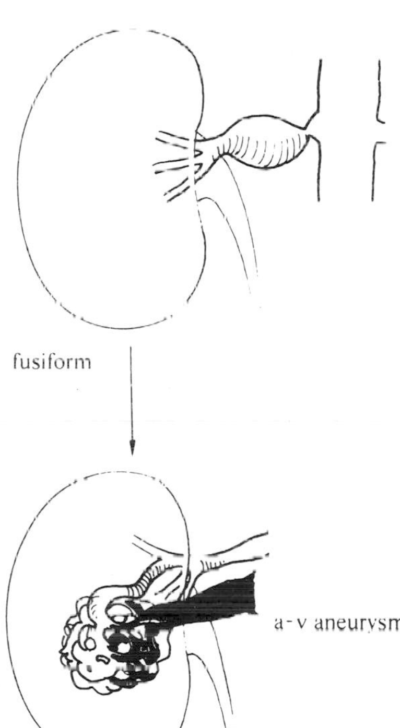

Fig. 10.3. Aneurysms of the renal artery.

urogram will show no contrast on that side but most of them will recover, given time. In adults the condition is very rare, sometimes occurring in acute glomerulonephritis.

ANEURYSM OF THE RENAL ARTERY

There are three types of aneurysm of the renal artery (Fig. 10.3): *saccular* and *fusiform*, each of which may involve the main renal artery or its main branches; and *arterio-venous* fistula. About 17% of aneurysms are intrarenal, and 50% involve the main artery. In 20% the condition is bilateral.

In about a quarter of the fusiform and saccular aneurysms there is calcification in the wall seen in a plain radiograph which may be mistaken for a stone. Arteriovenous aneurysms are common in malignant tumours, but they also occur after trauma, e.g. renal biopsy.

In any type of aneurysm there may be relative narrowing of the renal artery giving rise to ischaemia and so to hypertension. Sometimes a bruit may be heard over the kidney. The diagnosis depends upon good selective angiography (see p. 22).

Treatment

Saccular aneurysms have a risk of spontaneous rupture — sometimes estimated to be as high as 83% which may cause fatal internal haemorrhage, so that unless the patient is very ill it is safer to repair the aneurysm (if this is feasible) or remove the kidney. Fusiform aneurysms may extend up to the branches of the renal artery and be associated with hypertension. It is sometimes possible to reconstruct the whole system, using techniques to cool the kidney to provide a long period of safe ischaemia.

RENAL HYPERTENSION

Almost any disorder of the kidney may result in the release of renin and hypertension: this includes scarring, e.g. pyelonephritis, glomerulonephritis, tuberculosis, tumours, polycystic disease, aneurysms and hydronephrosis. Hypertension itself may damage the renal arteries, making things worse by causing further ischaemia.

The renin-angiotensin mechanism

Renin is a proteolytic enzyme made in the juxtaglomerular apparatus in response to lowered pressure in the afferent arteriole of the glomerulus.

Renin splits one of the α_2 globulins in the serum (*angiotensinogen*) to release *angiotensin I* which is a decapeptide. Angiotensin I is split again by another enzyme in the lungs to form *angiotensin II* (Fig. 10.4).

Angiotensin II is highly active: it raises the blood pressure by constricting peripheral blood vessels and stimulates the adrenal cortex to secrete *aldosterone* which makes the renal tubules conserve sodium and water and so increase the circulating volume.

There are feed-back controls which normally regulate the release of renin: thus an excess of aldosterone (as formed by the rare Conn's tumour) inhibits the release of renin, and in some disorders of the adrenals in which there is an impaired output of aldosterone, or where there is a low plasma sodium, more renin is released.

Investigation of renal hypertension

One should always seek a renal cause for hypertension in young patients because it can often be corrected. A simple IVU will demonstrate any

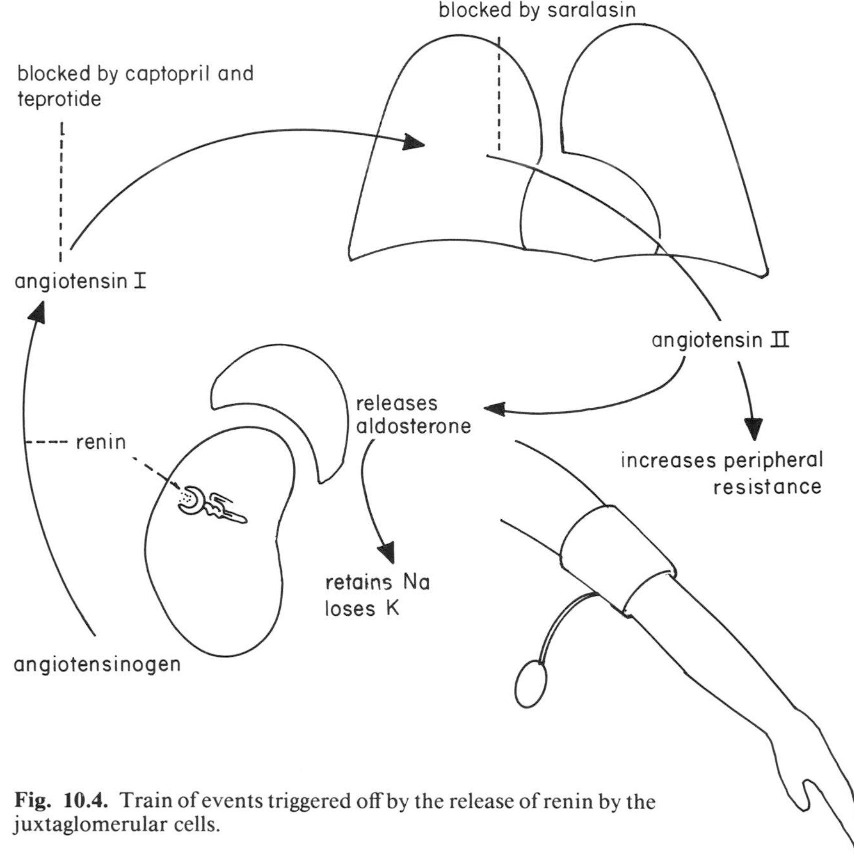

Fig. 10.4. Train of events triggered off by the release of renin by the juxtaglomerular cells.

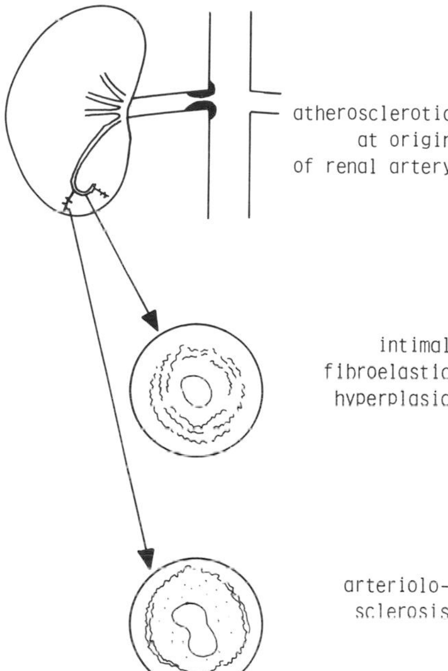

Fig. 10.5. Variations on the theme of arteriosclerosis. In the main renal artery and its major segmental branches, bulky plaques of atheroma may block it. In middle-sized arteries, e.g. the arcuate vessels, there may be intimal fibroelastic hyperplasia. In the vessels of glomerular afferent arteriole size, there is arteriosclerosis, with hyaline material laid down directly under the intima.

obvious mechanical disorder — a hydronephrosis or a small scarred kidney. In seeking evidence of impaired renal blood flow, isotope studies have today largely replaced other investigations (see p. 27). If these suggest an impairment of renal blood flow on one side, one can proceed to angiography using digital vascular imaging (see p. 23) to detect a stenosis of the renal artery.

It is possible to measure plasma renin, but it is easier to use indirect methods to detect its actions. Captopril and teprotide prevent angiotensin I from being converted to antiogensin II in the lungs, and saralasin blocks the action of angiotensin II, so if giving these substances lowers the blood pressure one can assume that renin was responsible for raising it.

Renal artery stenosis

There are two main disorders that can cause narrowing of the renal artery. The most common is *atheroma*, which forms a plaque at the origin of the main renal artery and may entirely block its lumen (Fig. 10.5). In the smaller blood vessels of the kidney the process takes a slightly different form — with a reduplication of the layers of the internal elastic lamina in the middle-sized vessels, and in the smallest ones (such as those entering the glomerulus) a deposit of eosinophilic hyaline material under the endothelium. Surgery can only usefully deal with the first type — where there is a single plaque occluding a short segment of the renal artery — and unfortunately this is rarely the case.

Renal artery dysplasia offers a more hopeful task for the surgeon (Fig. 10.6). The artery is deformed, narrowed irregularly like a string of

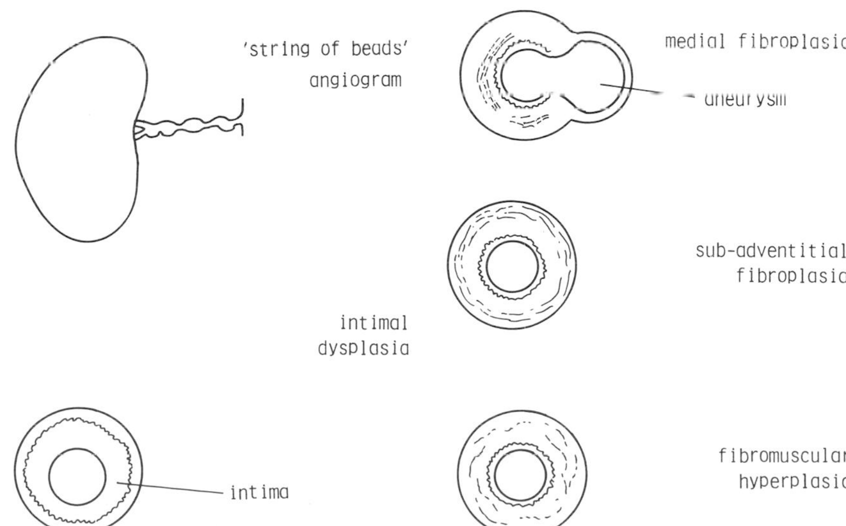

Fig. 10.6. Renal arterial dysplasia may give a 'string of beads' appearance in the angiogram, and take several histological forms: intimal dysplasia, medial fibroplasia, sub-adventitial fibroplasia or fibromuscular hyperplasia.

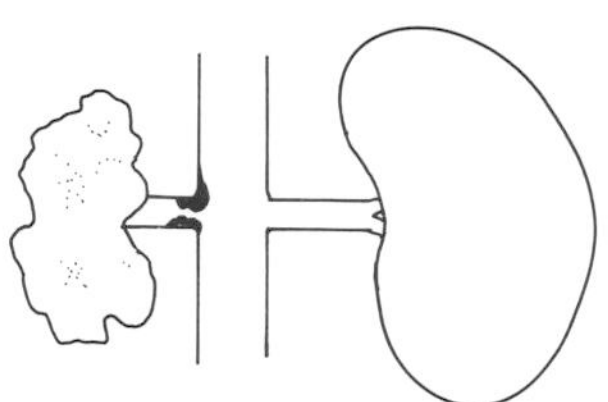

nephrectomy

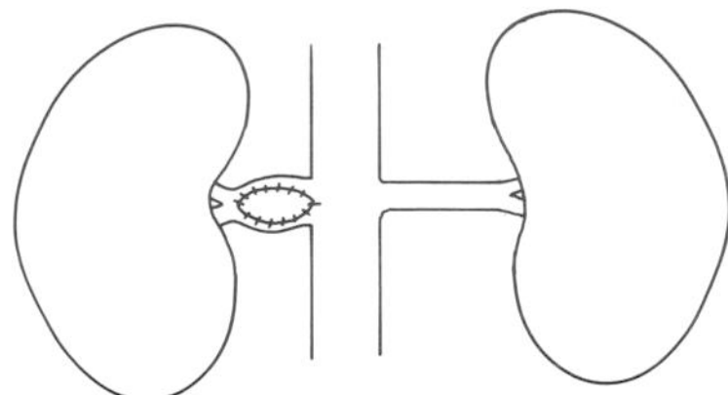

patch on stenosed renal artery

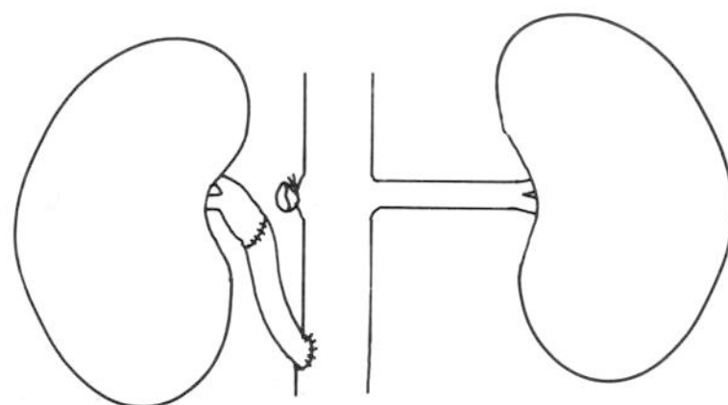

by-pass graft from aorta to distal healthy renal artery

Fig. 10.7. Renal artery stenosis causing hypertension may be treated by nephrectomy if the other kidney is normal, by letting in a patch (from a vein) onto the stenosed vessel, or by means of an arterial graft, by-passing the narrowed segment.

beads — here a thickening of the media and there a dilatation of its wall. When this disorder is confined to a short segment of the renal artery it can be bypassed with success.

Treatment of renal hypertension

Surgery is justified in relatively few cases even though the kidney is almost certainly causing the hypertension. Sometimes the remedy is obvious, e.g. there is a small contracted and functionless kidney or a gross hydronephrosis and little point in conserving the organ. The right operation is nephrectomy. If there is a relatively normal-sized kidney, and a proven renal artery stenosis, then it is worth attempting to restore its blood supply either by enlarging the narrow part with a patch (usually made of the wall of a vein) or bypassing it using a graft onto the aorta, the internal iliac artery, or the splenic artery (Fig. 10.7).

FURTHER READING

Atkinson AB, Brown JJ, Cumming AMM, Fraser R, Lever AF, Leckie BJ, Morton JJ & Robertson JIS (1982) Captopril in renovascular hypertension: long-term use in predicting surgical outcome. *British Medical Journal* **284**, 689–93.

Geyskes GG, Puylaert CBAJ, Oei HY & Dorhout Mees EJ (1983) Follow up study of 70 patients with renal artery stenosis treated by percutaneous transluminal dilatation. *British Medical Journal* **287**, 333–6.

Jamieson GG, Clarkson AR, Woodroffe AJ & Faris I. (1984) Reconstructive renal vascular surgery for chronic renal failure. *British Journal of Surgery* **71**, 338–40.

Ortenberg J, Novick AC, Straffon RA & Stewart BH (1983) Surgical treatment of renal artery aneurysms. *British Journal of Urology* **55**, 341–6.

11 The Adrenal Gland

SURGICAL ANATOMY

Each adrenal gland lies medial and adjacent to the upper pole of each kidney. On the right the adrenal vein drains into the vena cava through a short and delicate vein that is easily torn. On the left the adrenal vein enters the left renal vein (Fig. 11.1). The arteries that supply the adrenal are all small and arise from the phrenic and renal arteries as well as directly from the aorta. At operation the adrenal is easily torn and there may be persistent bleeding from its soft vascular medulla.

ADRENAL TUMOURS

There are two main types of adrenal tumour — those which secrete hormones, and those which do not. Those which secrete hormones include *phaeochromocytoma* (which secrete catecholamines), *Conn's tumour* (which secretes aldosterone) and the group of tumours found in *Cushing's syndrome* (which secrete cortisol). Those which do not secrete hormones include *neuroblastoma* and *non-functioning adrenal carcinomas*.

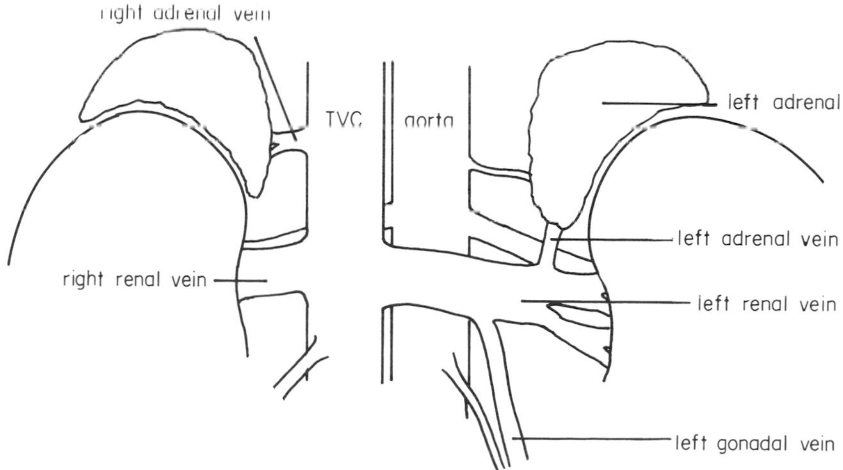

Fig. 11.1. Surgical anatomy of the adrenal glands.

PHAEOCHROMOCYTOMA

This is a tumour arising in the adrenal medulla. It may occur on its own, or in association with the *multiple endocrine neoplasia type II* — a familial disorder in which medullary carcinoma of the thyroid is a feature. It occurs either in the neighbourhood of the adrenals or in the organ of Zuckerkandl (on the aorta near the origin of the inferior mesenteric artery). Noradrenaline is converted to adrenaline by an enzyme and these tumours secrete one or the other — usually noradrenaline. The excess of these substances causes episodes or *paroxysms*, of headache, sweating, flushing, tremor, and pain in the chest.

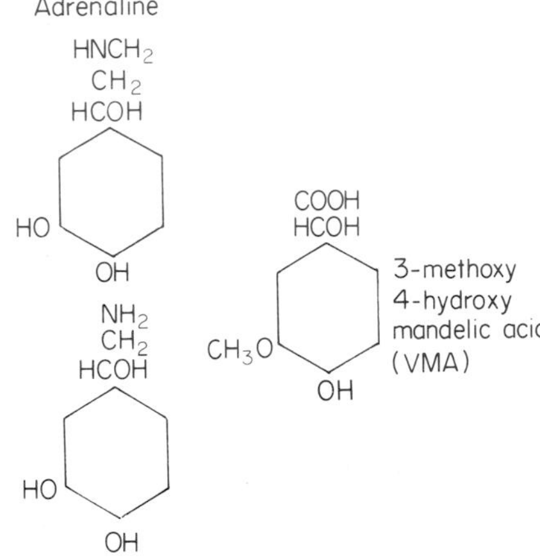

Fig. 11.2. Relationships between the structure of adrenaline, noradrenaline and their metabolic by-product, vanillyl-mandelic acid (VMA).

Diagnosis

The diagnosis of phaeochromocytoma demands a highly suspicious mind. To make the diagnosis, a 24 hour specimen of urine is collected and acidified with hydrochloric acid. This is then measured for adrenaline, noradrenaline and their metabolic product, VMA (Fig. 11.2). In doing this test the patient must avoid food containing vanilla (e.g. bananas, coffee etc.) for 24 hours. Since extra-adrenal tumours tend to make adrenaline rather than noradrenaline the quantity of each found in the urine may help to localize the tumour, but in practice one relies on radiological investigations. Formerly, angiography was the key to the localization of these tumours which are usually very vascular, but today CT scanning has largely replaced it.

Treatment

The treatment is to remove the tumour. To protect the patient from a sudden surge of hypertension the patient is prepared by phenoxybenzamine to block the alpha-receptors and propanolol to block the beta-receptors. Blood loss is kept to the very minimum and even though the patient is blocked, handling of the tumour is minimized until its main draining vein has been ligated. At this point the blood pressure may fall. How the tumour is approached depends on where it lies: tumours near the adrenal are easily reached through a 12th rib-bed incision, those near the organ of Zuckerkandl require a midline incision.

CONN'S TUMOUR

There may be single or multiple small, aldosterone-secreting tumours in one or both adrenals. Usually these are benign but as with any endocrine tumour, some prove to be malignant. Aldosterone secretion leads to sodium and water retention causing hypertension, and loss of potassium which causes weakness and even paralysis. Clinically the picture is one of hypertension associated with weakness, polyuria and thirst. The diagnosis is made by a low plasma [K], a high aldosterone, and a low level of renin. These findings are reversed by giving spironolactone.

Many cases can be satisfactorily managed with spironolactone, but it may cause unwanted side-effects — enlargement of the breasts, impotence, indigestion and constipation. In such cases, if the tumour can be localized with precision, it should be removed. At operation both tumours are exposed through 12th rib tip approaches with the patient prone. The dissection is controlled by frozen sections: if a single adenoma is found the entire adrenal on that side is removed. If both adrenals are involved the decision is more difficult, but probably it is better to remove both and give adrenal replacement therapy afterwards.

CUSHING'S SYNDROME

Here the cortex of the adrenal is secreting an excess of cortisol: the patient has the features of steroid overdosage — adiposity of the trunk and face, a buffalo hump of fat at the back of the neck, hirsutes, a red face, subcutaneous haemorrhages and cutaneous striae. There is often hypertension, steroid diabetes, and an osteoporosis which may lead to pathological fractures.

Pathologically there may be hyperplasia of one or both adrenals, or a single cortisol-secreting tumour. One difficulty in dealing with this condition is that although these tumours may arise out of the blue, they may occur as the result of ACTH produced by a basophil adenoma of the pituitary — or even by some other tumour such as a carcinoma of the bronchus.

The diagnosis is made by finding an increase in the various metabolites of cortisol — the *17-hydroxycorticosteroids* in the urine. If this is caused by ACTH stimulation, then giving ACTH intravenously will increase the plasma cortisol. If there is a primary adrenal cortical tumour, giving dexamethasone will lower the urinary level of 17-hydroxycorticosteroids.

If it seems that there is likely to be a primary adrenal cortical tumour, it is localized by means of CT scanning and angiography, and if localized, it is removed.

If it seems that there is hyperplasia of the adrenals, a careful search is made with CT for a pituitary tumour, and if none is found, the adrenals are explored. Exactly how much of each adrenal is removed is a matter for debate, but most surgeons will remove all of both glands, preferring to make up the deficiency with hormone replacement than risk a recurrence of the condition.

NEUROBLASTOMA

This is a tumour of toddlers. It grows to an enormous size and metastasizes early. It has to be distinguished from Wilms' tumour. Sometimes they secrete catecholamines and so elevated levels of VMA are found in the urine. In some cases there is spontaneous regression of the tumour.

NON-FUNCTIONAL ADRENAL CARCINOMA

These are usually large, presenting with weight loss and occasionally curious changes resulting from the secretion of steroids which give rise to gynaecomastia. By the time the diagnosis is made, they may have metastasized widely. If they are detected before they have spread, there is often some debate as to their malignancy, but in general it is felt that it is safer to remove them.

FURTHER READING

Ackery DM, Tippett PA, Condon BR, Sutton HE & Wyeth P (1984) New approach to the localisation of phaeochromocytoma: imaging with iodine-131-meta-iodobenzylguanidine. *British Medical Journal* **288**, 1587–91.

Donohue JP (1988) Diagnosis and management of adrenal tumors. In: Skinner DG & Liskovsky G (Eds) *Diagnosis and Management of Genitourinary Cancer.* WB Saunders, Philadelphia. pp. 372–404.

Ganguly A & Donohue JP (1983) Primary aldosteronism: pathophysiology, diagnosis and treatment. *Journal of Urology* **129**, 241–7.

Snell ME, Lawrence R, Sutton D, Sever PS & Peart WS (1983) Advances in the techniques of localisation of adrenal tumours and their influence on the surgical approach to the tumour. *British Journal of Urology* **55**, 617–21.

Swales JD (1983) Primary aldosteronism: how hard should we look? *British Medical Journal* **287**, 702–3.

12 Renal Failure

ACUTE RENAL FAILURE

Aetiology

There are many causes of acute renal failure (Fig. 12.1), and they fall into three main categories:

1 where there is underperfusion of the kidney;
2 where the renal tubules are poisoned;
3 where the tubules are blocked.

Sometimes there is an element of all three processes.

Poor renal perfusion

This is seen when there is excessive loss of blood or tissue fluid (as in major injury or burns, severe diarrhoea and vomiting), or in septicaemic shock, coronary thrombosis, or the period of anoxia suffered by the transplanted kidney between being removed from the donor and put into the recipient.

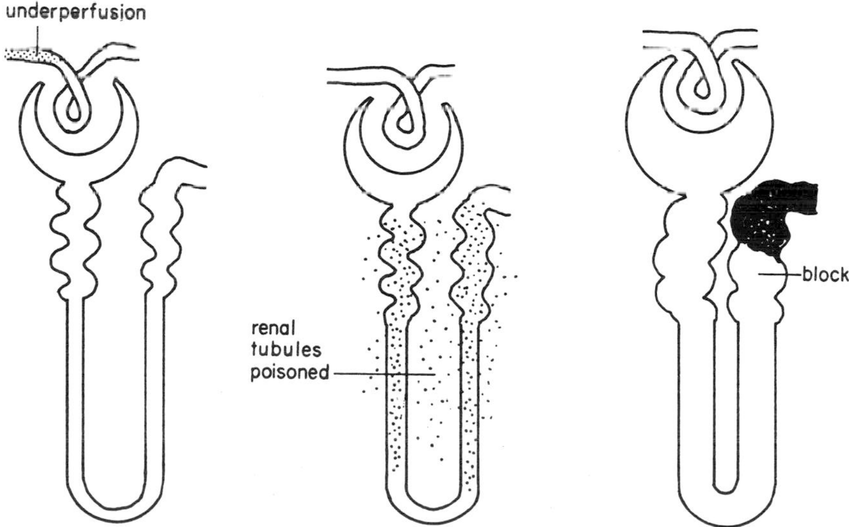

Fig. 12.1. The three main causes of renal failure: underperfusion, poisoning of the renal tubules and blockage of the renal tubules.

Renal tubular poisons

Many substances are known to poison the renal tubules, among them mercury, phenol, carbon tetrachloride, glycol and the toxin produced by *Clostridium welchii.*

Renal tubular blockage

The tubules may be blocked by myoglobin when there has been massive destruction of skeletal muscle (the crush syndrome), by porphyrins, bilirubin in severe jaundice, haemoglobin (following haemolysis in the TUR syndrome or mismatched transfusion), by sulphonamide crystals, and by uric acid in the tremendous catabolic response that follows successful treatment of tumours with chemotherapy.

Pathology

The gross appearances of the kidney vary from one case to another: usually it is large, oedematous and pale, the medulla is congested and the cortex pale (Fig. 12.2). The tubules are choked with debris from shed tubular cells giving the appearance of necrosis — hence the common term *acute tubular necrosis*, although the condition is often reversible. Some of the causes of poor renal perfusion can be prevented by prompt restoration of renal circulation combined with an alpha-blocker. If not reversed, blood is shunted from the cortex to the medulla via arterio-venous anastomoses leading to necrosis of the renal cortex from which there is no recovery — *cortical necrosis* (Fig. 12.3). After a little while calcification is seen at the inner and outer limits of the dead cortex — the so-called tramline calcification. When this is seen, the kidney is dead and will never recover.

Clinical features

In many patients the cause of the renal failure will be giving rise to its own particular symptoms, e.g. septic abortion, septicaemic shock or multiple injuries with loss of blood. But against this background one can distinguish three phases of renal failure: prodromal, anuria or oliguria, and recovery.

Prodromal phase

At first there is some glomerular filtration and so some urine continues to be formed but it is heavily clouded with debris and casts. This initial prodromal phase is useful in distinguish the later anuria of renal failure from that caused by accidental surgical obstruction to the ureters where the cessation of formation of urine is abrupt and total.

Anuria or oliguria

After the prodromal phase comes a variable stage when there may be either no urine at all, or a reasonable volume, but it is very dilute, and

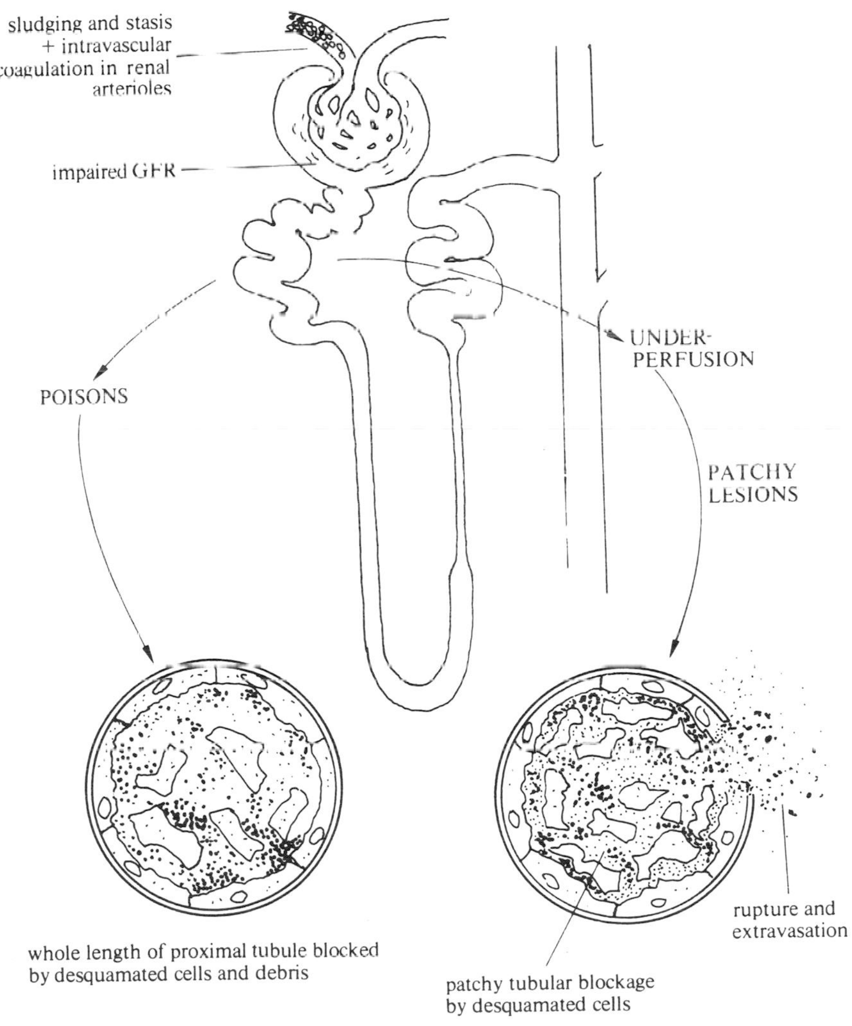

Fig. 12.2. Diagrammatic version of pathogenesis of acute renal failure.

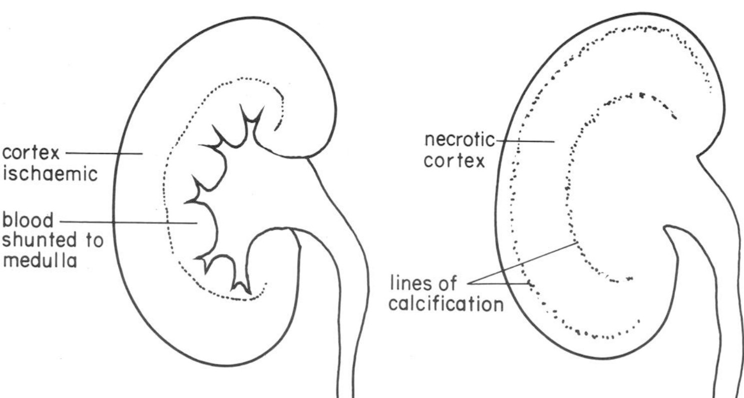

Fig. 12.3. Shunting of blood from cortex to medulla may be followed by ischaemic necrosis of the cortex with the appearance of parallel 'tramlines' of calcification. Renal failure is now irreversible.

there is insufficient glomerular filtration to excrete toxic wastes so the urea and creatinine rise, and the urine that is formed is unprocessed by the tubules, so it is isotonic and dilute. Urea, creatinine and other toxic waste products are not eliminated and increase day by day as protein continues to break down. The rate at which these waste products accumulate is accelerated in patients who have massive breakdown of tissue from sepsis or severe injury.

Recovery

Unless the renal cortex has become irreversibly ischaemic, there may be recovery. At first any urine that emerges is of low specific gravity and osmolarity, as if hardly processed in the tubules. Before long, a huge volume of this thin urine may be lost in the phase of obligatory diuresis. Many litres of fluid may have to be given — even intravenously, to keep the patient hydrated and replenished with sodium.

Management of acute renal failure

The aim of management is to keep the patient alive until the kidneys recover. This may take up to six weeks, during which time there is a continual breakdown of protein and accumulation of creatinine and potassium. During this phase there is a danger that giving too much water will lead to heart failure, and too much food which will add to the burden of protein catabolism. He can have only as much water as is lost each day in sweat and respiration plus what little urine is formed. About 1000 calories a day are given to minimize unnecessary catabolism of protein: there is no advantage in giving any more.

Some patients recover before the levels of creatinine or potassium have reached danger levels, but when they do it is necessary to remove them. Potassium liberated by cell breakdown is removed by giving glucose and insulin followed by ion-exchange resins. The other waste products are eliminated by dialysis (see below). The method of dialysis is chosen according to the cause of the renal failure: it may be necessary to use haemodialysis when there is intra-abdominal sepsis or when there is a very large amount of protein being broken down. In other cases it may be possible to use peritoneal dialysis.

CHRONIC RENAL FAILURE

In some patients the rate of deterioration of renal function is very slow — as in polycystic disease. In others the course is measured in weeks. When the rate of deterioration is very slow one may be able to keep the patient relatively well for a time by a diet low in protein: thus a patient with a creatinine clearance of 20 ml per minute can have his plasma creatinine halved by the modest restriction of protein input to 40 g per day. More severe dietary restriction of protein to 20 g per day can maintain a patient whose creatinine clearance is as little as 5 ml per minute.

Clinical features of chronic renal failure

In addition to the signs and symptoms of its cause, patients gradually develop *itching* and *pigmentation* of the skin.

Anaemia varies with the erythropoietin produced by the remaining renal tissue: it is seldom a feature of polycystic disease but can be very marked when the kidneys have shrunk in end-stage renal disease from other causes. It is worst of all when both kidneys have had to be removed prior to transplantation because they harbour infection or are causing uncontrollable hypertension. Fortunately a new remedy is now available in the form of synthetic erythropoietin.

Neuropathy is variable: loss of myelin from peripheral nerves results in weakness, loss of sensation and burning paraesthesiae especially in the feet.

Pericarditis occurs when a patient is being underdialysed and the creatinine has been allowed to rise too high.

Bone changes

There are two important changes in the metabolism of bone in renal failure: the bowel becomes less sensitive to the action of vitamin D, and there is secondary hyperparathyroidism (see p. 83). Because the bowel is less sensitive to vitamin D, less calcium is absorbed from it, and growing bone is imperfectly calcified — forming *osteoid* rather than true bone, and in adults this is seen around each trabecula in the bone which becomes weak and prone to fracture — *osteomalacia* (Fig. 12.4).

At the same time the accumulation of phosphate in renal failure lowers the plasma calcium, causing secondary hyperparathyroidism which leads to *osteoporosis*. Biopsy of the bones in renal failure show both these processes going on at the same time — the wide osteoid seams of osteomalacia covering the thinned out trabeculae of osteoporosis.

Because of the secondary hyperparathyroidism, calcium salts are added to the blood from the eroded bony trabeculae, and these are then deposited in soft tissues — *heterotopic calcification* — typically in the intervertebral discs where the alternate bands of decalcified bone and heterotopic calcification in the soft tissue give the characteristic *rugger-jersey spine* (Fig. 12.5). Of more importance, the heterotopic calcification stiffens the joints of the bones of the middle ear and causes deafness.

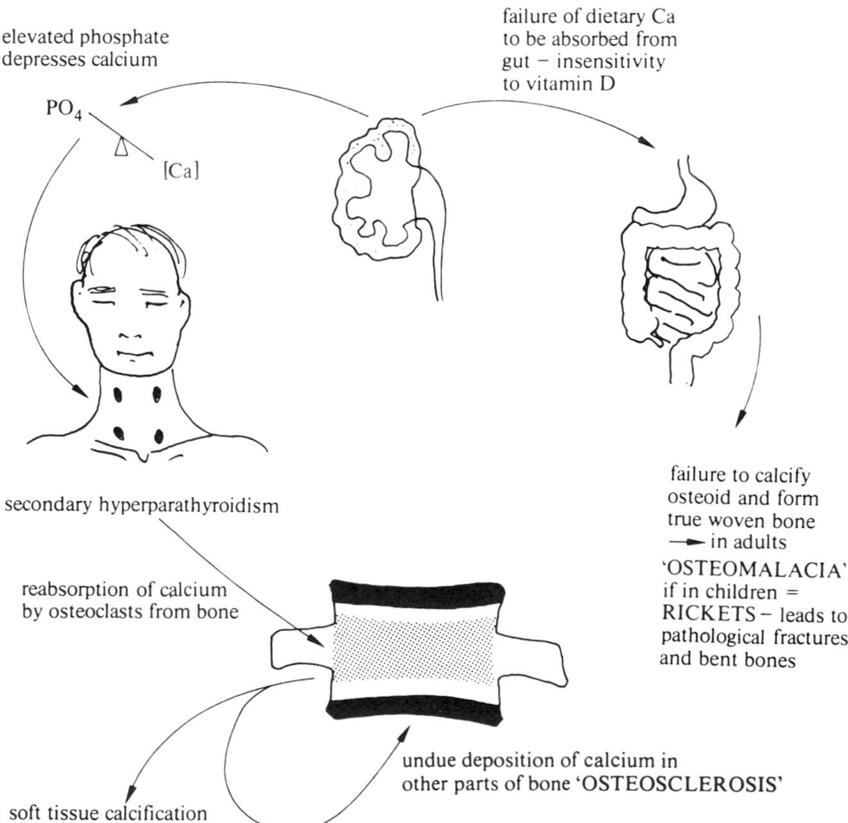

Fig. 12.4. Bone changes in renal failure.

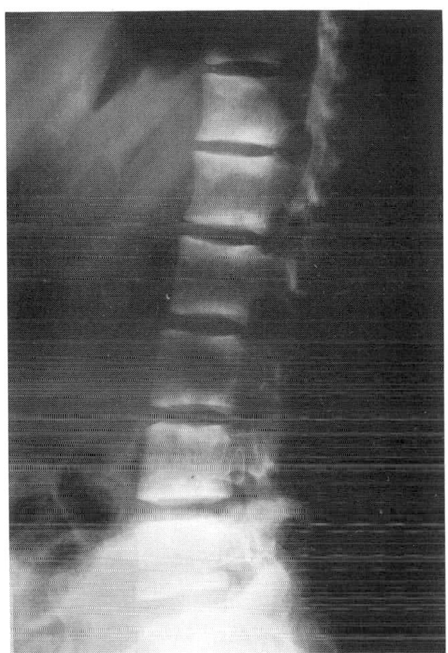

Fig. 12.5. Rugger jersey spine of secondary hyperparathyroidism.

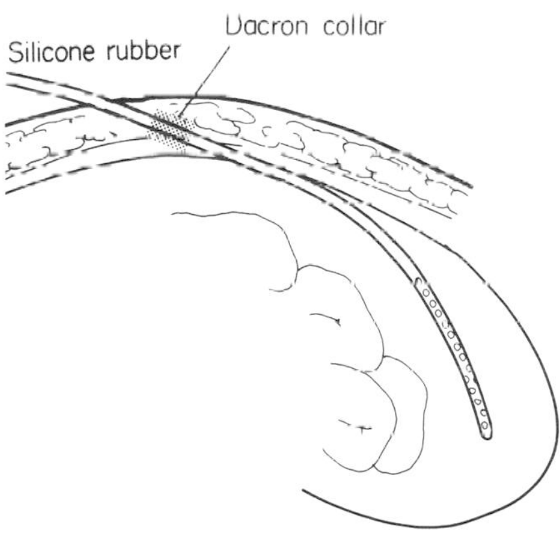

Fig. 12.6. Peritoneal dialysis by means of the Tenckhoff cannula.

Dialysis

Chronic Ambulant Peritoneal Dialysis (CAPD)

A silicone rubber catheter is inserted into the peritoneal cavity with its end, provided with multiple side-holes, lying in the pelvis (Fig. 12.6). Fluid is run into the peritoneal cavity and left there for several hours while the patient walks about and leads a relatively normal life. This allows creatinine and other products of catabolism to diffuse into the fluid. It is then allowed to run out, and is replaced. Patients soon learn to instill and remove the fluid themselves. The main complication of this system is, as one might expect, recurrent infection in the peritoneal cavity.

Haemodialysis

Blood from the patient flows over a thin membrane separating it from the dialysis fluid. Formerly the blood was pumped out of the patient through a long coil and back again. In recent years the pump has given way to methods which makes use of the patient's own blood pressure to do the work. There are many different systems in use: all make use of the same principle, unwanted products of catabolism diffuse into the dialysis fluid while protein and red cells are retained (Fig. 12.7).

The main difficulty with haemodialysis has been vascular access — how to get the blood out of the patient and back again. At first cannulae were tied into the radial artery and vein, but these quickly became blocked by thrombosis and inflammation and were unsuited to long-term use. Later they were replaced by inert silicone rubber cannulae which emerged through little holes in the skin — the *Scribner shunt* (Fig. 12.8).

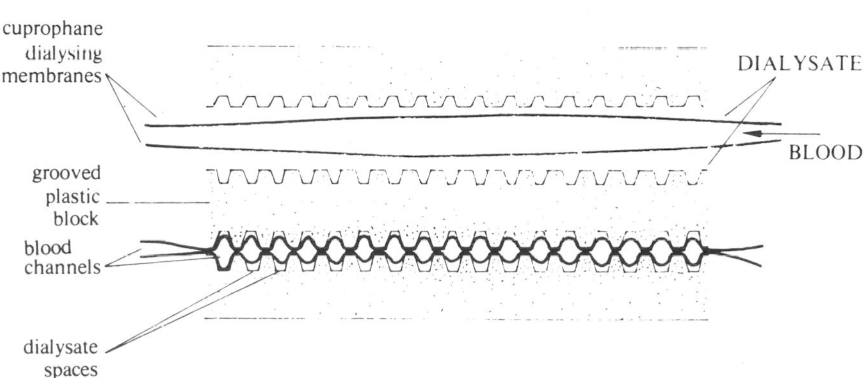

Fig. 12.7. Principle behind most 'artifical kidneys: blood circulates under its own blood pressure, or with the aid of a pump, over a thin membrane separating it from dialysate. Grooved plastic blocks form the channels in the Kiil design.

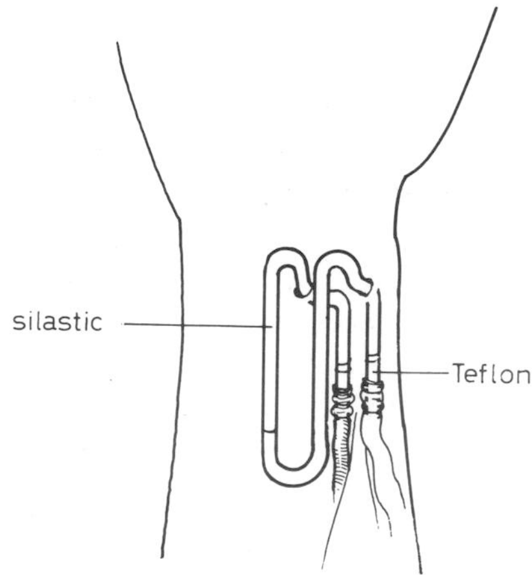

Fig. 12.8. Access to the blood stream may be obtained for short times using a Scribner shunt, where the cannulae are tied directly into (usually) the radial artery and cephalic vein.

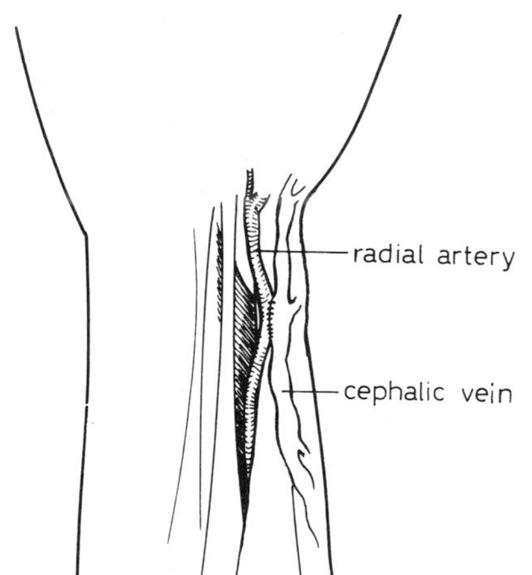

Fig. 12.9. Cimino fistula: the radial artery and the cephalic vein are anastomosed end-to-side or side-to-side.

These indwelling shunts are largely replaced by methods in which a large hypertrophied vessel is formed by anastomosing a peripheral artery to a vein, to form an artificial arteriovenous fistula — *Cimino fistula* (Fig. 12.9). The patient is taught to insert a large needle with two channels into the dilated vessel through which blood runs out, through the machine and then is returned to the vein. The trauma of the repeated needling may block these fistulae and every year more ingenious techniques are devised to provide suitable access for intermittent haemodialysis.

Renal transplantation

The operative steps of renal transplantation are now standard and successful. A kidney is obtained from a living related donor or a dead person. It is replaced in one or other iliac fossa. The renal artery is anastomosed either to the external or internal iliac artery and the renal vein to the external iliac vein. The ureter is anastomosed to the bladder through a long submucosal tunnel to prevent reflux (Fig. 12.10).

There are three major difficulties which continue to dominate the field: obtaining enough cadaver kidneys; rejection; and preservation of the donor organ.

Obtaining cadaver kidneys

It is always a tragedy when a pair of kidneys that could have saved two lives by transplantation, are left to decay in a dead patient. Very few relatives refuse to give permission for kidneys to be removed, and then as a rule only for some religious reason. The shortage of cadaver donors does not stem from the refusal of relatives to give their permission, but from failure on the part of doctors and nurses to ask for it.

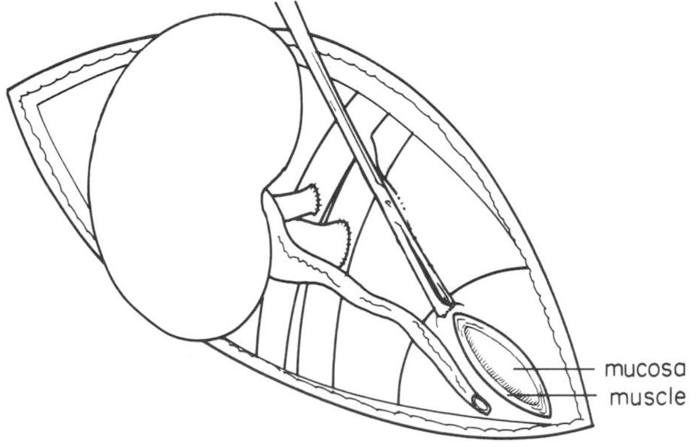

Fig. 12.10. Transplantation of the left kidney from the donor to the right iliac fossa: the recipient artery is anastomosed to the right external iliac artery, the vein to the external iliac vein and the ureter is about to be anastomosed through the submucosal tunnel to the bladder.

The donor

Suitable donors are those without cancer (except for a primary brain tumour), and without major sepsis. They should have extensive, irrecoverable brain damage (e.g. from severe head injury, intracranial haemorrhage or cardiac arrest or respiratory arrest that has led to anoxic brain damage). Such patients will be maintained on a ventilator, and it must have been established that they have suffered irreversible brain damage, for which strict guidelines have been laid down.

Many of these patients will have not only kidneys that can be used, but also other organs such as the heart, lungs, liver and corneae, and the opportunity should never be lost to consider the possibility of using more than one organ.

Rejection

When an unrelated transplant (*allograft*) is performed for the first time there is a latent period in which the anastomoses heal, the kidney perfuses and makes urine. After 10 to 14 days lymphocytes in the regional lymph nodes enlarge, divide, develop pyronin-staining deposits in their cytoplasm and start to swarm towards the graft. At the same time other lymphocytes are stimulated to produce immunoglobulins which are laid down on the intima of the vessels of the graft, which fix complement, attract platelets and soon set up thrombosis which blocks the vessels and leads to infarction of the kidney. This is the *first-set* reaction.

Another graft from the same donor put into the same recipient suffers the same process but much more quickly and with a much more severe inflammatory reaction: this is the *second-set* reaction: it signifies that the patient has become sensitized to antigens on the first graft. A graft from a different donor is handled in the sluggish manner of the first-set, i.e. the antigens that set up rejection are specific to each donor.

Grafts from *identical twins* provoke no transplant rejection, nor is there any rejection when tissue is taken from one part of the body to another in the same person. The most important of the antigens responsible for rejection are found on the surface of most cells in the body, and appear to be made by a group of genes in the 6th pair of human chromosomes — the *Major Histocompatibility System (MHS)* (Fig. 12.11).

The first of these antigens was discovered by the Nobel laureate Dausset as recently as 1958: since then many others have been discovered. Some are detected because they give rise to serum antibodies which fix complement (*Serum Detected — SD.*) Others can be detected

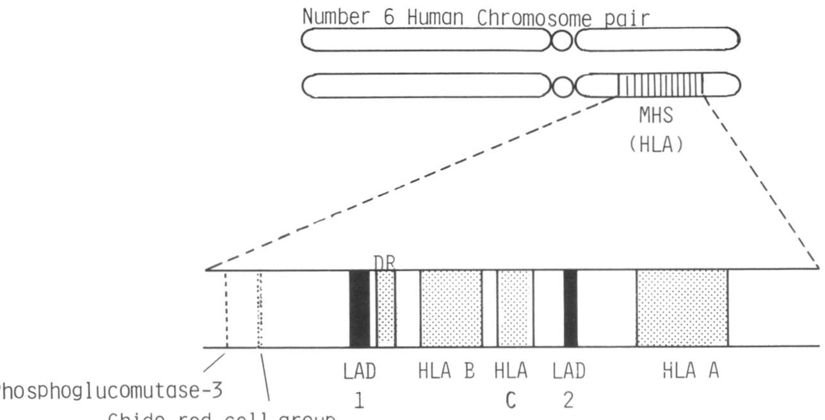

Fig. 12.11. Map of the Number 6 human chromosome pair showing the Major Histocompatibility System and where some of the genes are situated. (Modified from Festenstein & Démant 1979.)

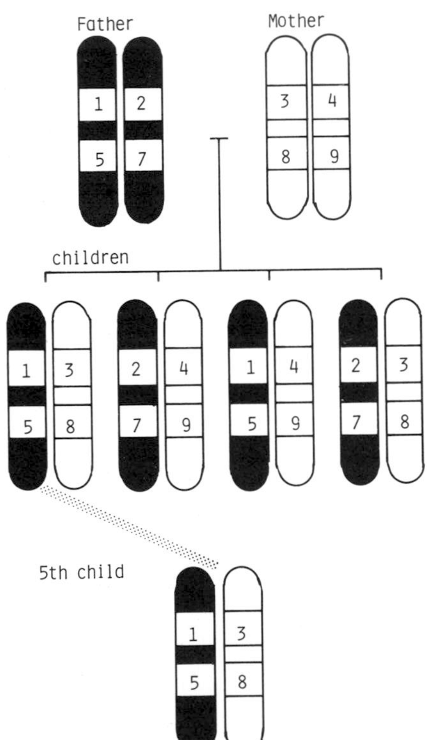

Fig. 12.12. Pattern of inheritance of the MHS. A fifth child must be HLA-identical with at least one of the other four siblings.

only in mixed lymphocyte culture when host lymphocytes recognize foreign lymphocytes, swell up and undergo division — (*Lymphocyte Activating Determinants — LAD*).

Some of these LADs provoke activity only in the lymphocytes that are derived from the thymus (*T-cells*) and others only in those derived from the bursa of Fabricius (*B-cells.*)

SDs can be detected within an hour or two by serological tests but the LADs may take two or three days of mixed lymphocyte culture, and can only be tested for in retrospect, or in proposed living donor transplants. Both the LADs and the SDs are sought on human lymphocytes, and are grouped together as *Human Lymphocyte Antigens* (HLA).

Rejection in response to incompatibility of these transplant antigens can be overcome by drugs which paralyse the various components of the immune system. Of these there are three which are in daily use: steroids, azathioprine, and cyclosporin A. In addition, various kinds of antisera directed against lymphocytes have been developed from time to time, but none are in routine use and all have appreciable side-effects. In most transplant units a combination of steroids and cyclosporin A is used, with azathioprine kept in reserve. With these combinations even complete incompatibility at the MHS can be overcome. They are all toxic. Azathioprine tends to suppress bone marrow and cyclosporin A is nephrotoxic and may cause epileptic fits.

The human MHS and the HLA system. Because of the way chromosome pairs are split up at meiosis and transmitted by haploid gametes from parents to children, each child must receive half its genetic programming from one parent and half from the other (Fig. 12.12). In any family with more than five children one pair of children must always be identical with respect to their MHS, and when these children exchange kidneys there should be virtually no rejection. In fact this is not the whole story: other less important antigens exist, and some immunosuppression is always needed except where children are truly identical twins. In cadaver kidneys, and kidneys from unrelated living donors, even if the HLA antigens are matched, these other factors are likely to be more important. Even with modern methods of immunosuppression, getting the SDs correctly matched can double the survival of transplants at 2 years.

For this reason most transplant units cooperate in schemes which enable kidneys to be moved around from one centre to another in order to ensure that the maximum number of HLAs are identical.

Living related donors. It follows from the inheritance of the HLA antigens that in very large families there will always be pairs of brothers and sisters who have identical MHSs, and a parent will always have at least one half of the MHS in common with a child. Because of this, rejection is less marked in living-related transplants and usually easier to treat. The donor kidney can be carefully investigated and proven to be healthy before it is taken out, and there is never any delay in sewing it into the recipient. For all these reasons transplants from living related donors do extremely well.

Rejection episodes. A recipient may unwittingly be sensitized to the donor antigens so that when the clamps are removed and blood enters the kidney there is an immediate second set reaction: within minutes the kidney becomes swollen and congested and thrombosis quickly follows, leading to infarction of the organ. Sometimes this is caused by pre-existing cytotoxic antibodies and so before any transplant, a cross-match is performed to test for these.

At any time afterwards there may be episodes of rejection: the kidney becomes swollen and the surrounding tissues tender: its function deteriorates as shown by a falling creatinine clearance and a reduced blood-flow in the DTPA scan. Fine-needle aspiration cytology from the graft may show that T- and B-lymphocytes have invaded it. Prompt action with high doses of Imuran, steroids and cyclosporin A usually reverses the episode, but when one episode succeeds another the kidney ends up by being completely infarcted and it must then be removed. The patient is returned to dialysis, and awaits another transplant.

The long-term results of renal transplantation

Over the last 20 years there has been a steady improvement in the results of transplantation: today one expects that > 80% of cadaver kidneys will be functioning at the end of a year, figures little different from those found in living related donors.

FURTHER READING

Flangian WJ, Gaston RS & Goeken NE. (1987) Clinical transplantation. In: Gonick HC (Ed) *Current Nephrology* (10). Year Book Medical Publication Inc., Chicago. pp. 377–418.

Morris PJ (1983) *Kidney Transplantation, Principles and Practice.* 2nd Ed. Grune & Stratton, London.

Nortman DF & Franklin SS (1984) Therapy and management of acute renal failure. In: Suki WN & Massry SG (Eds) *Therapy of Renal Diseases and Related Disorders.* Martinus Nijhoff Publishing, Dordrecht. pp. 47–62.

van Stone JC & Nolph KD (1987) Dialysis. In: Gonick HC (Ed) *Current Nephrology* (10). Year Book Medical Publishing Inc., Chicago. pp. 325–76.

13 The Renal Pelvis and Ureter

ANATOMY

The anatomical relations of the renal pelvis were described earlier (p. 30). The ureter descends on each side anterior to the psoas muscle. the iliohypogastric and ilioinguinal nerves, and behind the artery and vein of the testis or ovary. Each ureter is crossed anteriorly by a stout branch from the internal iliac artery which supplies the bladder and (in the female) the uterus — the superior vesical pedicle. This is continued up into the so-called obliterated umbilical artery. In males the ureter is crossed, just before it enters the bladder, by the vas deferens. The ureter then tunnels obliquely through the muscle of the wall of the bladder to open on the trigone (Fig. 13.1).

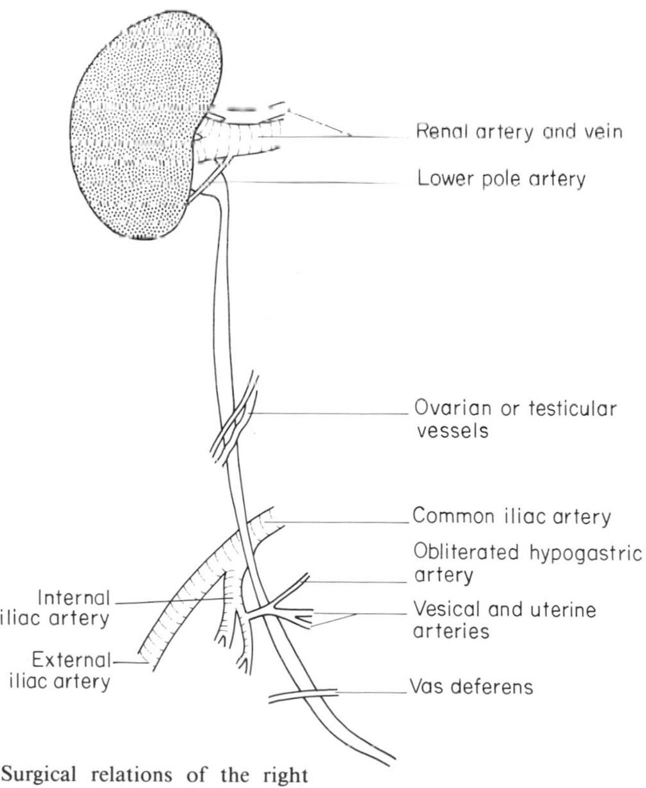

Fig. 13.1. Surgical relations of the right ureter.

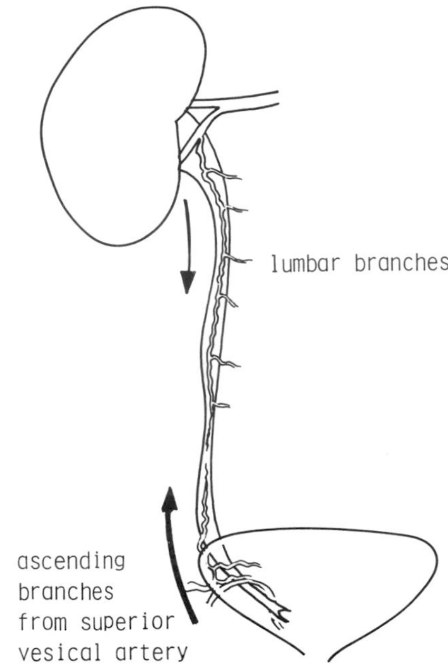

Fig. 13.3. The blood supply of the ureter.

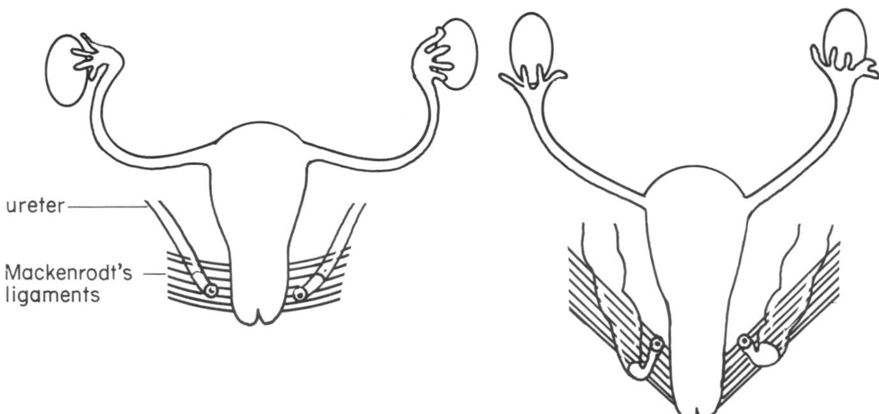

Fig. 13.2. The ureter runs through the suspensory ligament of the cervix. In prolapse, the ureters may be pulled down, kinked and obstructed.

In women the ureter has an important surgical relationship with the *cardinal ligament* of Mackenrodt — a tough band of fibrous tissue which holds up the cervix (Fig. 13.2). The ureter passes through the middle of this ligament and if the uterus descends, it can drag the ureter down with it. The ureter lies just above the lateral fornix of the vagina and is easily damaged in the course of operations on the uterus.

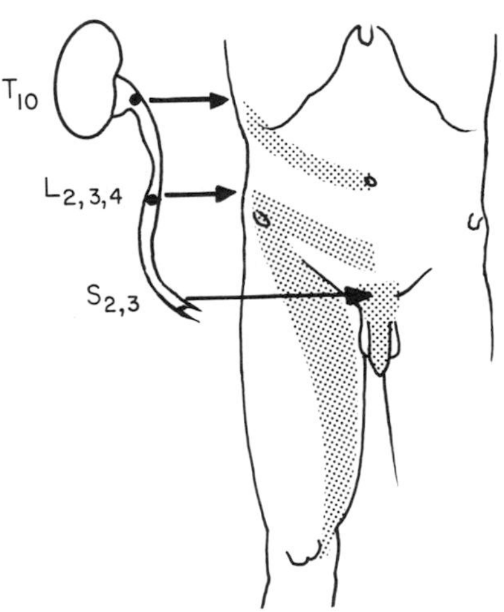

Fig. 13.4. Pain referred from a stone in the ureter is felt at different levels according to the affected dermatome.

Blood supply of the ureter

The renal pelvis has a profuse blood supply which makes it possible to construct flaps of almost any shape for the purposes of pyeloplasty. The ureter receives its main blood supply from the inferior segmental artery of the kidney (Fig. 13.3). This is reinforced at intervals by branches from the lumbar arteries, but its next important blood supply comes upwards from the superior vesical artery near the bladder. If the ureter is divided near the bladder this branch is cut, hence the poor results of attempts to anastomose the ureter near the bladder.

Nerve supply

The nerves of the ureter follow a segmental pattern: in its upper part like the kidney it is supplied by T10, hence pain is referred to the umbilicus (Fig. 13.4). Lower down pain is felt at progressively lower levels until irritation of the lowest part of the ureter may give pain referred to the tip of the penis or vulva (S3).

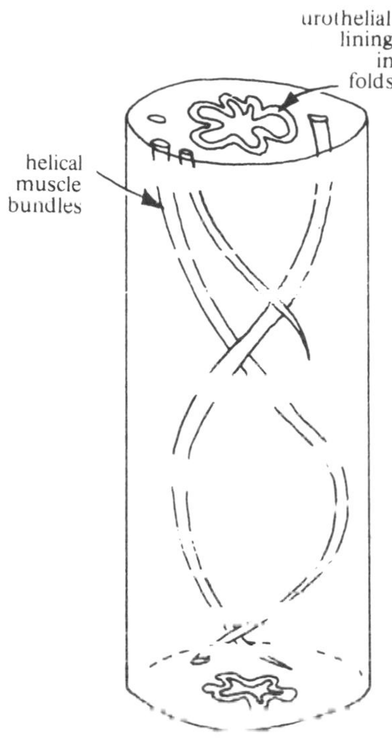

Fig. 13.5. Structure of the ureter.

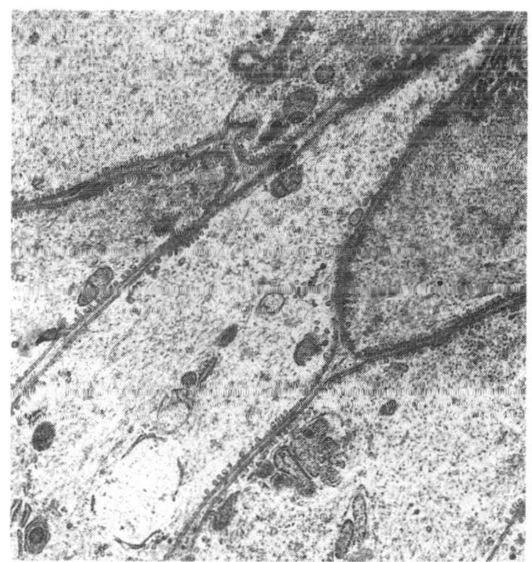

Fig. 13.6. Electron micrograph of the junction between ureteric muscle cells (×10 000). The jig-saw interdigitations are the *nexuses* which convey excitation from one cell to another without the need for any nerve supply. (Courtesy of Mr R. G. Notley.)

PHYSIOLOGY OF THE URETER

Peristalsis

The muscle of the ureter is formed of long helices, one intertwined with another, the whole tube being lined with urothelium on a thin layer of submucosa (Fig. 13.5). Each muscle bundle is composed of hundreds of smaller smooth muscle cells with jig-saw connections between them (*nexuses*) visible only on electron microscopy (Fig. 13.6). These allow electrical excitation to pass from one muscle cell to the next without the need for nerves or ganglia. The result is a slow writhing peristaltic motion of the ureter which is set off by distension or irritation (e.g. pinching with a forceps). A pacemaker which sets the tempo of this peristalsis lies in the renal pelvis (Fig. 13.7). Because nerves are not needed for this peristaltic activity the denervated transplanted ureter functions perfectly well.

Ureteric peristalsis normally adjusts to the rate of urine flow, going faster and faster until a point is reached when the ureter remains open like a drainpipe, and its walls no longer close to form compartments, and peristalsis becomes less efficient. The ureter has to be able to wriggle. When it is inflamed, surrounded by fibrous tissue or involved by the fibrosis of schistosomiasis it becomes stiff and inert, and even though it is not closed, there is a functional obstruction.

Investigation of ureteric function

Sometimes it is difficult to know if a dilated wide ureter seen in a radiograph is obstructed or widened for some other reason. A cannula is passed percutaneously over a guide-wire into the renal pelvis and contrast medium is run in at a constant rate while the pressure in the system is recorded. The rate is chosen to be the maximum likely to be seen in a diuresis, e.g. 10 ml/minute. If the pressure rises there must be obstruction downstream in the ureter: this is *Whitaker's test* (Fig. 13.8).

Congenital anomalies of the ureter

The embryology of the ureter (see p. 43) is the clue to its congenital anomalies. The ureter buds out from the Wolffian mesonephric duct towards the metanephros, but becomes angulated as the Wolffian duct is carried down in the urogenital septum. As the lower part of the Wolffian duct is absorbed into the trigone the ureter comes to enter upstream of the ejaculatory duct. When the ureteric bud branches early to form a duplex system, the ureter from the upper half-kidney enters the trigone caudal to that from the lower half-kidney (the Weigert-Meyer law).

Ectopic ureter

In girls, if the angle of the Wolffian duct is particularly long and acute, the ureteric bud may open caudal to the external sphincter (Fig. 13.9) and the ectopic ureter is found just to one side of the external urinary meatus. The anomaly often occurs together with a duplex ureter. The child may complain of incontinence but curiously this is seldom noticed until adolescence. The diagnosis ought to be easy, but the upper half-kidney is often very small, and the ectopic ureter so small as to be easily overlooked. The cure is easy: the upper half-kidney is removed.

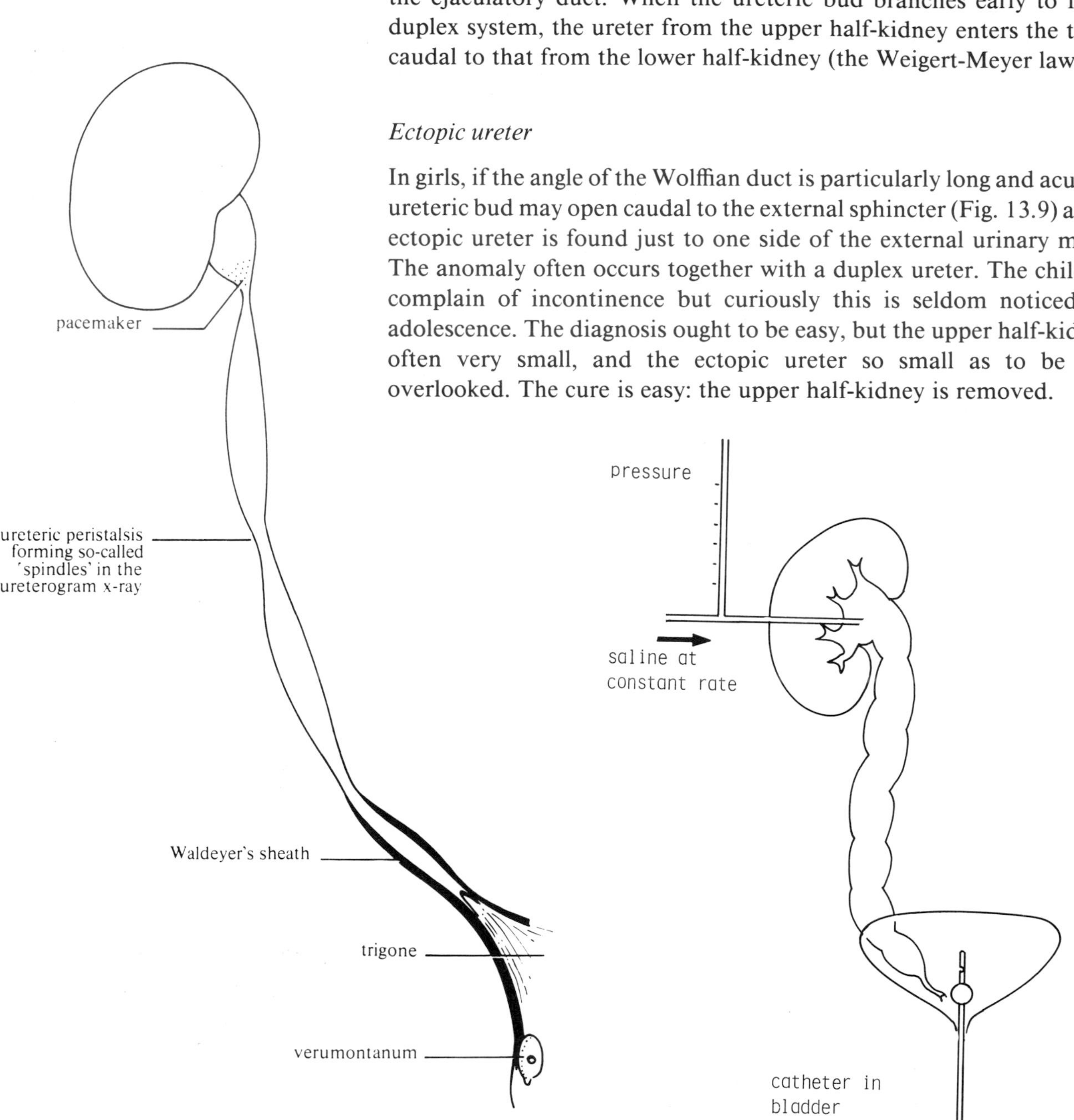

Fig. 13.7. Ureteric peristalsis probably originates in pacemakers in the calix or the renal pelvis.

Fig. 13.8. Whitaker's test: to determine whether a wide ureter is obstructed or merely floppy, fluid is run into it at a constant rate and the pressure measured.

Ureterocele

Sometimes the medial part of the Wolffian duct is not completely absorbed into the trigone and remains as a thick balloon-like covering for the ureter (Fig.13.10). This may obstruct the ureter, bulge into the bladder, or even become prolapsed through the urethra to appear at the external meatus as a bizarre cystic swelling. Sometimes a stone forms inside the stagnant urine in a ureterocele. Ureteroceles are usually treated at first by incision, but this may lead to reflux up the ureter which may then have to be reimplanted.

Reflux

This has been considered on p. 66 as one of the main causes of obstructive uropathy and scarring in the kidney. Some children are born

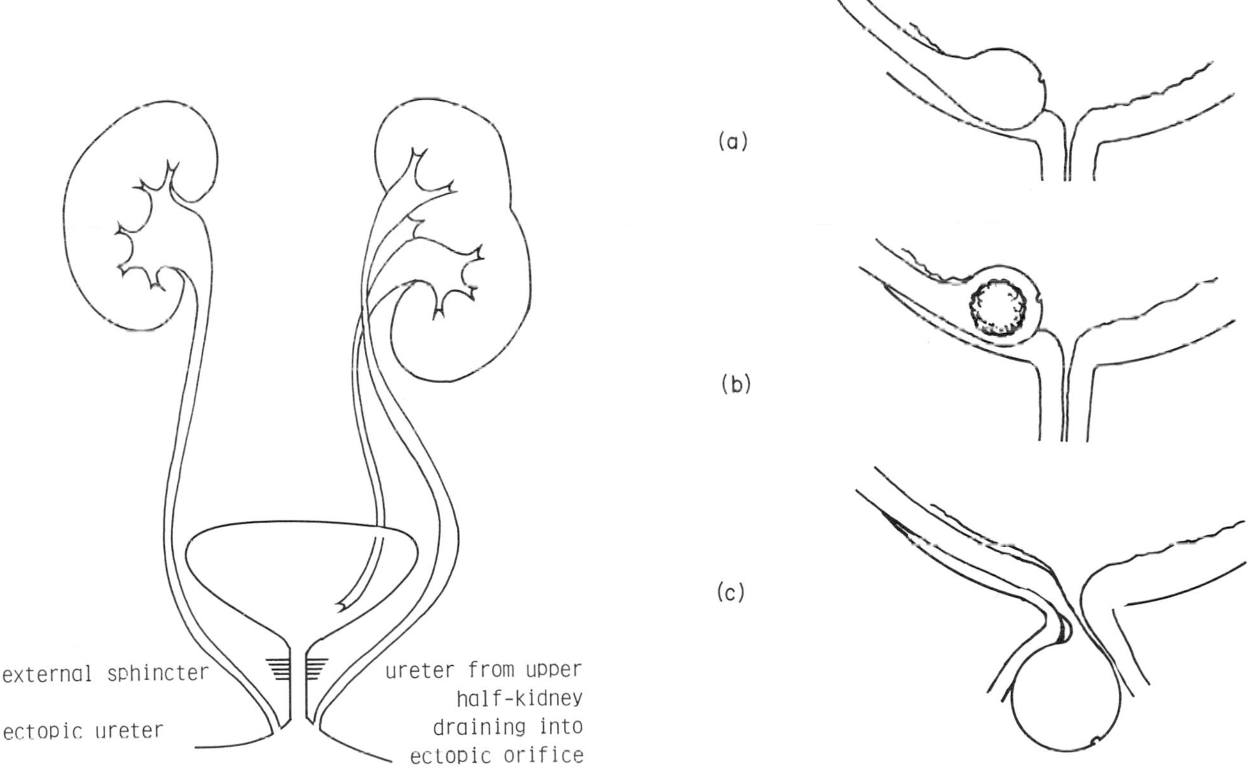

Fig. 13.9. The ectopic ureteric orifice that opens downstream of the external sphincter may give rise to persistent leak of urine.

Fig. 13.10. Most ureteroceles (a) cause no trouble at all. A stone may form in a ureterocele (b). A ureterocele may prolapse through the urethra in a female (c) and cause acute retention of urine.

with a very short intramural ureter, as if there had been too much absorption of the lower part of the Wolffian duct. These ureters are often rather wide apart and appear unusually large. The diagnosis is made by a micturating cystogram (p. 156) which may show intra-renal reflux. Three grades of reflux are recognized: Grade 1 where the lower ureter is filled; Grade 2 where the contrast reaches the kidney; Grade 3 where it fills the renal pelvis and probably enters the parenchyma as well (Fig. 13.11). Grades 1 and 2 can be expected to resolve spontaneously so long as infection can be controlled with antibiotics. In Grade 3, and in cases where the infection cannot be controlled, something must be done to stop the reflux.

Ureteroneocystostomy

There are many methods for reimplanting the ureter: all rely on the construction of a new long submucosal tunnel for the ureter (Fig. 13.12). A recent alternative is to inject a little Teflon or collagen paste just at the ureteric orifice by means of a child's cystoscope: this raises a little mound and is said to prevent reflux (Fig. 13.13).

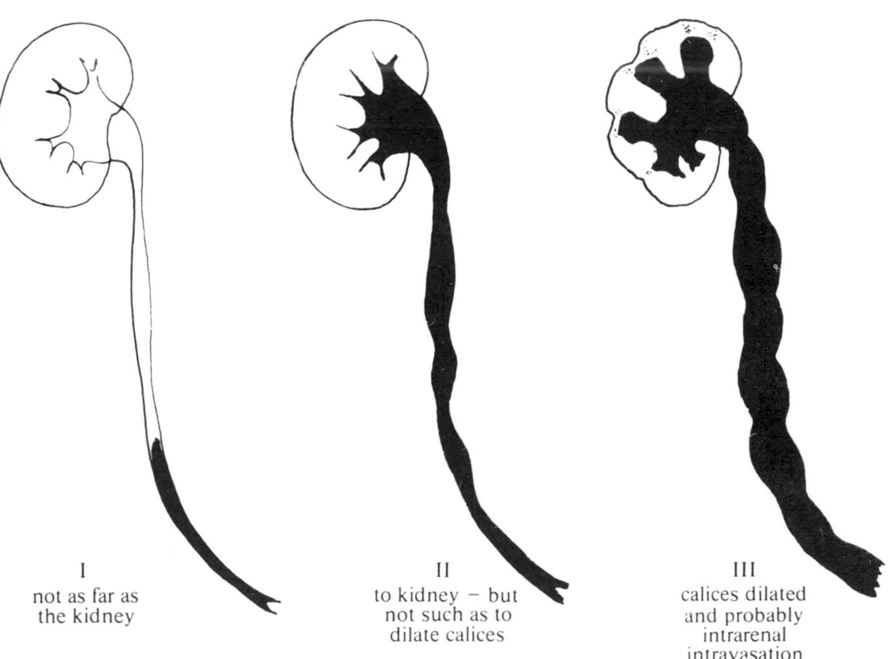

Fig. 13.11. Grades of reflux.

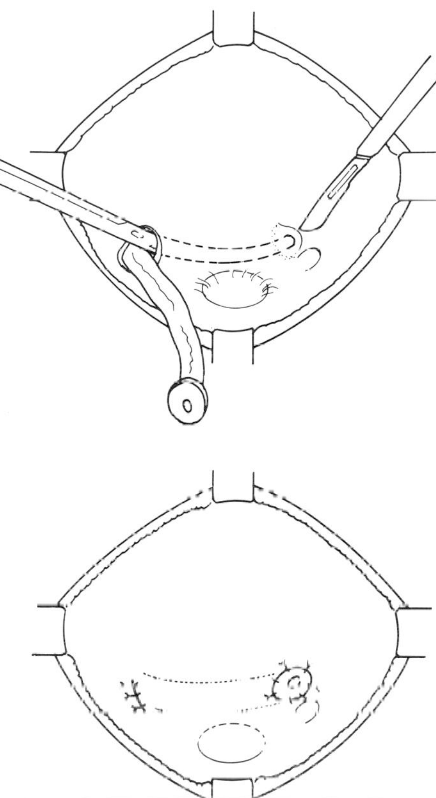

Fig. 13.12. Reimplantation of the ureter for reflux using Cohen's method.

Simple duplex kidney

Duplex kidneys and ureters are quite common and by themselves are of no account. Occasionally a patient is seen with severe intermittent pain, related to an unusual disturbance of flow in the ureters — the yo-yo reflux — where the more powerful pelvis of the lower half-kidney forces urine up the Y-junction into the smaller pelvis of the upper half causing dilatation and pain (Fig. 13.14). The condition, which is not common, can easily be diagnosed with a ureterogram and corrected by opening both upper stems of the Y and making them into one channel.

Blind ending duplex. Rarely, one of the buds fails to induce development of its part of the metanephros resulting in a ureteric 'diverticulum' (Fig. 13.15). Tiny versions of this are common near the very lowest end of the ureter. None of them need any treatment unless they can definitely be proved to be the cause of symptoms.

Ureteric atresia

Atresia of the ureter occurs in association with congenital dysplasia of the kidney (see p. 48).

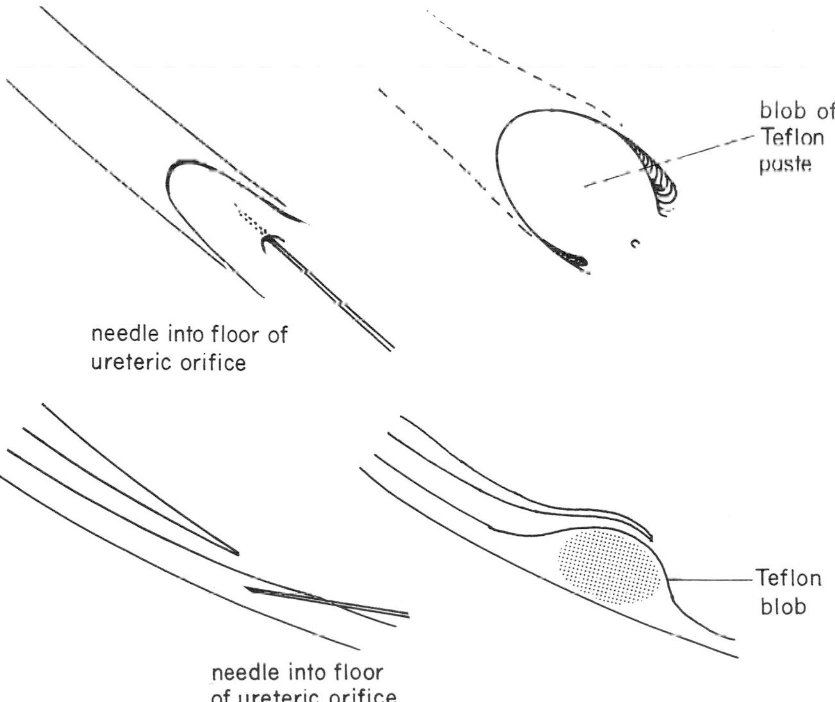

Fig. 13.13. Reflux may be prevented by injecting a small blob of Teflon or collagen paste beneath the ureteric orifice.

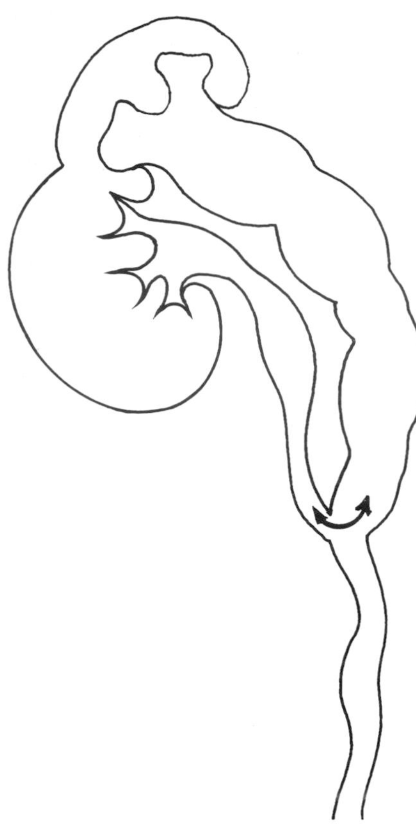

Fig. 13.14. Yo-yo reflux; urine from the more powerful lower half-kidney may be squirted up to the upper half-kidney to cause distension and pain.

Congenital wide ureter: megaureter

Some ureters are wide because they are obstructed and others are wide because they are floppy and inert thanks to a congenital defect in their muscle. Obstructed megaureter is seen when there is a congenital narrowing at the lower end of the ureter just before it enters the bladder (Fig. 13.16). The cause is not known. Once it has been proved that this is an obstructed ureter (e.g. with Whitaker's test) it is reimplanted after excising the narrow segment.

Another type of very wide ureter occurs with *vesicoureteric reflux* (see p. 45).

A common cause of dilated ureters is seen when there are *congenital urethral valves* (see p. 247). These give rise to outflow obstruction and a grossly dilated bladder. A bizarre exaggeration of this gives rise to the curious condition called the *prune-belly syndrome*: here the valves have given rise to such severe and persistent distension of the bladder in the fetus that the muscle of the wall of the abdomen fails to develop. These little boys have a thin wrinkled abdomen, bilateral undescended testes, grossly dilated ureters and bladder, and (usually) the remnants of congenital urethral valves — though these are sometimes missed.

Pelviureteric junction obstruction

In this common condition there is a ring of fibrous tissue just where the renal pelvis joins the ureter. Its cause is unknown. It may be detected by ultrasound scanning *in utero*, or it may not appear until adult life. The result is that the renal pelvis becomes grossly dilated (Fig. 13.17).

At first the obstruction may be intermittent, and patients only have pain when they drink a lot. Later the pressure continues to remain high in the renal pelvis and the parenchyma begins to atrophy. Symptoms are usually of pain, but infection or stone formation may complicate the picture.

Often the dilated renal pelvis bulges forwards above the lower pole renal vessels, giving the impression that these 'anomalous' vessels are causing the obstruction (Fig. 13.18). The vessels are not anomalous and they are not causing the obstruction.

Diagnosis. Sometimes an IVP may show what seems to be a large baggy pelvis but there are no obvious signs of obstruction. To show whether these are obstructed or not a renogram is performed with a diuresis produced by an injection of frusemide. In real obstruction, the isotope continues to accumulate in the renal pelvis: in those which are merely

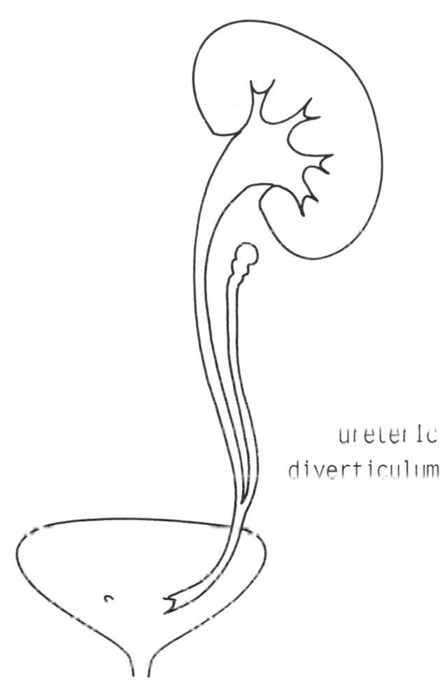

Fig. 13.15. Ureteric diverticulum.

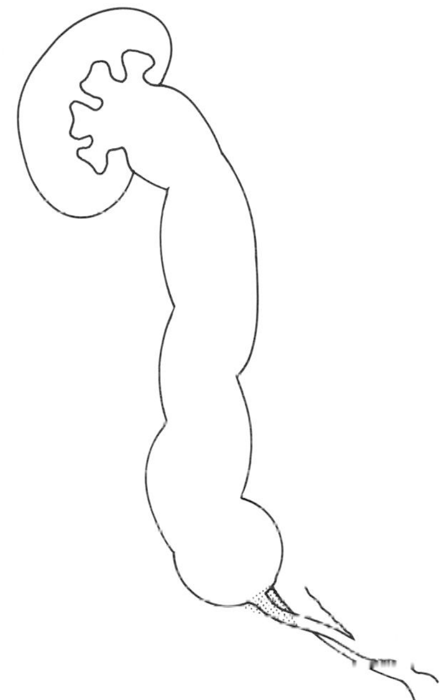

Fig. 13.16. Obstructed megaureter. There is a fibrous band surrounding the lower end of the ureter.

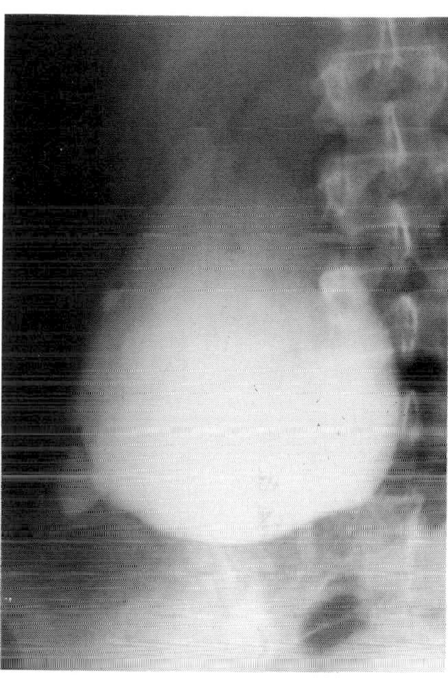

Fig. 13.17. Giant hydronephrosis caused by obstruction at the pelviureteric junction.

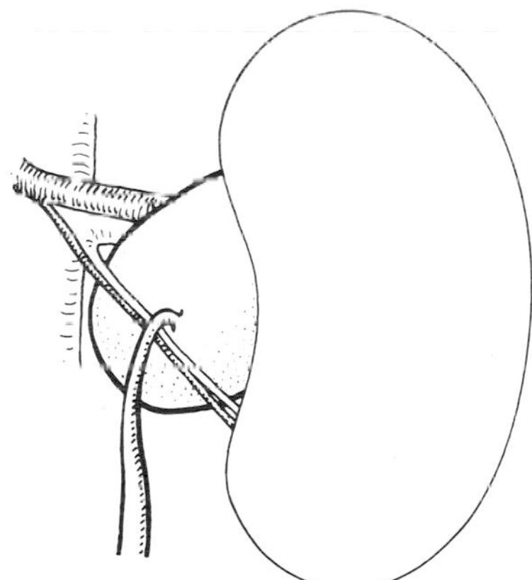

Seen from behind the lower polar vessels appear to be causing the PUJ obstruction

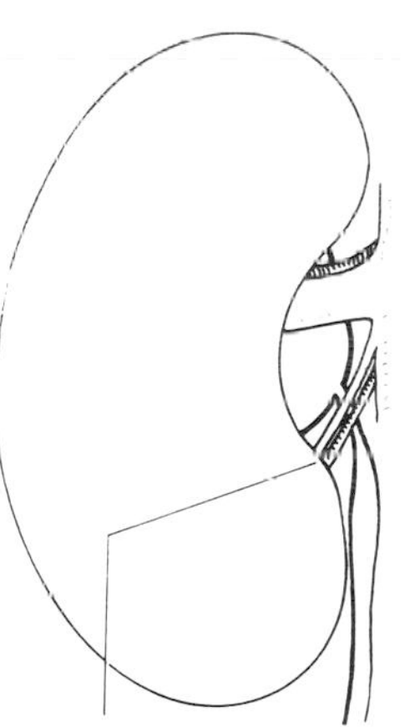

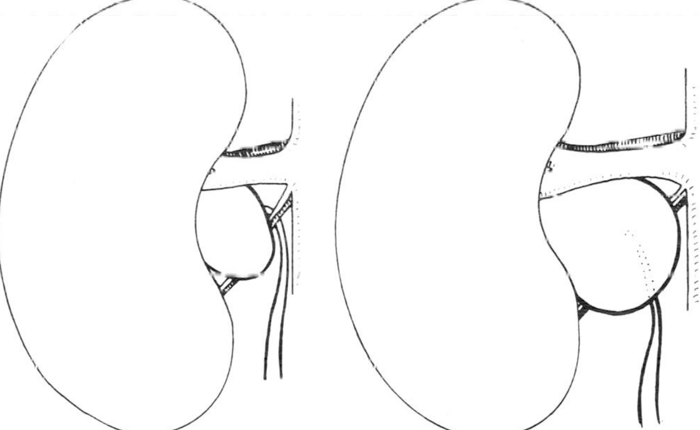

Fig. 13.18. Idiopathic hydronephrosis. Beginning with a stiff ring of fibrous tissue at the pelviureteric junction, the obstructed pelvis balloons out over the lower pole segmental artery.

Anterior view. With increasing enlargement the pelvis bulges forward over the lower pole segmental vessels

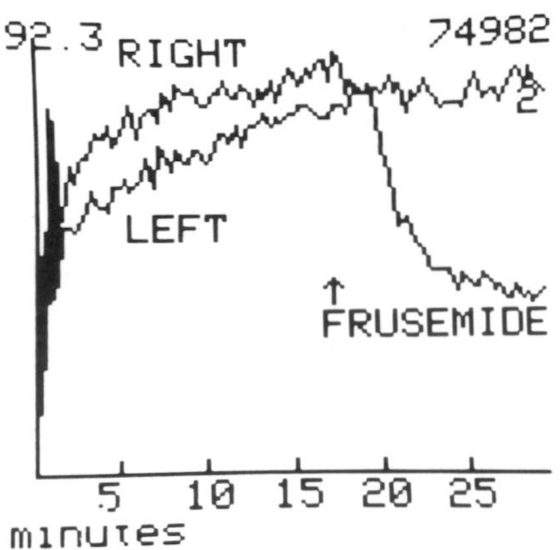

Fig. 13.19. Renogram with frusemide. On the right side the isotope is quickly washed out of the kidney; on the left it continues to accumulate, signifying obstruction.

rather large baggy (but otherwise normal) pelves, the isotope is washed away in the diuresis (Fig. 13.19).

Sometimes it is doubtful whether it is worth trying to save the kidney when it is very distended. A DTPA scan is performed (p. 38) to measure how much useful renal tissue remains.

Pyeloplasty. A preliminary ureterogram (p. 21) is performed before proceeding to pyeloplasty to make sure that the rest of the ureter is normal. The kidney is approached, usually through an anterior transverse incision. The junction of the ureter and renal pelvis is separated from the lower pole vessels (if these happen to be nearby) and a U-shaped flap is constructed from the surplus renal pelvis, and let into the slit-up end of the ureter as a long gusset. If there is a longer thin segment to the upper end of the ureter the gusset is made a little longer by borrowing from more of the renal pelvis (Fig. 13.20). The anastomosis is protected by a suitable splint (e.g. Cummings tube) which is left in position for about 10 days and then clamped. If there is no discomfort or fever the tube is removed.

Retrocaval ureter

A very rare congenital anomaly is caused by persistence of the postcardinal veins of the embryo: instead of running in front of the inferior vena cava, the ureter winds round behind it (Fig. 13.21). The urogram is

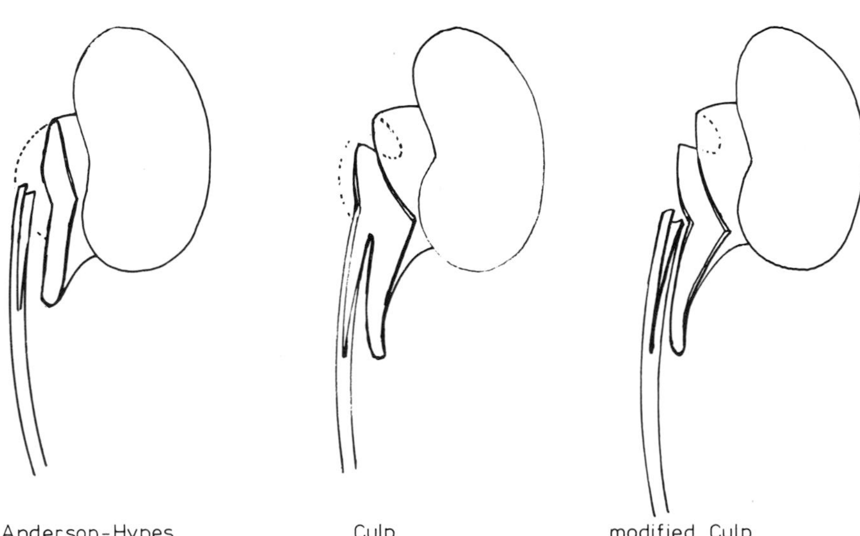

Fig. 13.20. The three standard pyeloplasty methods all have in common the insertion of a long, dependant, ∩-shaped flap into the spatulated, upper end of the ureter.

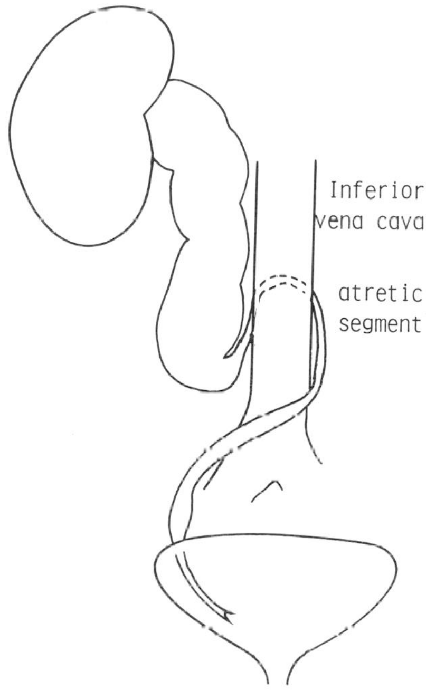

Fig. 13.21. Retrocaval ureter.

characteristic. The part of the ureter behind the vena cava is useless, and need not be touched. The lower end of the ureter is joined to the upper baggy part with a long oblique anastomosis.

URETERIC INJURY

Closed injuries of the ureter are very rare unless the kidney is injured too (see p. 54). Penetrating injuries with a knife or low-velocity gun-shot injury are easily overlooked at the time the wound is explored, and may only be noticed when there is a leak of urine from the wound. If noticed at the time the ureter can be anastomosed over a suitable splint so long as it is not severely damaged.

Surgical injuries of the ureter

The ureter is at risk in any operation in the pelvis, especially in hysterectomy or in operations on the rectum or ovary. Usually the ureter is injured where it is crossed by the superior vesical and uterine arteries but it can also be caught up in a suture used in closing the peritoneum (Fig. 13.22).

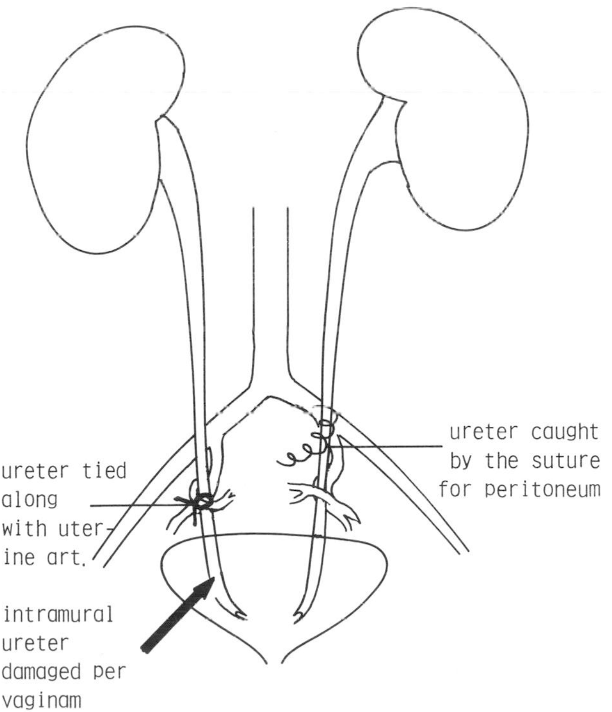

Fig. 13.22. Common site of ureteric injuries in pelvic surgery.

When the injury is noticed at operation, and the ureter is uninflamed and healthy, it may be repaired by end-to-end anastomosis but when the injury is near the bladder it is safer to reimplant it using the Boari flap (see below).

More often the injury to the ureter is not noticed at the time of the operation. If the ureter is obstructed the patient may develop pain in the loin, and often a high fever if the urine is infected. If both ureters are obstructed, the patient will be anuric. Here the difficulty is that the kind of surgical operation where the ureters are both mistakenly caught up by a ligature is also just the kind of operation when there will have been shock from loss of blood leading to underperfusion of the kidney and acute tubular necrosis (see p. 121).

In acute tubular necrosis from underperfusion of the kidney a small volume of urine, rich in granular (tubular) casts is often produced before there is complete shut-down. In obstruction an ultrasound scan, or an IVU using a large dose of contrast, will show that both the ureters are dilated.

Far more often nothing seems to be wrong for several days after the operation, until fluid is seen to escape from the vagina (after hysterectomy) or the perineal wound (after excision of carcinoma of the rectum). The first and urgent task is to confirm whether or not the fluid is urine: this is easily done by aspirating a few drops and having its creatinine and urea measured in the laboratory (Fig. 13.23). If these are higher than those in the blood the fluid cannot be anything other than urine.

The next investigation is an excretion urogram which will usually show some obstruction when a ureter has been injured (Fig. 13.24).

In former days it was taught that these injuries should be left alone for 6 weeks or so before repair was attempted. It has been shown that this is incorrect, and that (in general) the sooner they are repaired the easier and the better the result, so there is some urgency in making the exact diagnosis.

To do this a ureterogram is performed at cystoscopy which will show the precise site of injury to the ureter. The cystoscopy will also show if there is a coincidental injury to the bladder.

Reimplantation of the ureter with a Boari flap

Once the diagnosis has been confirmed, the previous incision is reopened. The ureter is traced down to the site of injury, divided, and implanted into a U-shaped flap made from the wall of the bladder (Fig. 13.25). This reimplantation uses a tunnel to prevent reflux

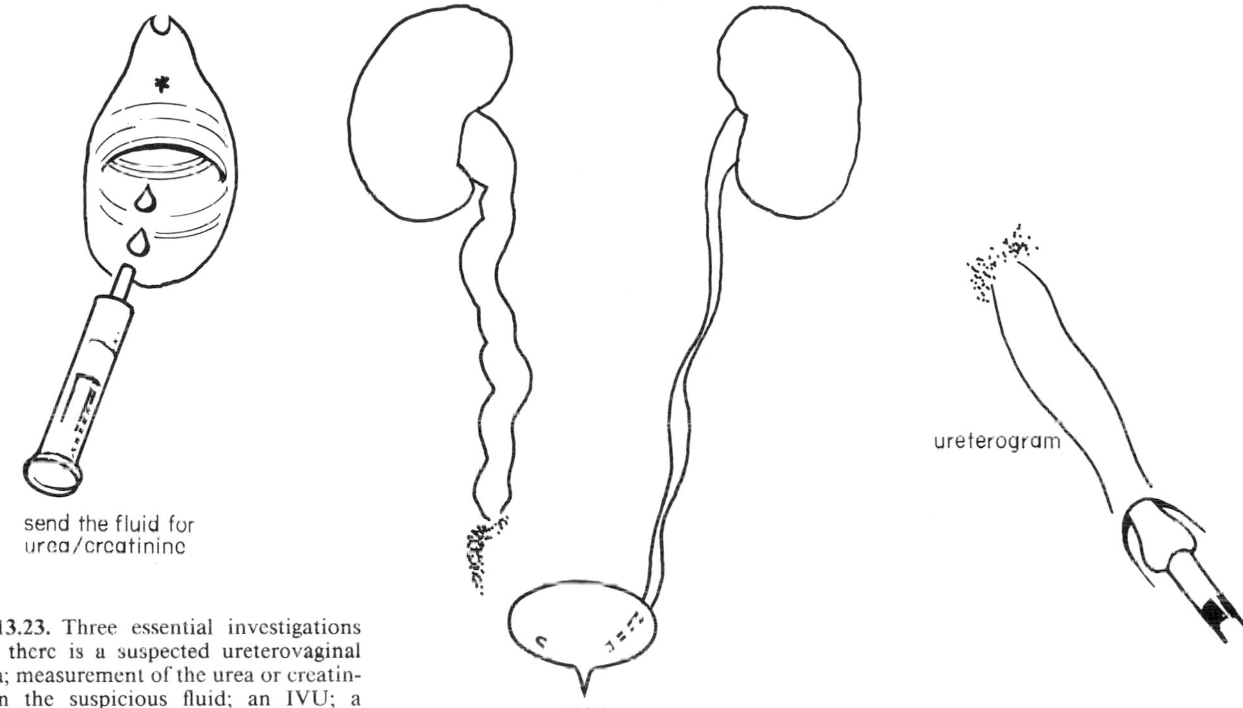

Fig. 13.23. Three essential investigations when there is a suspected ureterovaginal fistula; measurement of the urea or creatinine in the suspicious fluid; an IVU; a ureterogram on both sides.

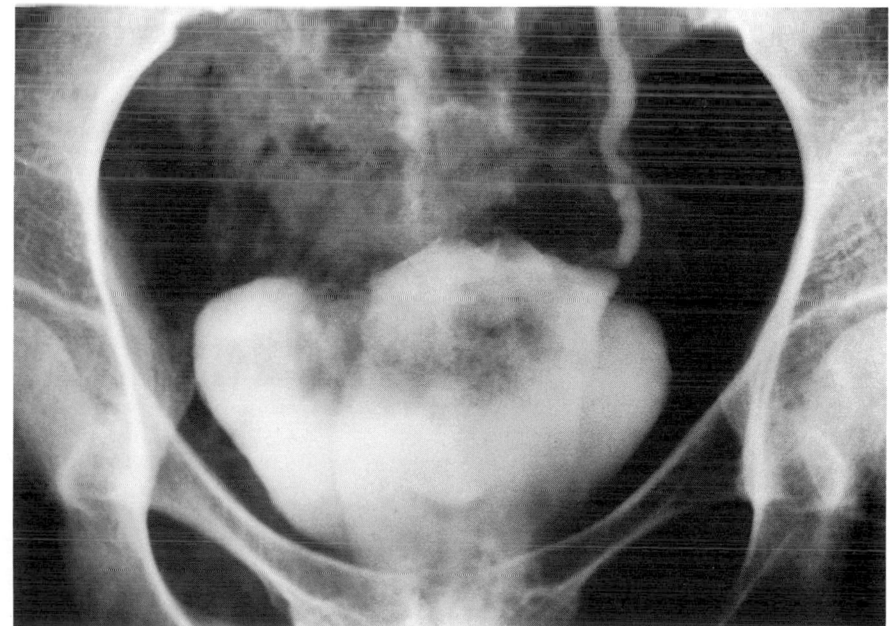

Fig. 13.24. Excretion urogram from a woman whose left ureter was injured at hysterectomy. The left ureter is slightly dilated and contrast in the vagina clearly distingishes it from the bladder.

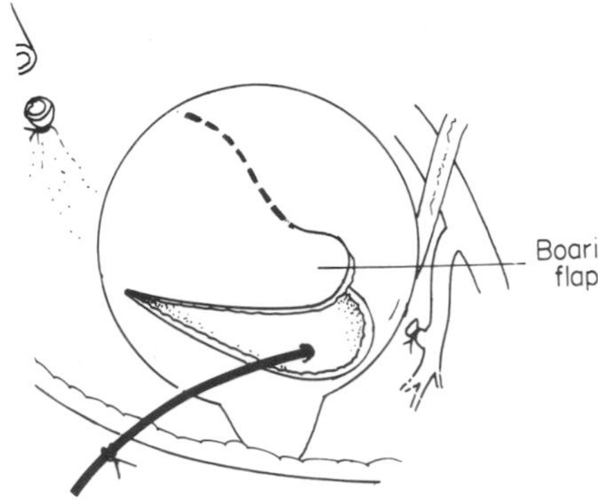

Fig. 13.25. Reimplantation of the ureter with a Boari flap: first step, making the flap of the detrusor muscle.

(Fig. 13.26). The end result is a ureter and bladder which are indistinguishable from normal.

Nephrectomy

There are some circumstances in which the ureter is injured in the course of removing a large tumour: the outlook is poor, and it is important to shorten the patient's stay in hospital. In such a patient a nephrectomy may well be a simpler and kinder remedy.

INFLAMMATION OF THE URETER

Ureteritis

Acute inflammation of the ureter probably accounts for much of the pain so often experienced by patients with acute urinary infections who have rigors and pain in the loin. It is accompanied by oedema of the wall of the ureter which may permit reflux to take place up the ureter from the bladder. It resolves completely with antibiotics and time.

Chronic ureteritis

Following a severe acute inflammation of the ureter the urogram may show multiple rounded filling defects in the ureter and renal pelvis: this is

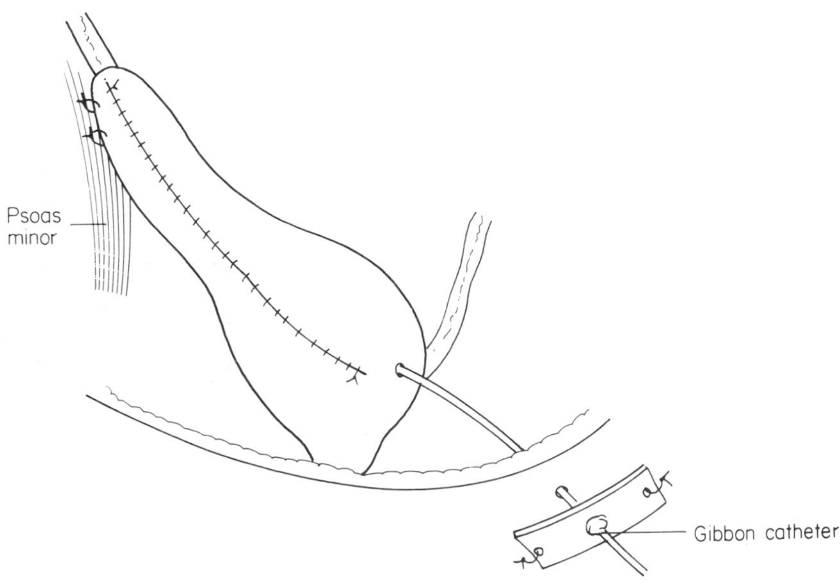

Fig. 13.26. Anastomosis of the ureter to a Boari tube over a suitable splint.

ureteritis cystica, and is caused by chronic inflammation where little nests of epithelium are buried under the healing lining of the ureter and swell up into tiny cysts (Fig. 13.27). This change resolves itself in time and needs no treatment: it is important to recognize it otherwise unnecessary investigations may be done to rule out cancer.

The ureter is always involved in *genitourinary tuberculosis* (see p. 75). In the early stages the ureter is oedematous and shortened: later it may become narrow and obstructed, calling for pyeloplasty or reimplantation into the bladder.

In *bilharziasis* (see p. 177) the wall of the ureter is infested with copulating pairs of *Schistosoma* worms in its submucosal veins. Their eggs work their way into the lumen of the ureter and as they die, set off a granulomatous inflammation which turns the ureter into a stiff swollen tube which is at the same time dilated, obstructed and often secondarily infected and accompanied by stones (Fig. 13.28).

Retroperitoneal fibrosis

There are three types of retroperitoneal fibrosis. In *malignant* retroperitoneal fibrosis a mass of fibrous tissue accompanies the spread of

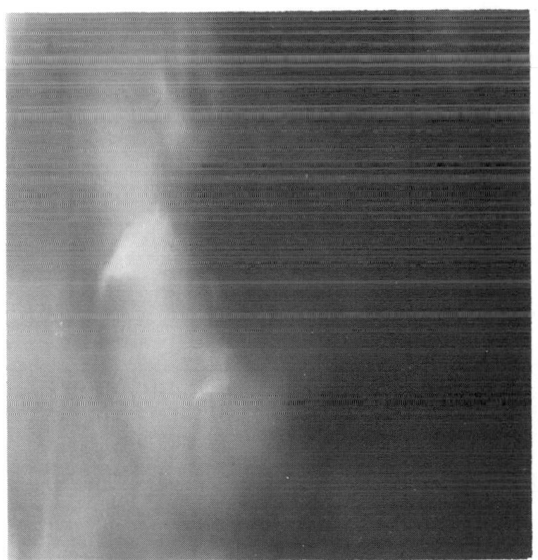

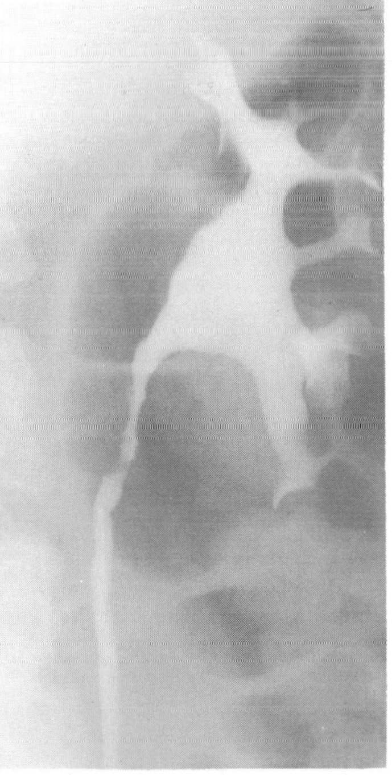

Fig. 13.27. Ureteritis and pyelitis cystica following a severe episode of urinary infection.

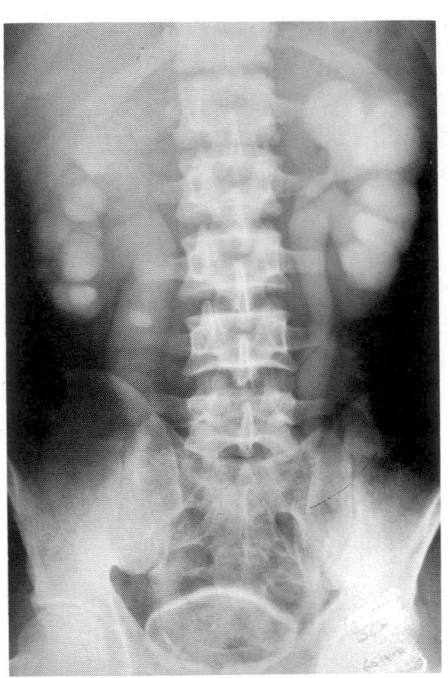

Fig. 13.28. Schistosomiasis. The wall of the bladder is outlined with calcification and both ureters are grossly dilated. There is a stone in the middle third of the right ureter.

metastatic tumour in the retroperitoneal tissues. The primary may be the prostate, stomach, breast or even lung. In *inflammatory* retroperitoneal fibrosis there is some obvious cause for the inflammation — e.g. Crohn's disease, appendicitis or diverticular disease.

More often no cause can be found, and the disease is labelled *idiopathic retroperitoneal fibrosis*. It is a very remarkable condition. Patients have vague ill-defined backache, they sweat, have a fever, and lose weight. Their sedimentation rate is raised and they are invariably hypertensive. The ureters are encased in a stiff corset of fibrous tissue (Fig. 13.29) which prevents them from moving, and produces severe obstruction even though, paradoxically, it is easy to inject contrast up them or pass a catheter. Frequently, they are profoundly uraemic by the time the diagnosis is made. The condition is not limited to the ureters: the vena cava and aorta are similarly encased, and the fibrous tissue may surround the tissues in the mediastinum or the porta hepatis. Its cause is entirely unknown.

The first task is to relieve the obstruction, and this is usually done

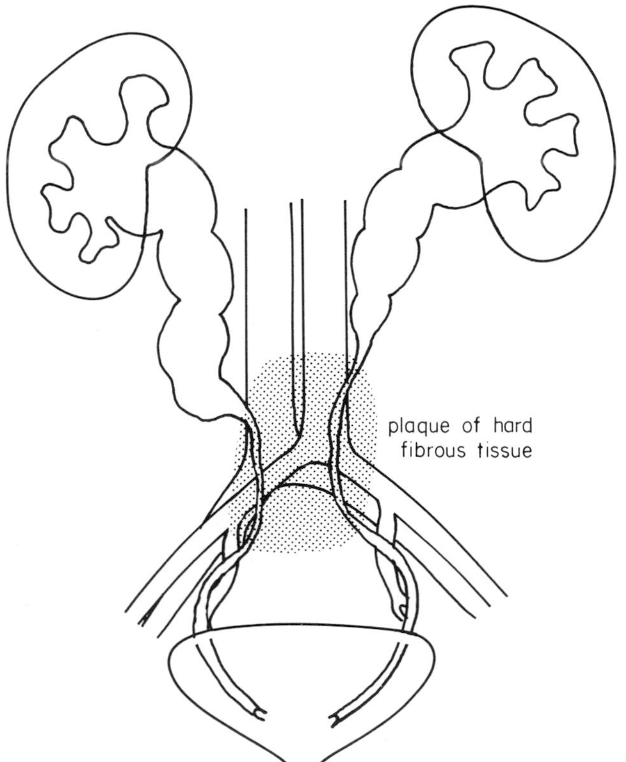

Fig. 13.29. Retroperitoneal fibrosis.

with a percutaneous nephrostomy (see p. 21). When the patient has recovered from the uraemia, the ureters are delivered from their surrounding fibrous tissue by *ureterolysis*. To prevent the fibrous tissue returning, the ureters are wrapped in omentum (Fig. 13.30). In people who are too ill for any operation, steroids may be given and in some cases these cause the fibrous tissue to resolve.

UROTHELIAL CARCINOMA OF THE URETER

The ureter is lined with urothelium which forms transitional cell tumours which are exactly similar to those of the kidney and bladder. They present with haematuria, or with pain from obstruction to the ureter upstream of the tumour (Fig. 13.31).

Diagnosis

The diagnosis is made in the urogram, confirmed by finding malignant cells in the urine, and defined by a retrograde urogram.

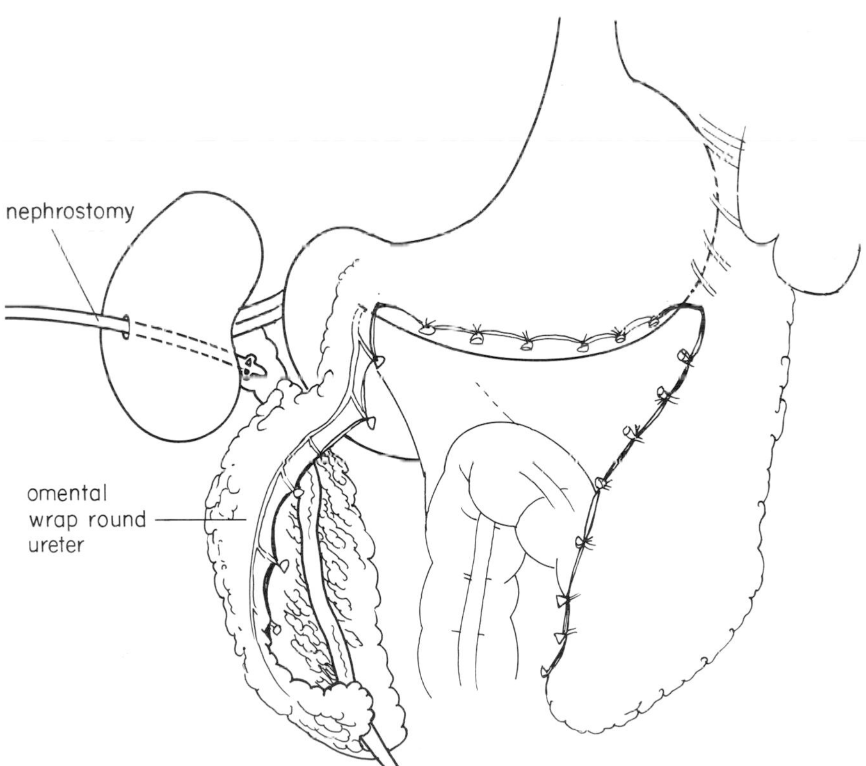

Fig. 13.30. The ureters are wrapped in omentum to prevent recurrence of the fibrosis.

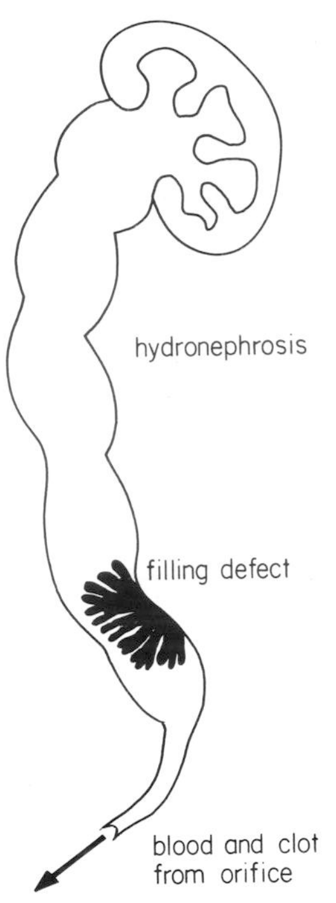

Fig. 13.31. Clinical features of carcinoma of the ureter.

Treatment

As with other urothelial cancers they are classified in three grades of malignancy, G1, G2 and G3. They may be single or multiple. For single G1 tumours a conservative removal is sufficient: but unfortunately these are not common, and it is usually necessary to remove the entire ureter and kidney.

STONES IN THE URETER

The commonest pathological condition of the ureter is undoubtedly a stone. About 20% of doctors can look forward to having at least one episode of ureteric colic: the diagnosis and management of this very common and important condition is dealt with on p. 96.

FURTHER READING

Badenoch DF, Tiptaft RC, Thakar DR, Fowler CG, Blandy JP (1987) Early repair of accidental injury to the ureter or bladder following gynaecological surgery. *British Journal of Urology* **59**, 516–8.

Bean WJ, Daughtry JD, Mullin DM & Rodan BA (1987) Ureteral balloon dilatation: a technique for retrograde ureteral stone removal and relief for ureteral strictures. *Journal of International Radiology* **2**, 27–32.

Chang R & Marshall FF (1987) Management of ureteroscopic injuries. *Journal of Urology* **137**, 1132–5.

Mufti GR, Gove JRW, Badenoch DF, Fowler CG, Tiptaft RC, England HR, Paris AMI, Singh M, Hall MH & Blandy JP (1981) Transitional cell carcinoma of the renal pelvis and ureter. *British Journal of Urology.*

Murphy DM, Fallon B, Lane V & O'Flynn JD (1982) Tuberculous stricture of ureter. *Urology* **20**, 382–4.

Richie JP (1988) Carcinoma of the renal pelvis and ureter. In: Skinner DG & Lieskovsky G (Eds) *Diagnosis and Management of Genitourinary Cancer.* WB Saunders, Philadelphia. pp. 323–36.

Tiptaft RC, Costello AJ, Paris AMI & Blandy JP (1982) The long-term follow-up of Idiopathic Retroperitoneal Fibrosis. *British Journal of Urology* **54**, 620–4.

Vaughan ED & Mills C (1983) Carcinoma of the ureter: natural history, management and 5 year survival. *Journal of Urology* **129**, 275–7.

14 The Bladder — Structure, Function and Investigation

SURGICAL ANATOMY

The bladder changes with age: in children it is mainly an abdominal organ, easily felt and easily needled, but in adults the bladder is difficult to feel unless it is distended. It lies deep in the pelvis and is protected by the symphysis. Above, the bladder is partly covered by the peritoneum, against which rest loops of small bowel and the sigmoid colon. A long tail of urachus tethers the dome of the bladder to the umbilicus — representing the fetal allantois (Fig. 14.1).

Anteriorly the empty bladder lies behind the symphysis, rising as it fills, mainly in the midline, but sometimes a little to one or other side. The bladder may bulge out into a defect in the inguinal canal to form the 'bladder ears' so common in the cystograms of children (Fig. 14.2). In

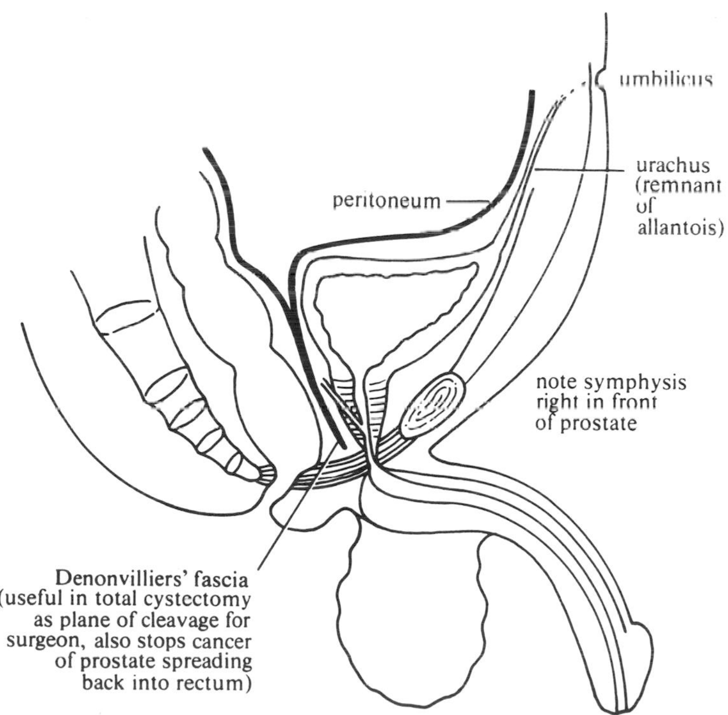

Fig. 14.1. Surgical anatomy of the bladder in the male.

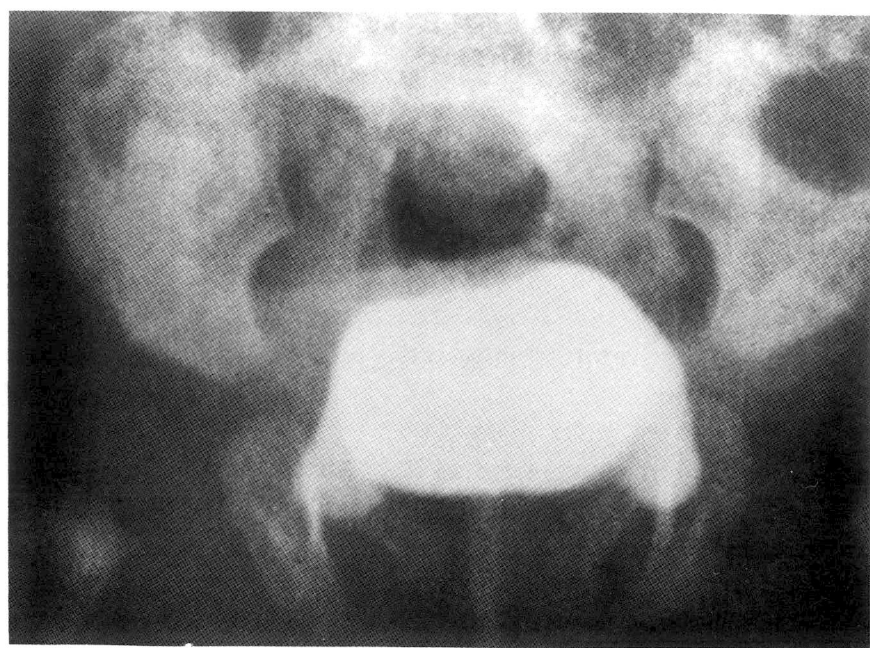

Fig. 14.2. Bladder 'ears'. These protrusions of the bladder into the groin are normal in babies.

adults the bladder is an important medial relation to an inguinal or a femoral hernia, and a diverticulum of the bladder just behind the sac of a large hernia is a notorious trap for the unwary.

Posteriorly the bladder is separated from the rectum by the important, though thin, fascia of Denonvilliers which is made of the fused layers of the peritoneum, and provides a very helpful plane of cleavage in the operations of radical prostatectomy and cystectomy. It also offers a remarkably impenetrable biological barrier to the spread of carcinoma of the bladder or prostate into the rectum.

Inferiorly the bladder rests (in the male) on the prostate gland below which the pelvic diaphragm, made of the levator ani muscle sandwiched in two layers of fascia, supports the contents of the pelvis. In females the bladder rests on the anterior wall of the vagina which is supported by the levator ani (Fig. 14.3).

Structure of the bladder

The fibres of the detrusor muscle of the bladder are arranged not in layers, as in the bowel, but like felt or basketwork. Its muscle fibres sweep around the wall of the bladder, passing from its outer part to its innermost layer and back again. Outside the muscle there is no true

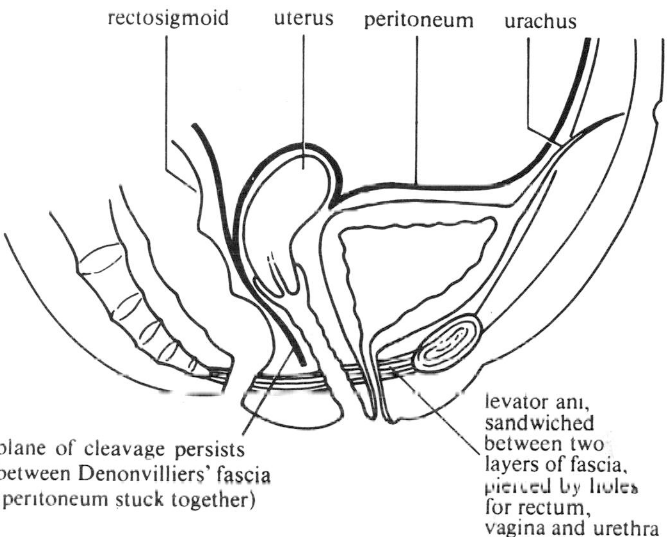

Fig. 14.3. Surgical anatomy of the bladder in the female.

capsule: where the muscle ends, there is fat, connective tissue and a plexus of huge veins (Fig. 14.4).

Within the detrusor muscle is a thin layer of submucosa which supports the waterproof *urothelium*.

Blood supply

The bladder has a rich blood supply and its arteries interconnect freely. This makes it possible to construct grafts and tubes from its wall with bases that are relatively very narrow compared with those required in the skin. This also means that the bladder can bleed profusely, either from disease (such as cystitis) or during surgical operations. There are three main branches of the internal iliac artery which supply the bladder (Fig. 14.5): the superior vesical pedicle (under which runs the ureter); a second leash of arteries supplying the base of the bladder and prostate; and a third group at the caudal end of the prostate.

From the bladder, a very rich plexus of veins passes to the internal iliac veins. In addition, there is a second 'backstairs' system draining into the veins of the pelvic bones, femora and vertebral bodies. Coughing or the Valsalva manoeuvre — or indeed anything that raises the intra-abdominal pressure will force blood from the pelvis into these bony plexuses so metastases from carcinoma of the prostate and bladder are often found there.

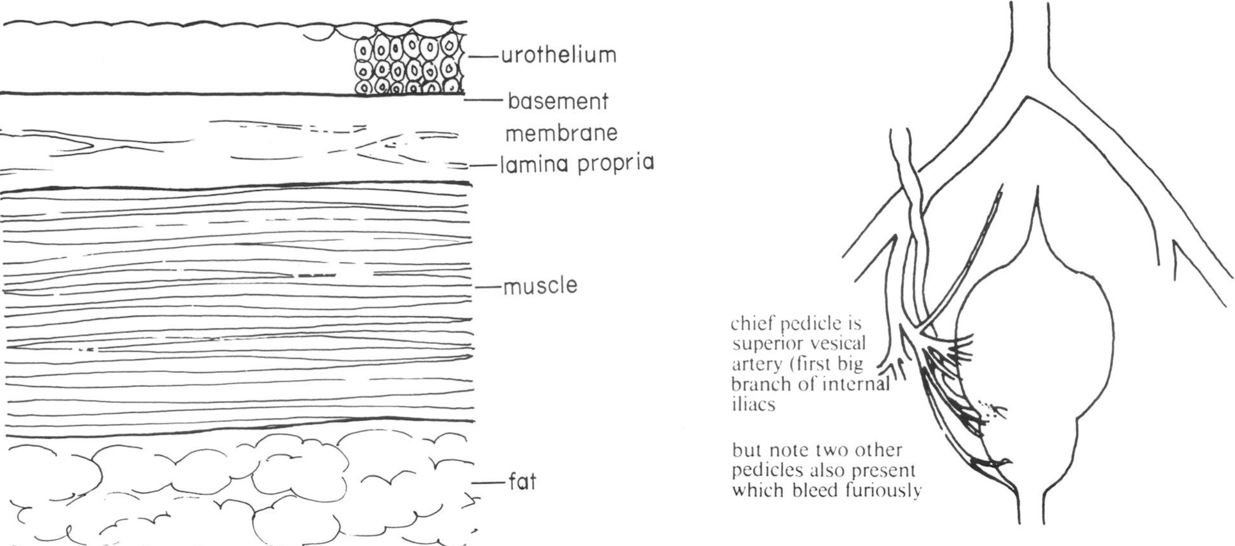

Fig. 14.4. Diagram of section through the bladder.

Fig. 14.5. Rich blood supply of the bladder from branches of the internal iliac artery.

Lymphatic drainage

Lymphatics are sparse in the innermost layers of the bladder since the bladder is designed to hold urine rather than absorb it. But the outer layers of the detrusor have a rich supply of lymphatics which drain directly into the lymph nodes of the pelvis, and also through a 'backstairs' system, like the veins, to the lymph spaces in the bones of the pelvis and upper ends of the femora through which metastases may spread.

Nerve supply of the bladder

The nervous system of the bladder is a very complicated one: not only is it supplied with sympathetic and parasympathetic nerves, but it has its own private curve network and its own secret ganglia. So for practical purposes it is difficult to determine whether a disorder is due to a fault in the intrinsic system or to outside influences.

The reflex arcs of the bladder

The main *afferent* impluses from the bladder pass up in the parasympathetic fibres of the nervi erigentes to the S2 and S3 segments of the spinal cord. There are, however, also afferent impulses which probably convey sensation of pain, which pass up in sympathetic nerves in the presacral plexus. The sympathetic and parasympathetic filaments reach the bladder in company with its arteries (Fig. 14.6).

Pain impulses from the bladder can reach unexpectedly high levels in the spinal cord: in order to block all pain from the bladder a spinal anaesthetic must reach as high as T6.

The reflex arc handling most of the work of the bladder is situated in the tip of the spinal cord in the S2 and S3 segments which lie at the junction of the thoracic and lumbar spine—the vulnerable part of the backbone-easily injured in traffic or industrial accidents.

Messages reach the bladder along three sets of fibres:

1 pelvic parasympathetic fibres which convey impulses to ganglia in the wall of the detrusor causing it to contract:

2 other pelvic parasympathetic fibres convey impulses to the supramembranous sphincter and bladder neck;

3 somatic efferent fibres in the pudendal nerve supply the striated muscle of the levator ani and pelvic floor.

Micturition

When the bladder fills, afferent fibres which are sensitive to stretch are stimulated. On completion of the reflex arc, efferent fibres cause the detrusor to contract. It is an essential ingredient of the reflex action that the efferent impulses to the supramembranous, internal and external sphincters should be inhibited when the detrusor is trying to empty the

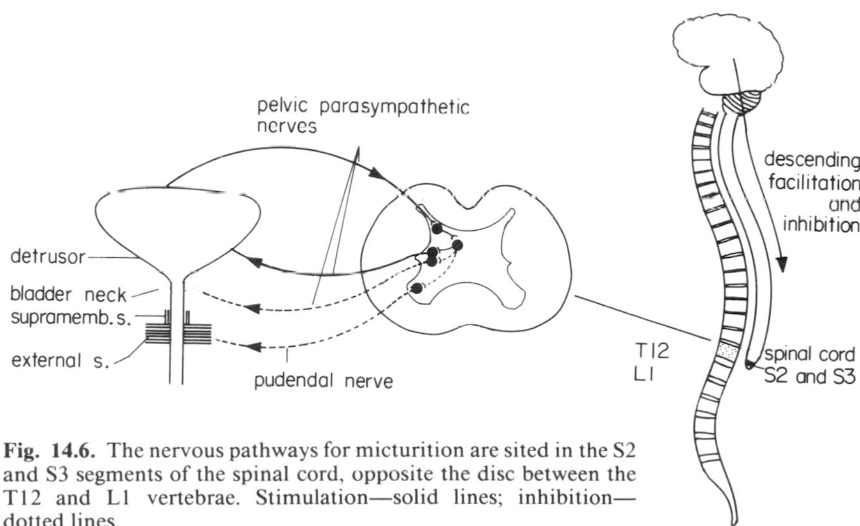

Fig. 14.6. The nervous pathways for micturition are sited in the S2 and S3 segments of the spinal cord, opposite the disc between the T12 and L1 vertebrae. Stimulation—solid lines; inhibition—dotted lines.

bladder. The motor nerves to the internal and supramembranous sphincter run in parasympathetic fibres: those to the levator ani are myelinated, and run in the pudendal nerve. Both are inhibited to allow the urine to leave the bladder. When it has all gone the external sphincter contracts, then the supramembranous sphincter milks the urine back and finally the internal sphincter shuts to close the bladder (Fig. 14.7).

As with any reflex arc this is influenced by higher centres: they may either facilitate or inhibit the reflex (Fig. 14.6). These influences are represented at every level of the central nervous system. It is a common observation that the urge to empty an overdistended bladder may drive all other thoughts from consciousness. Equally — when anxious or frightened — one may have an overwhelming urge to empty a bladder that is barely half-full.

In many clinical conditions the normal functioning of the human bladder is altered by disturbances of its innervation.

INVESTIGATION OF BLADDER FUNCTION — URODYNAMICS

Static cystometry

This is the oldest and most simple method of investigating the function of the bladder (Fig. 14.8). A fine catheter is passed: water is run slowly into the bladder and the pressure is continually measured.

Dynamic or voiding cystometry

More information is obtained by measuring the pressure in the bladder during micturition. To do this a small cannula may be passed into the

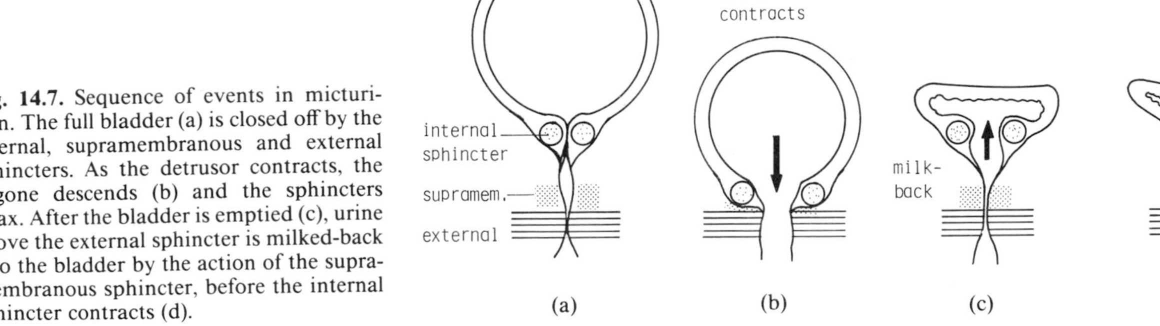

Fig. 14.7. Sequence of events in micturition. The full bladder (a) is closed off by the internal, supramembranous and external sphincters. As the detrusor contracts, the trigone descends (b) and the sphincters relax. After the bladder is emptied (c), urine above the external sphincter is milked-back into the bladder by the action of the supramembranous sphincter, before the internal sphincter contracts (d).

bladder suprapubically, or a second catheter passed alongside the first to measure the pressure (Fig. 14.9).

One of the difficulties in practice is that many patients tend to strain so as to help empty the bladder by increasing the intra-abdominal pressure. To allow for this, a third small catheter records the intra-abdominal pressure from inside the rectum, and an electronic gadget subtracts the rectal from the bladder pressure to give the *subtracted* pressure.

Simultaneous X-rays — voiding cystometrogram

If, instead of water, radio-opaque contrast medium is run into the bladder, one can observe and record the movement of the bladder at the same time as these pressure measurements are obtained. Such a system provides the *videocystometrogram*.

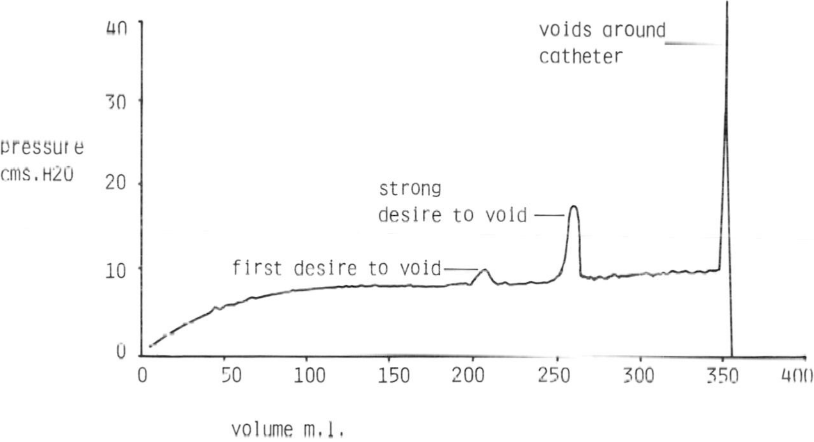

Fig. 14.8. Static cystometrogram.

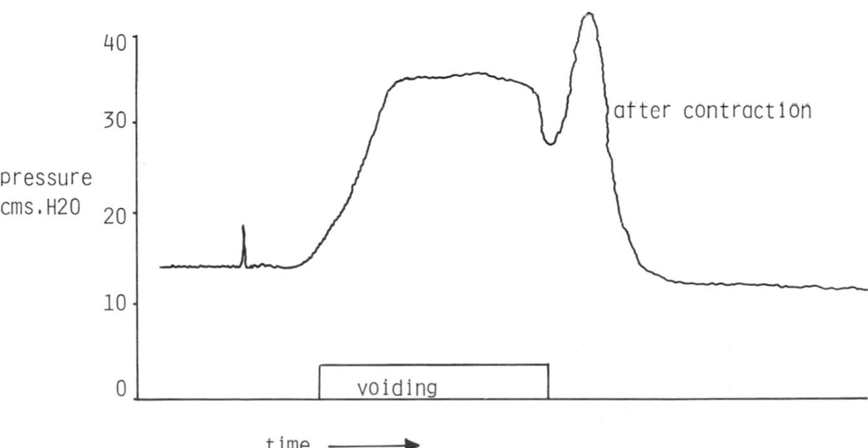

Fig. 14.9. Dynamic or voiding cystometrogram.

Electromyography (EMG)

If a very fine needle electrode is placed in the external sphincter, the electrical activity of the levator ani muscle can be recorded on an *electromyogram.* At rest there is a constant level of activity. When the bladder is emptying this is shut off. The EMG can be recorded on the same video screen as the cystogram and the true and subtracted bladder pressures (Fig. 14.10).

Flow-rate

If the detrusor is weak, or the urethra narrowed by stricture, then the jet of urine is a thin one. Much can be learned by the careful doctor who is prepared to spend time watching his patient pass water: but this only gives subjective information, is marred by numerous artifacts (including those arising from shyness), and cannot be recorded. Accurate methods of measuring the flow-rate are now available, and this too can be added to the record of the videocystometrogram.

Urethral pressure profile

A cannula with a side hole is used to record the pressure in the urethra as

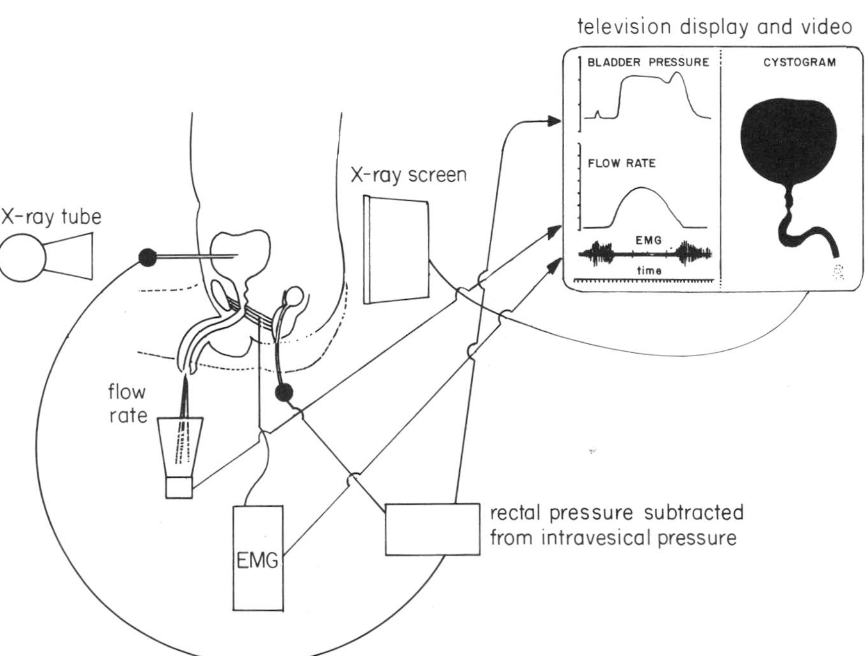

Fig. 14.10. Diagram of the elements of the videocystourethrogram (VCU). The true intravesical pressure (the measured bladder pressure *minus* intrarectal pressure) is recorded as well as the flow-rate and electromyogram while the radiographic image of the bladder filled with contrast medium is shown on the same television screen and recorded on videotape.

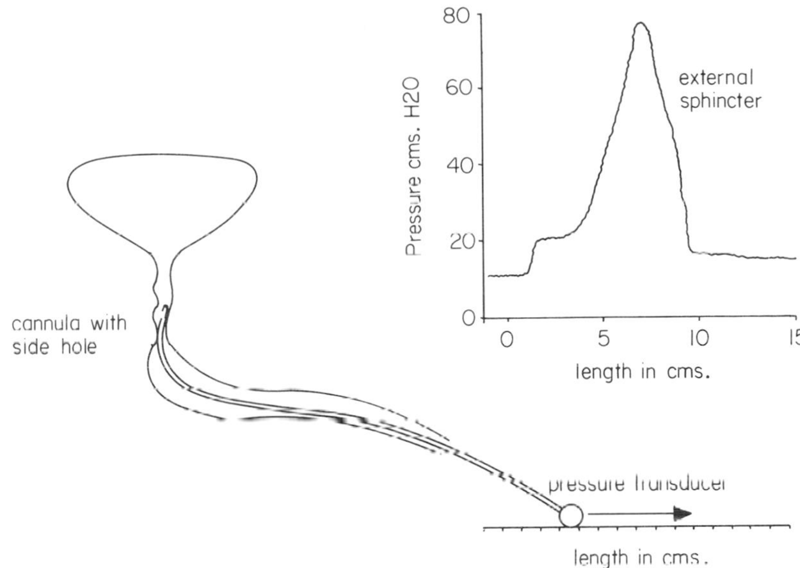

Fig. 14.11. The urethral pressure profile is the plot of the intraurethral pressure against the distance travelled by the cannula down the urethra. Not shown in the diagram is the slow continuous perfusion of the cannula.

the cannula is slowly withdrawn along the length of the urethra, recording the rise and fall of the components of the sphincter — the bladder neck, supramembranous and striated external sphincter. The system plots the distance from the lumen of the bladder against the pressure (Fig. 14.11).

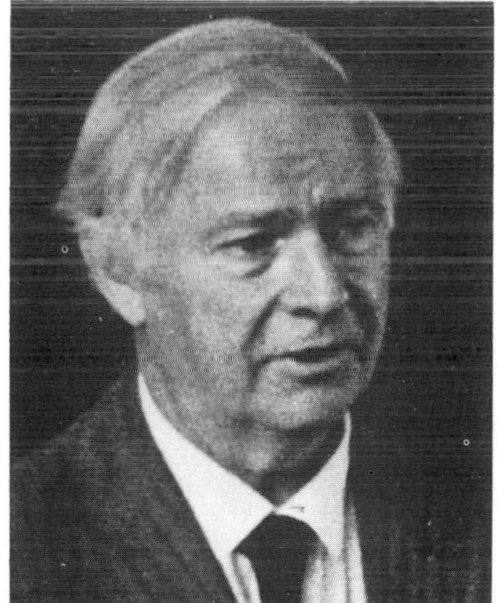

Fig. 14.12. Professor Harold Hopkins FRS, father of modern endoscopic surgery in all its branches.

INVESTIGATION OF THE STRUCTURE OF THE BLADDER — CYSTOSCOPY

Modern urology owes nearly all its instruments to the inventive genius of one man — Professor Harold Hopkins (Fig. 14.12).

Flexible endoscopy

The invention by Hopkins of the co-ordinated glass fibre bundle was as simple as it was brilliant. If a rod of optical glass is coated with glass with a different refractive index there will be total internal reflection, and all the light shone in one end will emerge from the other (Fig. 14.13). The rod can be heated and drawn out into long thin fibres. If these are now wound on a large wheel, glued together, and cut across (Fig. 14.14) an image, made up of hundreds of tiny dots, can be transmitted along a thin flexible tube. This is the basis of all modern diagnostic endoscopy which has revolutionized gastroenterology and coloproctology. Its effect upon urology has been no less important. The modern flexible cystoscope has channels for the image, for light, and for the passage of ureteric catheters, laser fibres, or biopsy forceps (Fig. 14.15). Passing the flexible cystoscope is entirely painless, and it has become the standard diagnostic method for almost every case where it is necessary to inspect the urethra and bladder.

No special preparation is necessary. The patient lies supine. A waterproof paper towel is placed round the penis which is cleaned with cetrimide. The urethra is filled for 5 minutes with 1% xylocaine gel. The

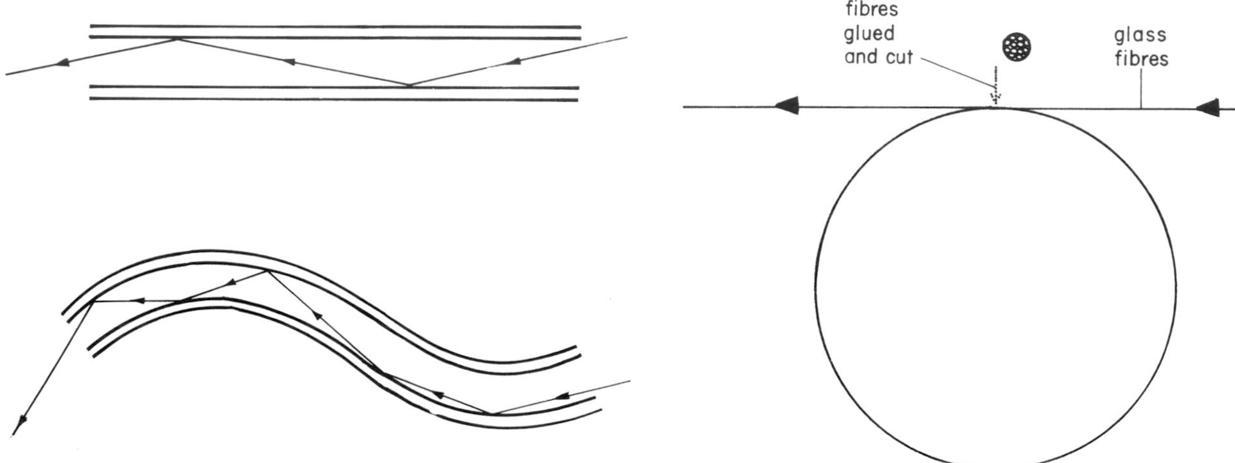

Fig. 14.13. Flexible fibre-lighting. Each thin glass fibre is coated with glass of different refractive index, ensuring total internal reflexion. Very powerful light sources can thus be sited at a distance from the patient.

Fig. 14.14. By winding the glass fibres on a wheel, glueing them together, and cutting them across, Hopkins was able to ensure exact alignment of the fibres at each end.

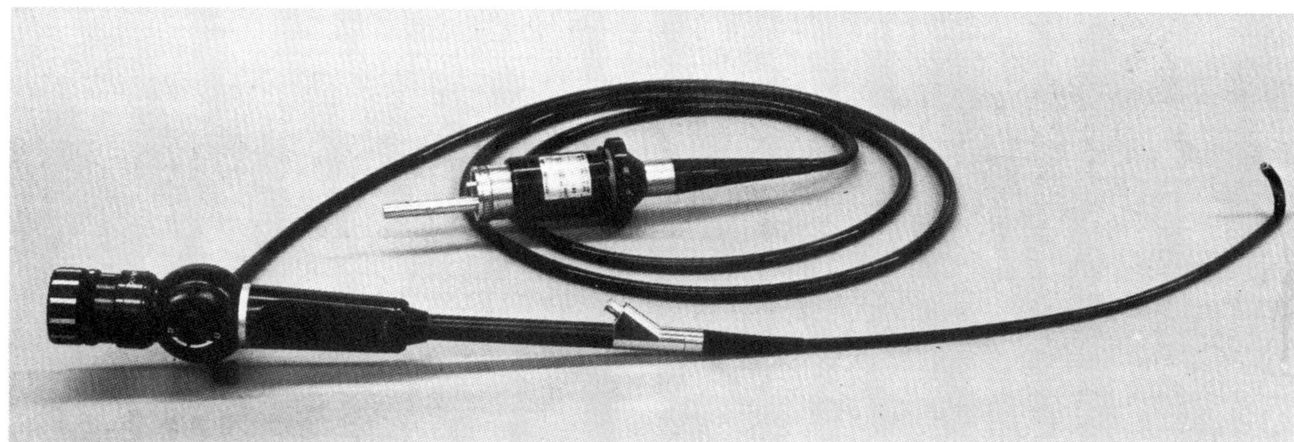

Fig. 14.15. Flexible cystoscope. (Courtesy of Mr C. G. Fowler.)

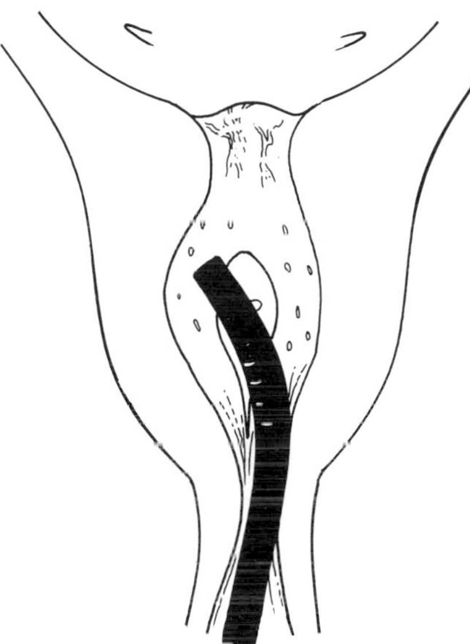

Fig. 14.16. The flexible cystoscope gives a clear view of the interior of the entire urethra including the prostatic part.

instrument is then gently advanced along the urethra, while water is slowly run in to keep the view clear. This shows the entire urethra, the sphincters, the prostatic urethra and the bladder neck (Fig. 14.16). The inside of the bladder is then carefully examined, and finally, by advancing the cystoscope and bending it back upon itself, the bladder neck and prostate can be examined (Fig. 14.17).

The rigid cystoscope

The modern rigid cystoscope also makes use of Professor Hopkins' inventions. First, Hopkins' rod-lens telescope uses glass rods for its spaces and air for the lenses (Fig. 14.18) — thus allowing the rods to be held on an optical axis, ground and bloomed with the precision of a modern microscope. The bladder is illuminated by his fibre-light system — using a bundle of glass fibres to admit light to the bladder (Fig. 14.19).

Endoscopic instruments

A very wide variety of instruments is now available for use with the rigid cystoscope: these make it possible to take a biopsy, resect a tumour with the cutting diathermy or control bleeding vessels with the coagulating current (Fig. 14.20). The ureters may be catheterized. Stones may be pulverized with the ultrasonic or electrohydraulic lithotriptor. There is almost no limit to what can be achieved through these instruments.

Preparation for rigid cystoscopy

Although it is perfectly possible to perform rigid cystoscopy using only

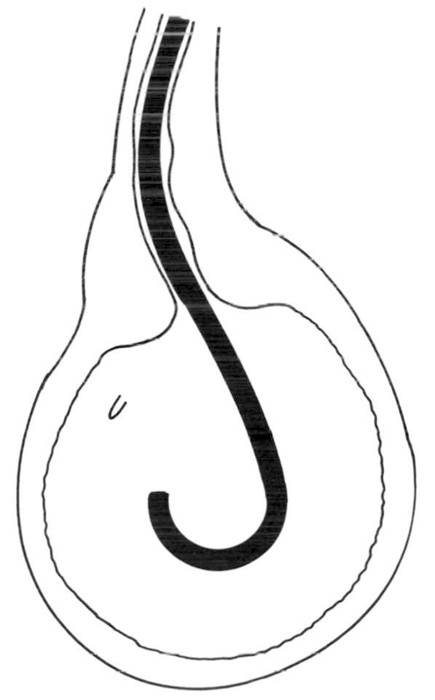

Fig. 14.17. By bending the flexible cystoscope on itself, a unique view of the internal meatus and prostate can be obtained.

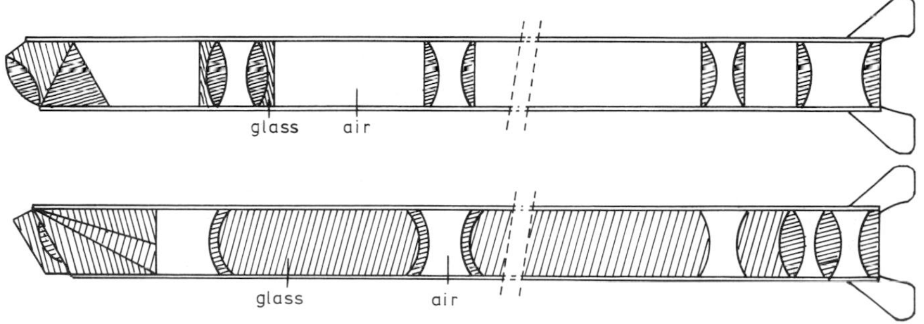

Fig. 14.18. The Hopkins' rod-lens telescope. Hopkins replaced the air spaces of the conventional cystoscope with glass and the glass with air, thus enormously improving the optical properties of the system.

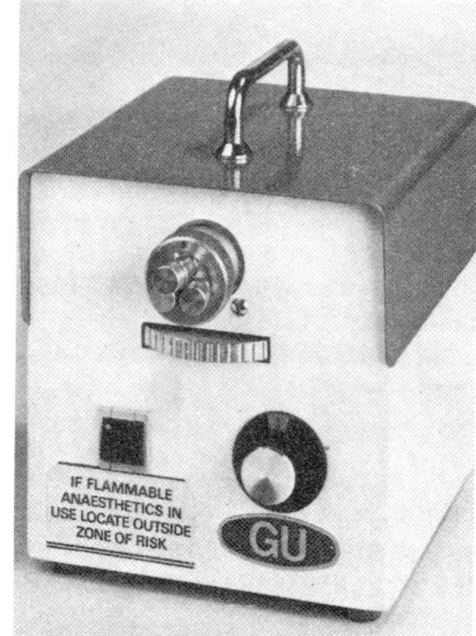

Fig. 14.19. Modern light source for use with flexible light cable. (Courtesy of Genitourinary Mfg Co.)

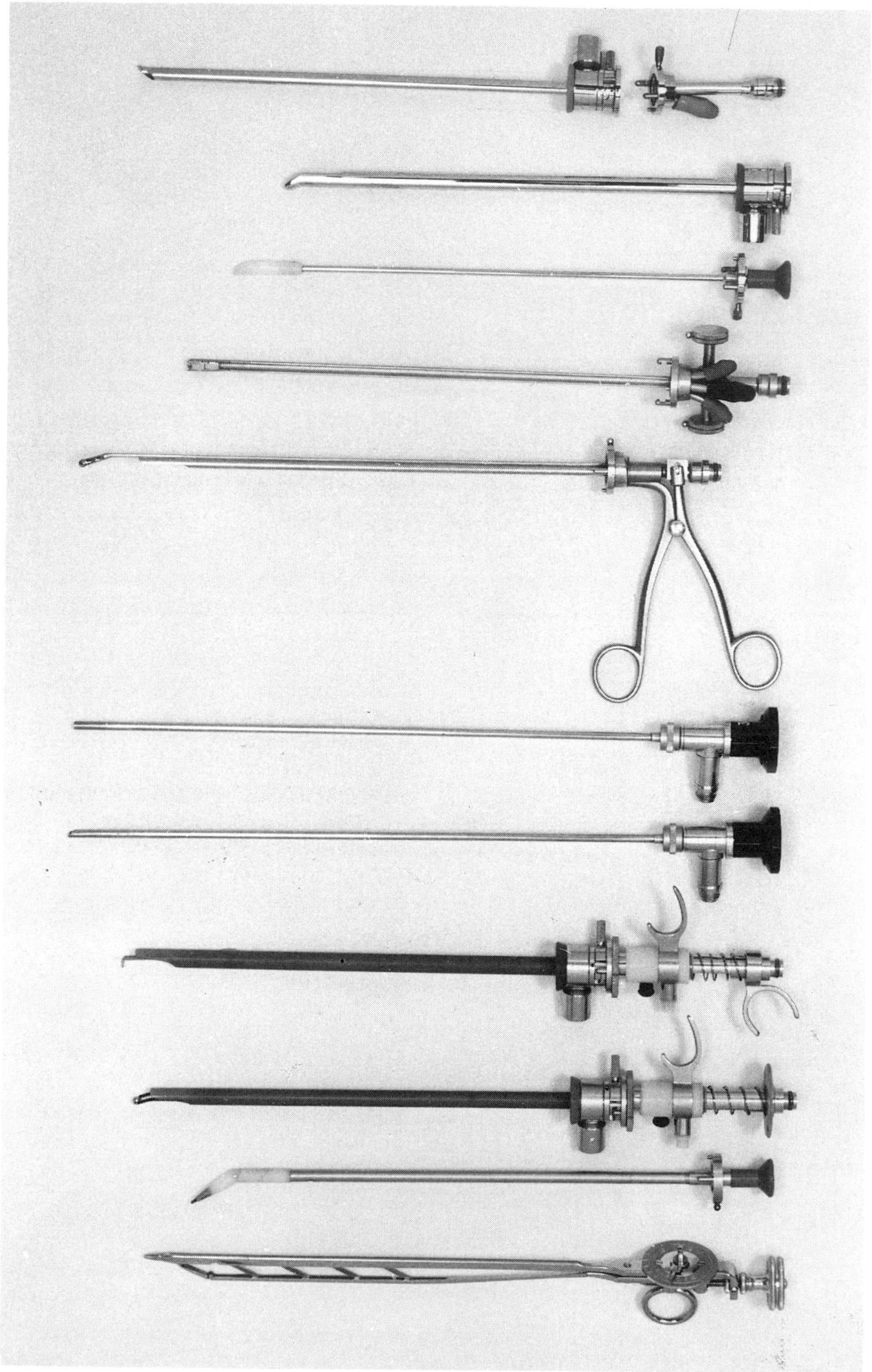

Fig. 14.20. Modern urologists 'kit' of endoscopic instruments which are interchangeable with each other. (Courtesy of Genitourinary Mfg Co.)

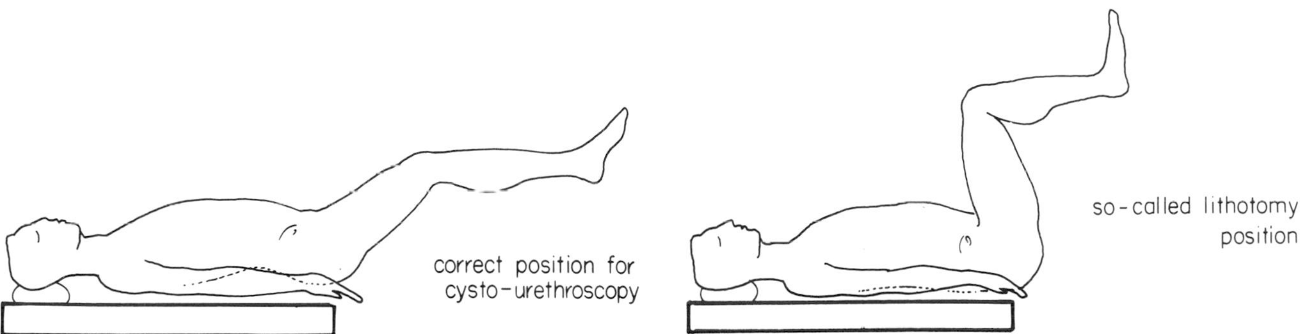

Fig. 14.21. Cystoscopy position.

local anaesthetic, most patients find it unpleasant and today prefer the flexible instrument: regional or general anaesthesia is necessary when a stone must be crushed or a tumour resected. For cystoscopy the patient is placed in the *cystoscopy* position (which is different from that used in *lithotomy*) (Fig. 14.21), and special tables with leg-supports are generally used.

FURTHER READING

Barrington FJF (1914) The nervous mechanism of micturition. *Quarterly Journal of Experimental Physiology* **8**, 33–41.

Fidas A, Galloway NTM, McInnes A & Chisholm GD (1985) Neurophysiological measurements in primary adult enuretics. *British Journal of Urology* **57**, 635–40.

Fowler CJ, Kirby RS, Harrison MJG, Milroy EJG & Turner-Warwick RT (1984) Individual motor unit analysis in the diagnosis of disorders of urethral sphincter innervation. *Journal of Neurology, Neurosurgery and Psychiatry* **47**, 637–41.

McGuire EJ, Shi-Chun Z, Horwinski ER & Lytton B (1983) Treatment of motor and sensory detrusor instability by electrical stimulation. *Journal of Urology* **129**, 78–9.

Mundy AR, Stephenson TP & Wein AJ (1984). *Urodynamics, Principles Practice and Application.* Churchill Livingstone, Edinburgh.

Mundy AR & Stephenson TP (1985) 'Clam' ileocystoplasty for the treatment of refractory urge incontinence. *British Journal of Urology* **57**, 641–6.

Ryall RL & Marshall VR (1982) Point of view: laws of urodynamics. *Urology* **20**, 106–7.

Shepherd AM, Blannin JP & Feneley RCL (1982) Changing attitudes in the management of urinary incontinence — the need for specialist nursing. *British Medical Journal* **284**, 645–6.

Snooks SJ & Swash M (1984) Abnormalities of the innervation of the urethral striated sphincter musculature in incontinence. *British Journal of Urology* **56**, 401–5.

15 The Bladder — Congenital Anomalies

EMBRYOLOGY

In the fetus the hind-gut — the cloaca — curls round, so that its tip connects with the umbilicus. The downgrowth of the urogenital septum separates the future bladder from the rectum, and drags down with it the Wolffian ducts which are partly absorbed into what will become the trigone (Fig. 15.1).

The urethra is formed by inrolling of folds on either side of the midline. In this whole complicated process there is ample scope for innumerable congenital mistakes to occur (Fig. 15.2). The following are some of the more important ones.

Agenesis

Rarely, the cloaca is not formed at all: usually in this condition both ureters are obstructed and so the disorder is incompatible with survival.

Duplication

The bladder may be divided either by a median, or a transverse septum, which gives it an hour-glass appearance.

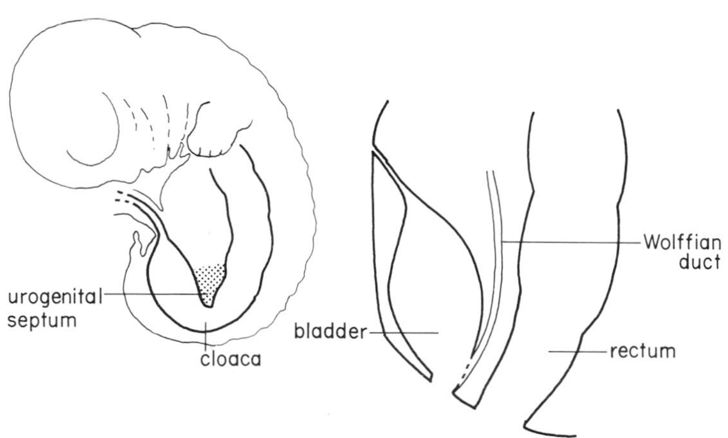

Fig. 15.1. Steps in the embryological formation of the bladder: the urogenital septum which separates the cloaca into the bladder and the rectum brings down the Wolffian mesonephric duct, part of which is absorbed into the future bladder.

Patent urachus

The allantois may remain patent and allow urine to leak through the umbilicus (Fig. 15.3). There is usually an associated obstruction at the neck of the bladder or the urethra. Sometimes the urachal remnant may form small cysts which become secondarily infected. Since it is derived from hind-gut, the urachus is lined with columnar epithelium: this can give rise to an adenocarcinoma. This type of tumour (which is very rare) causes haematuria. There is a small angry red lump at the apex of the bladder, and an unexpectedly large mass outside the bladder. The outlook is very poor because these tumours have usually spread into the peritoneum.

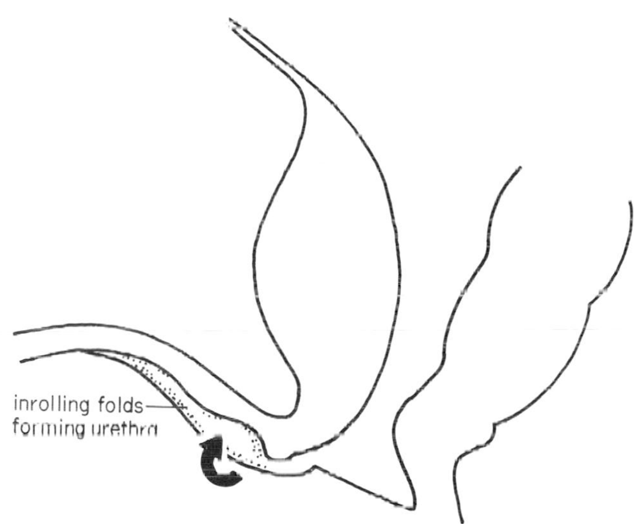

Fig. 15.2. The urethra is enclosed by rolling in the tissues from each side.

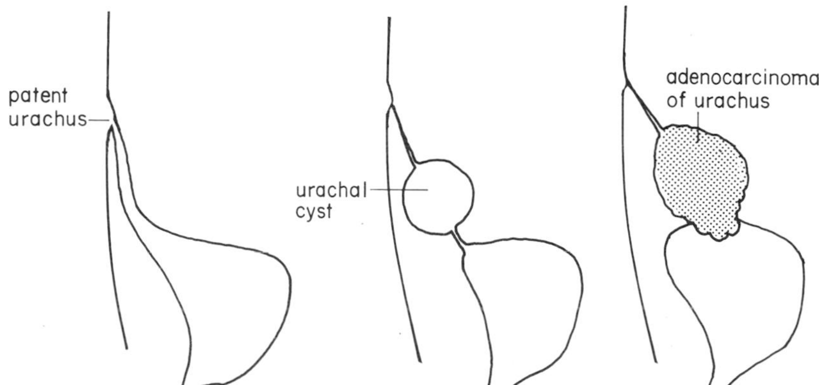

Fig. 15.3. Clinical problems sometimes associated with the urachus.

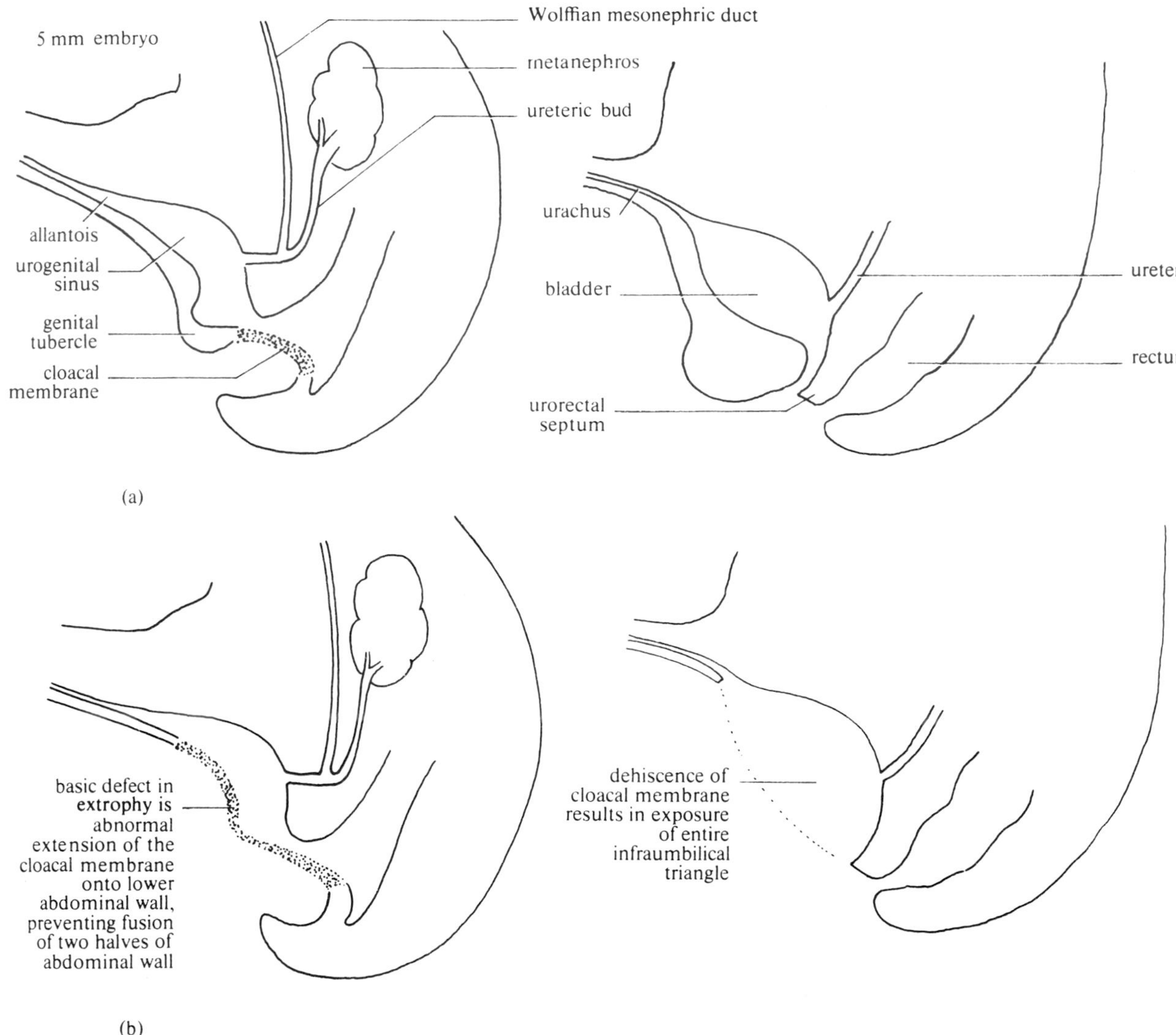

Fig. 15.4. (a) Normal development of the bladder. (b) Exstrophy: the error in development.

Exstrophy

In early fetal life there may be an abnormally large cloacal membrane which extends towards the umbilicus and prevents ingrowth of the tissue destined to form the muscle and skin of the abdominal wall (Fig. 15.4). It is normal for the cloacal membrane to dissolve in places to open up the anus, vagina and urethra but in *exstrophy* the dissolution of the extra-large cloacal membrane leaves exposed the whole triangle of tissue below the umbilicus: this gap may vary in extent. At its least there may be only a dorsal cleft in the penis — *epispadias* — at its worst the entire primitive cloaca may be exposed. In the usual type of exstrophy the bladder opens like a flat red ulcer on the abdomen, onto which the ureters discharge urine. Exstrophy is associated with prolapse of the rectum, undescended testes and a wide separation of the symphysis pubis (Fig. 15.5).

The exposed urothelium undergoes constant irritation and infection, followed by squamous or glandular metaplasia and after many years, squamous or adeno-carcinoma. The sufferers are continually incontinent.

Exstrophy is such a rare condition that the baby should at once be referred to a specialist paediatric urological centre. There are likely to be only one or two groups of surgeons in any one country with sufficient experience to offer the best results. On encountering this distressing condition the first duty of the doctor is to reassure the anxious parents that the child can be made to look normal, and then to refer him or her to a specialist centre. There, an operation will be performed almost as an emergency, as soon as possible after birth. The bladder mucosa is freed from the surrounding skin, rolled up, and sewn into a sphere. To close the abdominal wall over it the iliac bones may be divided near the sacroiliac joint to allow the pelvis to be closed like an oyster-shell (Fig. 15.6). Later on further operations may be required to reconstruct the bladder neck

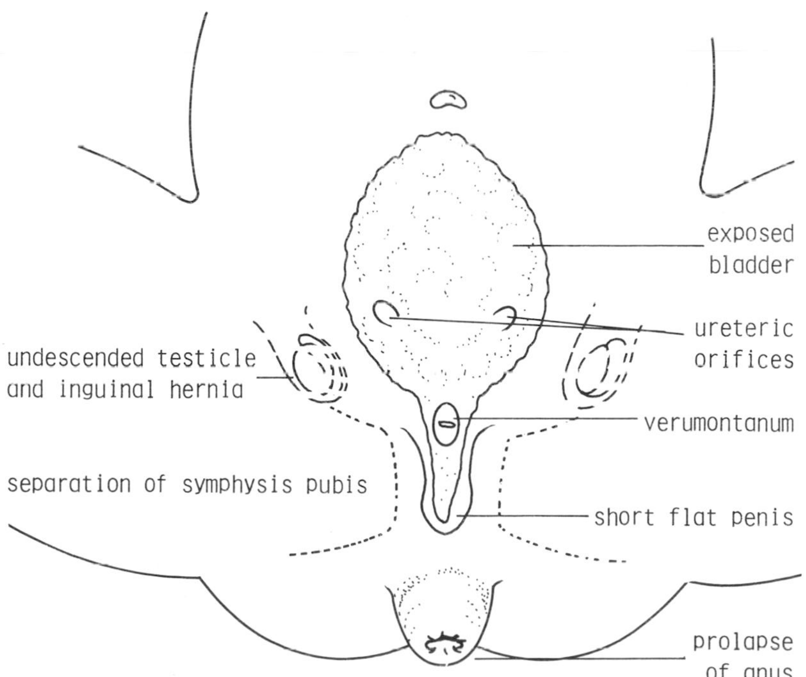

Fig. 15.5. Exstrophy of the bladder — the typical combination of deformities.

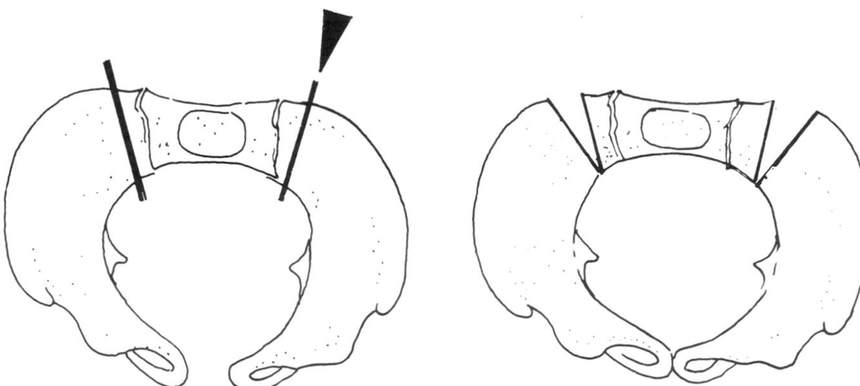

Fig. 15.6. Iliac osteotomy allows the pelvis to be closed together to assist in the closure of an exstrophied bladder.

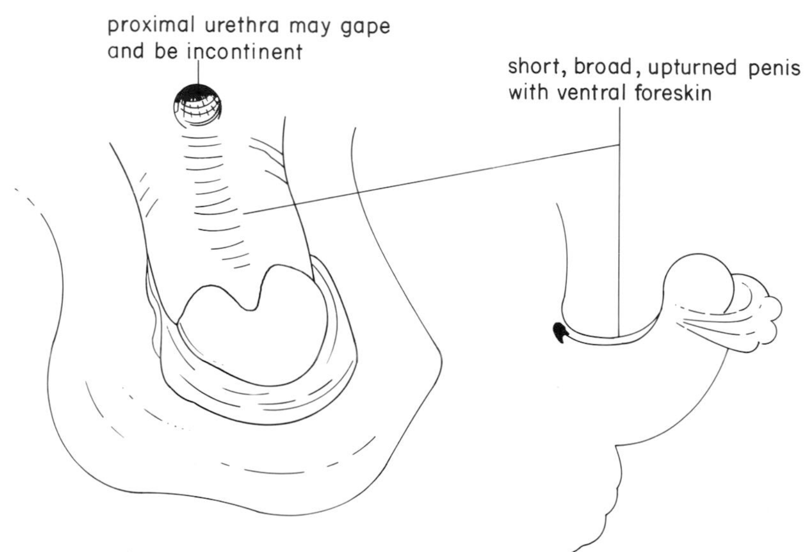

Fig. 15.7. Epispadias.

and, in boys, to bring down the testicles. Sexual function is often normal in these children: the boys grow up able to penetrate and ejaculate and the girls can have children.

Epispadias

This is a minor version of exstrophy (Fig. 15.7) in which the urethra opens on the proximal end of the dorsum of a short flat penis which curves upwards. The reconstruction is done in stages: first a new urethra is made and later on the neck of the bladder is reconstructed.

FURTHER READING

Arey LB (1986) *Developmental Anatomy.* 7th Ed. WB Saunders, Philadelphia. pp. 295–341.

Moore KL (1982) *The Developing Human.* 3rd Ed. WB Saunders, Philadelphia. pp. 255–97.

Smith D, Egginton JA & Brookfield DSK (1987) Detection of abnormality of fetal urinary tract as a predictor of renal tract disease. *British Medical Journal* **294**, 27–8.

Stephens FD (1963) *Congenital Malformation of the Rectum, Anus and Genitourinary Tracts.* Churchill Livingstone, Edinburgh.

16 The Bladder — Inflammation

ACUTE CYSTITIS

Acute cystitis is so common that in one study it was found that more than 70% of the wives and mothers accompanying their families to the doctor's surgery had experienced its characteristic symptoms. Infection is usually from one of the organisms in the bowel, e.g. *Escherichia coli, Klebsiella, Proteus mirabilis,* or *Streptococcus faecalis.* Recurrent infections may be due to reinfection by the original strain of micro-organism or a different one. Not all cystitis is caused by bowel flora: infection by *Herpes virus hominis, Chlamydia* and even *Neisseria gonorrhoeae* may at times be responsible.

Bacterial infection occurs when something has lowered the local resistance to infection, e.g. diabetes mellitus. In some patients the attacks of cystitis are always preceded by an upper respiratory infection, in others the minor trauma of sexual intercourse is followed by an attack. Chemical cystitis may occur from detergents added to the bath-water or deodorants applied to the vulva. Substances secreted in the urine may cause chemical cystitis, e.g. cyclophosphamide or even large doses of mandelic acid used in treating urinary infection.

Pathology

Whatever its cause the macroscopic features of the acute inflammation are those of inflammation elsewhere: the mucosa of the bladder is red, swollen and painful (Fig. 16.1). The afferent arc of the micturition reflex is intensely stimulated: the patient keeps wanting to empty the bladder even though it is barely half-full. Exfoliated pus and urothelial cells make the urine turbid and the bacterial fermentation of urea into ammonia gives it a fishy smell. When the inflammation is severe there may be haematuria. The cystoscopic appearances of the bladder are very striking: the mucosa is red, ulcerated in places, and bleeds when touched with the instrument.

Clinical features

There may be a sudden onset of suprapubic pain, frequency and scalding on micturition. The patient may sit for hours on the toilet with the urge to

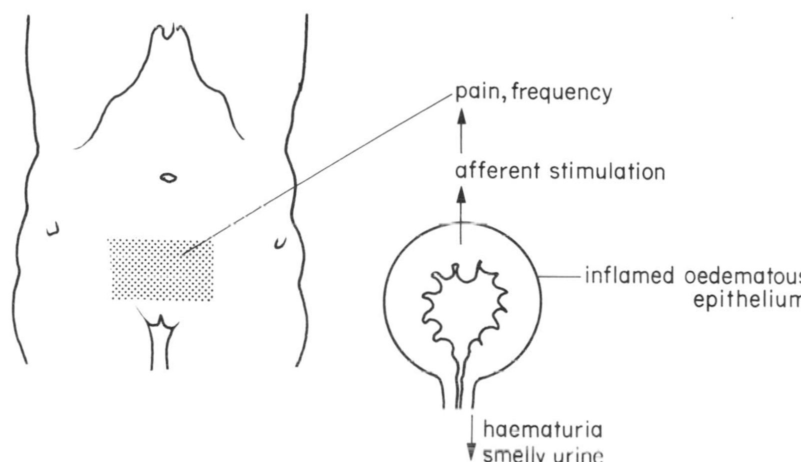

Fig. 16.1. Clinical features of cystitis.

void every few minutes, often passing blood. When the infection is confined to the bladder there may be no fever. Later, as the infection spreads up the ureters to the kidneys there is pain in the loin, fever and rigors.

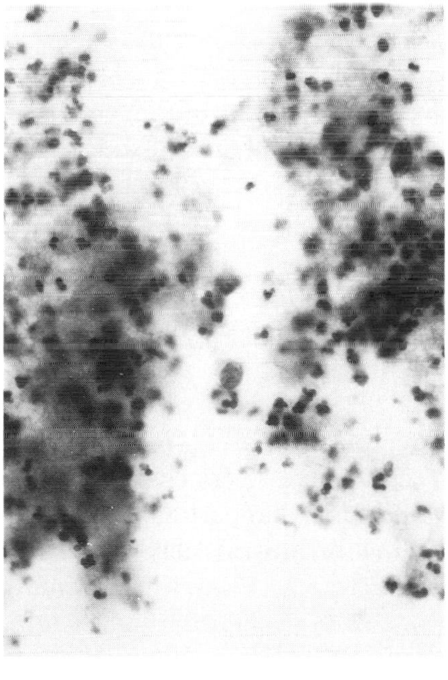

Fig. 16.2. Pus (polymorphonuclear leucocytes) in urine. (Courtesy of Dr Jo Martin, London Hospital Institute of Pathology.)

Investigations

There are seldom any physical signs apart from some tenderness in the suprapubic region. The diagnosis is made by examination of the urine. Simple inspection of the urine is a very useful test: urine that is crystal clear is seldom infected, whereas in cystitis the urine is usually turbid and has a fishy odour. Microscopy reveals many pus cells and bacteria can be seen under the high power (Fig. 16.2). The urine is cultured at once using a dip-slide, or placed in a refrigerator prior to being taken to the laboratory.

Treatment

At first one can only guess at the causative organism but when a patient has suffered many previous attacks of acute cystitis she will know which antimicrobial agent made her better, and it is a good rule to start off with the same one, pending sensitivity studies from the laboratory. Choose a safe and cheap antimicrobial, e.g. trimethoprim, nalidixic acid, a sulphonamide or nitrofurantoin. Reserve expensive, wide-spectrum antibiotics for severe cases, and use them only under microbiological control. Given promptly at the beginning of an attack, a short course — for 2 to 3 days — works as well as a long one.

It usually takes 24 hours for the antimicrobial treatment to kill the organisms and perhaps another 24 hours for the inflammation to resolve. Making the urine alkaline may make passing urine more comfortable (e.g. by giving up to 6 g sodium bicarbonate per day or a similar dose of potassium citrate). It may help to keep the urine dilute, and patients should be encouraged to drink as much fluid as possible. Alcohol may make the bladder more uncomfortable. (In Britain it is customary to give patients barley water. This is a very ancient tradition. The barley water looks like infected urine and therefore *must* do good according to the immutable Laws of Magic: at least it does no harm.)

Follow-up investigations

Acute cystitis is so very common that the doctor needs to keep a sense of balance in choosing which cases to investigate. In males, acute cystitis often signifies some underlying disorder, e.g. urinary stasis or a stone. In women, it is seldom worth investigating the first attack unless it has been accompanied by haematuria, but recurrent episodes, and all episodes in children, must be gone into. A plain KUB film to rule out a calculus is followed by an ultrasound scan of the kidneys and bladder. In patients with haematuria the urine is examined for malignant cells and when the attack has settled down, a flexible cystoscopy must be performed to rule out a bladder tumour.

One feature is always to be taken very seriously. If the specimen of urine shows pus, but no organisms have been grown in the dip-slide or the laboratory, then one must think of the other more serious causes of sterile pyuria — *tuberculosis* and *bladder cancer.*

CHRONIC CYSTITIS

Aetiology

Many patients have repeated attacks of acute cystitis often from the same intestinal organism. If the intestinal flora have been changed by a prolonged course of a broad-spectrum antibiotic, and particularly if they have been in hospital, then the invading organisms may be highly pathogenic and resistant to common antimicrobials. From time to time a patient who has undergone repeated courses of antibiotic therapy may end up with a persistent vaginal infection that is resistant to every medication, and the recurrent cystitis will only stop when all antibiotics are stopped and the normal vaginal flora is re-established.

In other patients the cystitis is not so much relapsing as persistent.

Sometimes there is a specific organism of which *Mycobacterium tuberculosis* is the most important and must never be forgotten.

The natural defences of the bladder

The bladder is like a dustbin which must be emptied regularly if it is to be kept clean (Fig. 16.3). If one tries on purpose to infect the healthy bladder with an inoculum of micro-organisms, and the patient empties the bladder regularly, it is impossible to establish an infection. Given that *Escherichia coli* takes 15 minutes to divide, it needs no great mathematician to calculate that at the end of 3 hours 10 organisms will have become > 28 000 (see p. 63). If they are now emptied out, they must start all over again. On the other hand, the patient who holds her urine for 6 hours will have accumulated > 8 million organisms and the residual inoculum may be enormous. Frequent and complete emptying of the bladder is the most important defence against infection. To ensure this, the patient must drink plenty of water. This may have the added benefit of diluting the nutrient on which the micro-organisms live.

In a healthy bladder some bacteria always cling to the urothelial cells after it has been emptied (Fig. 16.4), but these are killed off by the natural bactericidal action of the urothelium. This natural protection may be impaired in diabetes and in the disordered cells of a bladder tumour.

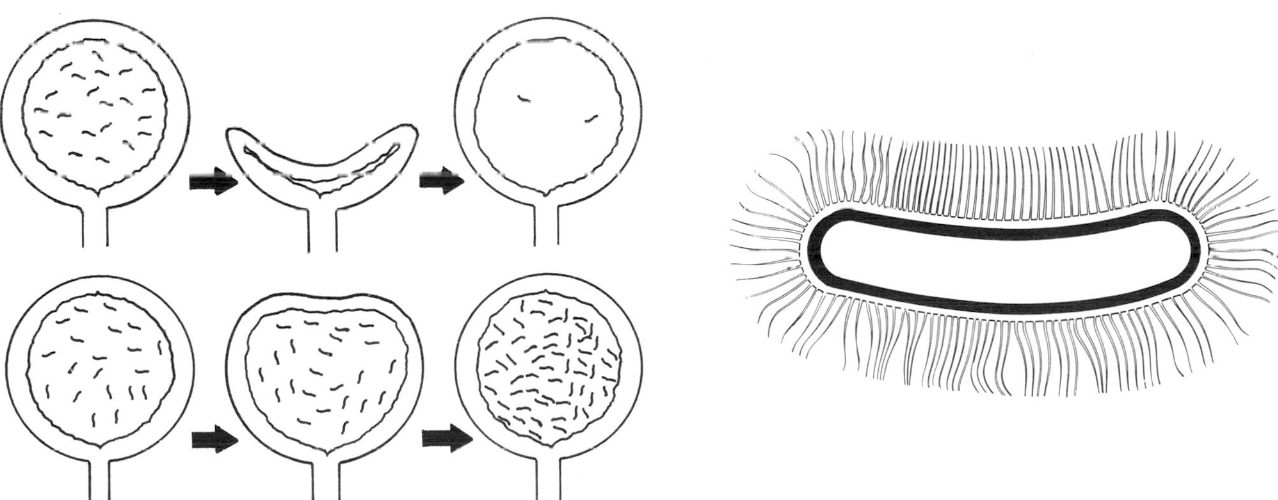

Fig. 16.3. The chief natural defence of the bladder against infection is to keep itself regularly emptied out.

Fig. 16.4. Diagram of an enterobacillus showing the 'pili' which help the bacillus to stick to urothelial cells like a hairy caterpillar.

Pathology of chronic cystitis

Cystitis follicularis

Repeated infections may give rise to chronic inflammatory changes in the mucosa of the bladder. Cystoscopy shows little pimples (*follicular cystitis*) and on biopsy these reveal collections of lymphocytes some of which are large enough and active enough to have germinal follicles.

Cystitis cystica

In severe infections the urothelium may be shed, leaving little islands of cells here and there (Fig.16.5). As the mucosa heals again these islands become buried, divide and form little cysts under the mucosa (*von Brunn's nests*). These look like little glistening bubbles under the urothelium on cystoscopy hence the term *cystitis cystica.* In most cases cystitis cystica is entirely innocent and resolves when the infection has been cured by prolonged antibiotic treatment, but in other cases if it persists the buried cysts change. They start to form mucus inside the cysts, and eventually the lining of the cysts alters to resemble the lining of the intestine — *adenomatous metaplasia* — and this, in some cases, is the precursor of an adenocarcinoma.

Malakoplakia

Another variation on this theme is *malakoplakia* where collections of lymphocytes and macrophages form large soft brownish plaques in the mucosa in response to persistent or relapsing infection. These may bleed, and they resemble carcinoma on cystoscopy.

Squamous metaplasia

Persistent infection, especially associated with a stricture in the urethra, a calculus, or infestation with *Schistosomiasis* is followed by metaplasia of the urothelium into squamous epithelium. This is a very dangerous condition and in many cases will be followed by a squamous carcinoma (see p. 184).

Alkaline encrusted cystitis

In association, as a rule with stones and persistent *Proteus* infection, chronic inflammatory changes infiltrate right into the muscular wall of

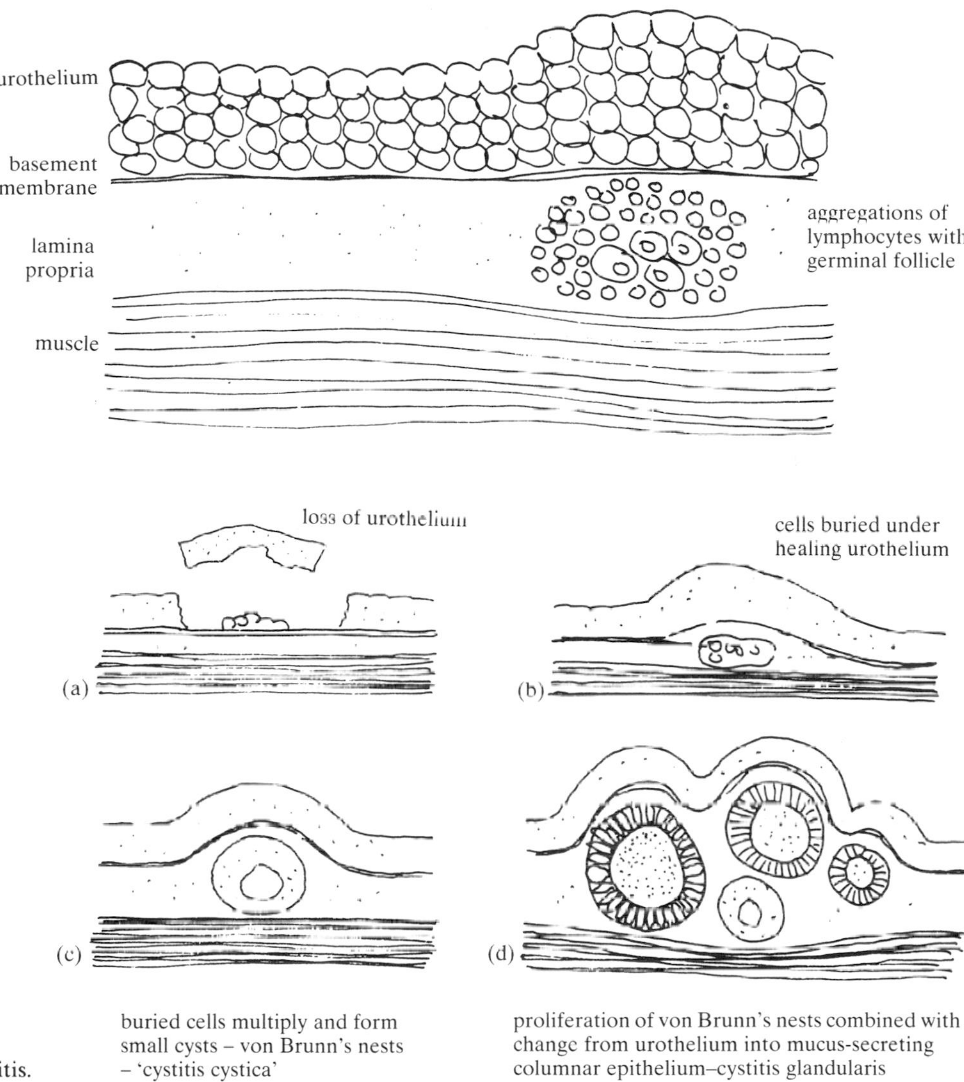

Fig. 16.5. Changes in chronic cystitis.

the bladder converting it into a stiff, rigid sphere. The wall of the bladder may become partly calcified, and on cystoscopy is found to be covered with flakes of stone. The urine smells of ammonia.

Hunner's ulcer

This is a condition with no known cause. Clinically the patient (who is usually a woman) has intense pain when the bladder is half-filled. The pain is felt in one part of the bladder. The patients have severe frequency.

On cystoscopy cracks appear in the mucosa as the bladder is filled and when emptied, they bleed. It is said that a biopsy of the mucosa will show an excess of mast cells. Every year a new remedy is proclaimed for this condition. Some patients get relief from the instillation of dimethylsulphoxide and others are relieved by overdistension of the bladder, but for some the only way to stop the pain is to remove the entire bladder and replace it with caecum — *caecocystoplasty* (see p. 76).

Investigations

Patients with chronic cystitis are investigated (a) to see if there is some specific organism and (b) some mechanical cause for the persistence of the infection. In the West, the chief specific organism to be considered is *Mycobacterium tuberculosis* and in all patients three early morning specimens of urine will be sent for Ziehl-Neelsen staining and Loewenstein-Jensen culture (see p. 74).

A plain radiograph is necessary to detect stones — a common cause of persistent infection because organisms lurk in the soft crumbly inner layers of stones and cannot be reached by antibiotics in the urine. An ultrasound scan or an IVU is performed to detect collections of stagnant urine which cannot be emptied out and so never become completely sterile. In children reflux must be excluded by a micturating cystogram (see p. 66). Cystoscopy and urethroscopy may give the diagnosis, e.g. a stricture in the urethra, a diverticulum, the changes of follicular cystitis or the rough necrotic surface of a tumour. Stones may be found that have been missed in the X-ray.

Treatment

Treatment is determined by the investigations. Tuberculosis calls for its own management (see p. 75). Carcinomas are dealt with according to their grade and stage (see pp. 184 and 186). Stagnant urine caused by outflow obstruction from prostatic disease requires prostatectomy. Diverticula may need to be removed. A hydronephrosis may require pyeloplasty. There remain a large number of patients who have none of these obvious causes for their recurrent infections. What can be done for them?

First, they must get into the habit of drinking a very large amount of fluid, and of emptying their bladder very often. A good rule is to watch the clock and make sure they go to the lavatory every 2 hours whether they want to go or not, and to drink a glass of water (or a cup of tea) each time they go.

This simple advice will cut down the number of relapses very considerably, but never completely. When their resistance is low, there will be a reinfection. Patients who have had many attacks know at once when another one is coming on. They also know which medication is likely to cure it. Rather than delay treatment until the laboratory has confirmed what the patient already knows, it is more sensible and more effective to keep the patient armed with a supply of some simple antimicrobial (e.g. trimethoprim or a sulphonamide) which she can take whenever an attack comes on. She will usually find that within 24 hours the episode has been terminated, and there is no need to continue the medication any longer.

When this simple system does not work patients may be given long-term methenamine mandelate or hippurate to reinforce their natural defences.

SCHISTOSOMIASIS

The trematode flukes *Schistosoma haematobium, mansoni* and *japonicum* belong to the order *Digenea,* flatworms whose complex life-cycles involve one stage in vertebrates and one stage in molluscs. In man there are three main species. *S. haematobium* and *mansoni* in Africa, the West Indies, north-east Brazil, southern Portugal and Spain and *S. japonicum* in China and Indo-China.

The adult flukes are about 5 mm in length and live inside human veins, attached to the endothelium by a sucker (Fig. 16.6). The male enfolds the female in a long slit down his belly, hence the name *schisto* (split) *soma* body. As they were first discovered in the portal vein of Egyptian children with portal hypertension, hepatosplenomegaly and ascites, by the great German pathologist Theodor Bilharz, then working in Cairo, the disease is rightly called *Bilharziasis.* The females continually lay eggs which have terminal spines, differing slightly in shape according to the species.

When the adult flukes happen to be living in the submucosal veins of the bladder, their eggs work their way through the urothelium causing haematuria, and provoking a granulomatous reaction which eventually causes a 'bilharzial polyp'. The calcified dead eggs can be seen to glisten like grains of sand under the mucosa of the bladder on cystoscopy. Later, ulcers are formed, the surrounding mucosa shows squamous metaplasia, and eventually a squamous-cell carcinoma develops (Fig. 16.7).

The millions of dead calcified ova outline the submucosa of the bladder (Fig. 16.8) and the lower ureters in a plain X-ray as if with a pencil. The ova are shed in the urine, hatch in slowly moving rivers or irrigation ditches and tiny *miracidia* emerge from them. The miracidia

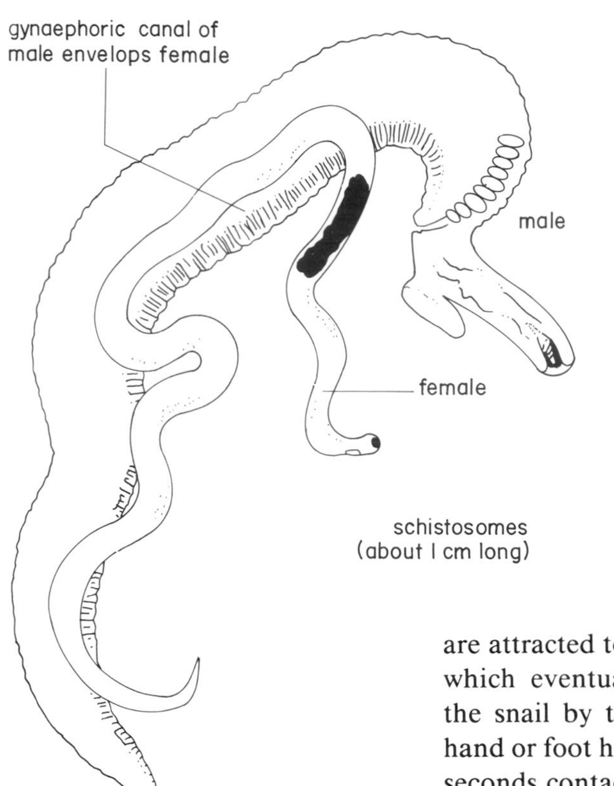

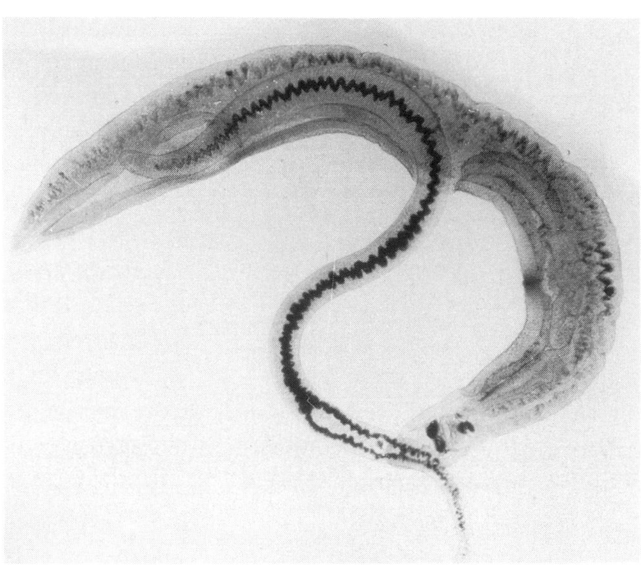

Fig. 16.6. Pair of adult Schistosome worms removed from a vein (diagram on left: photograph on right).

are attracted to fresh water snails, invade them, develop into sporocysts which eventually give rise to minute flukes *(cercariae)* which leave the snail by thousands, and penetrate the skin of any human whose hand or foot happens to be in the water at the right time. It only takes 10 seconds contact for this penetration by the cercariae to take place (Fig. 16.9).

In the skin, the cercariae can cause an itching rash — *swimmers' itch* — but they are soon carried in the lymphatics into the systemic circulation where they may give rise to a fever. They are carried all round the body, and may settle in any suitable vein, including the spinal cord and cerebral cortex. In little children masses of the flukes cause obstruction in the portal vein. Many of them infest the veins of the pelvic organs, especially the bladder, ureters and rectum, to begin the life-cycle all over again.

Schistosomiasis is one of the major scourges of mankind, second only

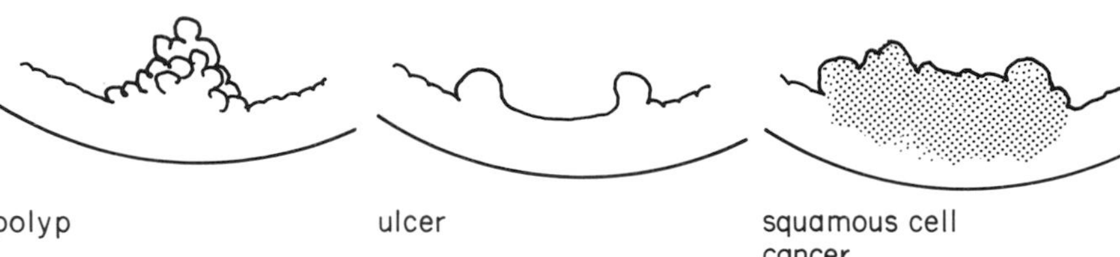

Fig. 16.7. Progress of bilharzial inflammation in the bladder.

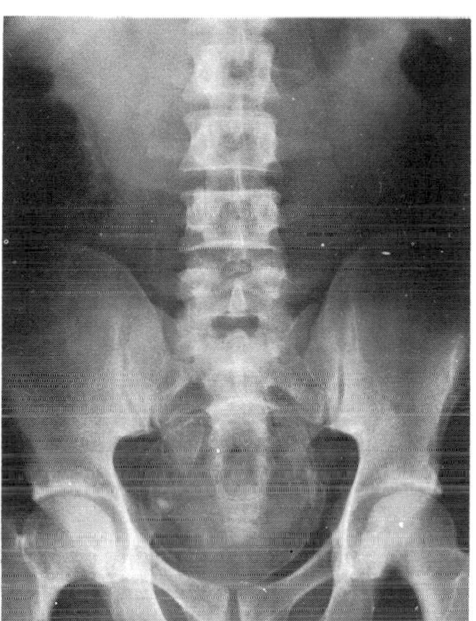

Fig. 16.8. Schistosomiasis: the bladder is outlined with calcification from the dead calcified ova of Schistosoma haematobium.

to malaria as a cause of suffering. Its eradication depends on a supply of clean water and effective disposal of urine and faeces.

Treatment

It is futile to treat infestation if the patient must return to the source of his original infection, but there is highly effective treatment with sodium or potassium antimony tartrate, niridazole, lucanthone, hycanthone and metrifonate all of which are somewhat toxic. Efficacy of treatment is judged by measuring the numbers of eggs shed in the urine.

Surgical relief of the obstruction in the ureter may require reimplantation of the ureter and treatment of secondary infection. Stones often need to be removed, and the typically dilated ureter seen in bilharziasis lends itself to the use of the ureteroscope.

The carcinoma of the bladder which occurs in bilharziasis is nearly always squamous, resistant to radiotherapy, but if treated early with radical cystectomy, carries a good outlook. Sadly, this is one form of cancer which is entirely preventable.

STONE IN THE BLADDER

Vesical calculi are common in some parts of the world, e.g. Thailand, the Yemen, and Turkey, but today they are rare in Europe except when there is outflow obstruction from the prostate. They are sometimes found on non-absorbable sutures used in pelvic surgery which have migrated into the bladder or as fragments of stone forming outside a catheter. Neglected stones may in time set up squamous metaplasia and any suspicious part of the bladder should be examined by biopsy.

Clinical features

Classically, patients with stone in the bladder have pain when they are walking about rather than when lying down: the pain radiates to the tip of the penis, and little boys with this condition constantly tug at their foreskin to try to relieve the pain (Fig. 16.10).

Investigations

The stone is easily seen in a plain radiograph (Fig. 16.11), but this should be confirmed by cystoscopy. As with all stones in the urinary tract, the routine tests for stone disease should not be omitted (see p. 86).

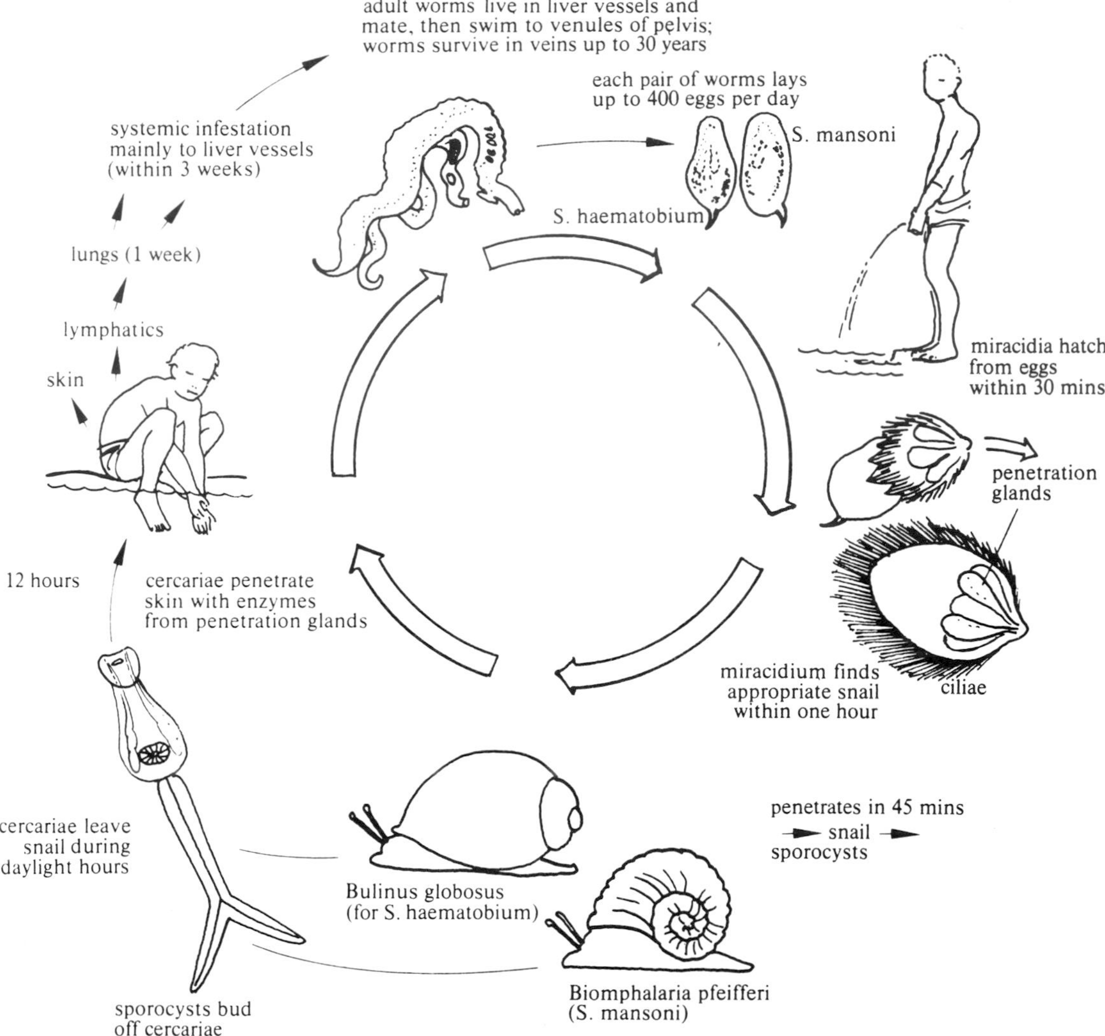

Fig. 16.9. Bilharzia life cycle.

Treatment

Stones in the bladder are crushed with the classical lithotrite — *litholapaxy* (see p. 98). Surgeons inexpert in its use may prefer a modern ultrasonic or electrohydraulic lithotriptor, but they take a good deal longer and are less reliable. Stones which are too large to be encompassed by the jaws of the classical lithotrite, and stones in little boys whose urethras may be damaged by the instrument, are removed by suprapubic lithotomy (Fig. 16.12).

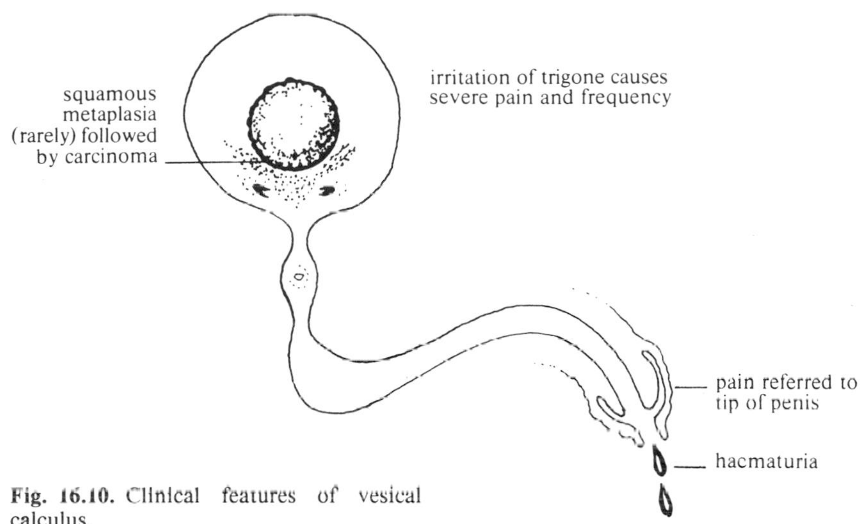

Fig. 16.10. Clinical features of vesical calculus.

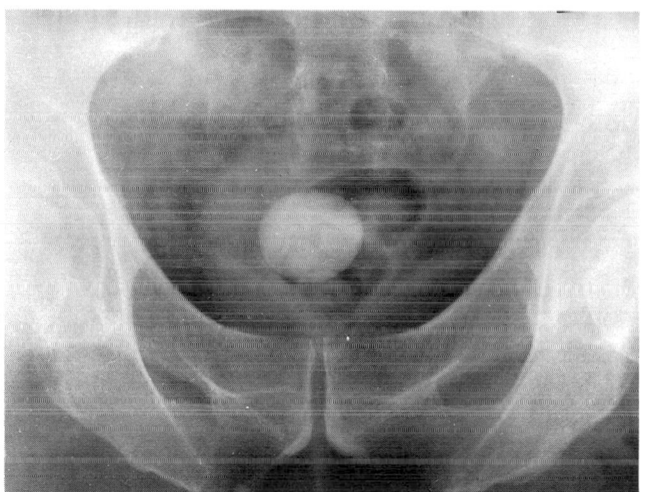

Fig. 16.11. Vesical stone.

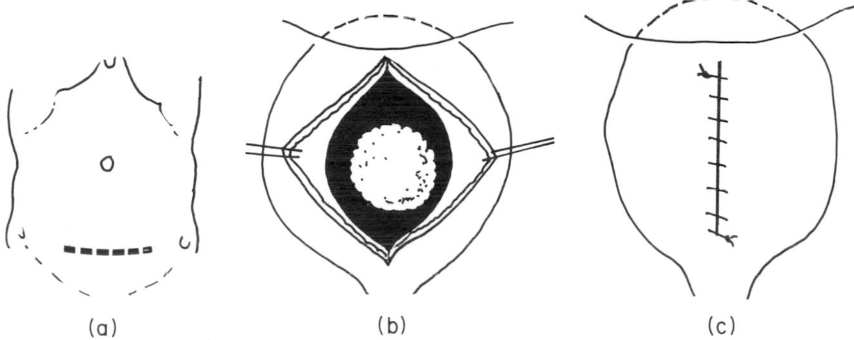

Fig. 16.12. Suprapubic lithotomy. Through a Pfannenstiel incision (a) the bladder is opened between stay sutures (b) and the stone removed. The bladder is closed with catgut (c).

FURTHER READING

Cronberg S, Welin C-O, Henricksson L, Hellsten S, Persson KM-S & Stenberg P (1987) Prevention of recurrent acute cystitis by methenamine hippurate: double blind controlled crossover long term study. *British Medical Journal* **294**, 1507–8.

Levison DA (1985) Pathology of urinary tract infections. In: Whitfield HN & Hendry WF (Eds) *Textbook of Genitourinary Surgery*. Churchill Livingstone, Edinburgh. pp. 469–76.

Parivar F & Bradbrook RA (1986) Review: interstitial cystitis. *British Journal of Urology* **58**, 239–44.

17 The Bladder — Neoplasms

The bladder is lined by urothelium and its neoplasms are usually urothelial (transitional cell carcinomas) but urothelium may undergo metaplasia into squamous or glandular epithelium which gives rise to squamous-cell or adeno- carcinoma. Very rarely, neurofibroma, sarcoma and even phaeochromocytoma is seen in the bladder. Secondary carcinoma may occur by direct invasion from a primary tumour in the colon, rectum or uterus.

CARCINOMA OF THE UROTHELIUM

Aetiology

In 1894 Rehn noticed that workers in the aniline dye industry were developing an undue proportion of cancer of the bladder. Investigations showed that it was neither aniline nor the finished dyestuffs that caused the trouble, but a group of nitrophenols (Fig. 17.1) of which the most dangerous were 2-naphthylamine and benzidine. Industries using these and similar compounds included chemical works, dyeing, rubber moulding, cable covering, pitch, gasworks, the optical industry (where pitch was used to hold the lenses steady for grinding and polishing), hairdressing, nursing, leather work, and medical practice. In the upper tract, analgesic abuse and Balkan nephropathy were implicated (see p. 68). Smoking is certainly a contributory factor — year by year the list of known or suspected hazards grows longer. Relatively few patients are notified as suffering from a prescribed industrial disease, largely because it may take some 20 years or more between exposure to a carcinogen and the development of bladder cancer in which time records are lost and memories fade. Epidemiologists toiling in this field of research keep

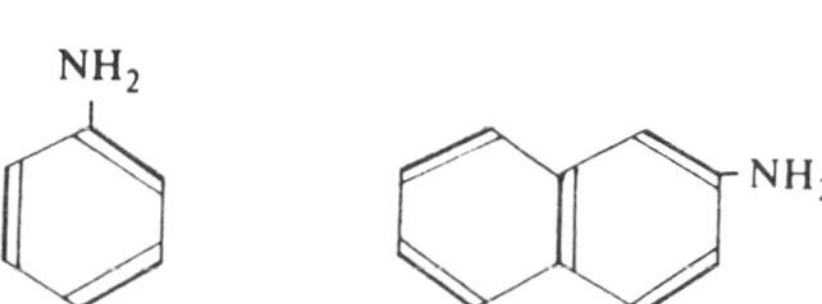

Fig. 17.1. Structural formulae of some carcinogens.

closing stable doors from which the horses have long since bolted. World-wide, the main cause of bladder cancer is schistosomiasis (see p. 177) where prolonged irritation from living and dead ova gives rise to squamous metaplasia and squamous cancer.

Pathology

Macroscopic features

Bladder tumours may be single or multiple. On cystoscopic examination they take the form of a (papillary) cauliflower, a solid lump or an ulcer (Fig. 17.2).

Microscopic features

Papilloma is a term which should hardly ever be used: one ought to say carcinoma. Truly benign papillomas in the bladder are so rare (less than 1%) that the diagnosis should always be questioned and a second opinion on the section always obtained. Even so the patient should be strictly followed up.

Grades

There are three grades of malignancy, G1, G2, G3, where G3 is the worst and G1 the most well-differentiated (Fig. 17.3).

Squamous carcinoma

Some squamous metaplasia is a common feature of G3 tumours of the bladder (and is of importance since it denotes resistance to radiation treatment, see below). But in true squamous carcinoma there is a thick layer of keratinized 'skin' over the tumour with epithelial pearls.

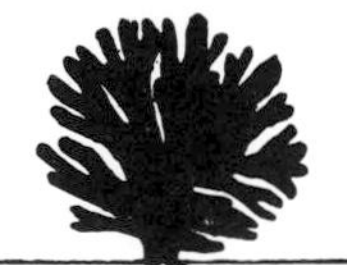

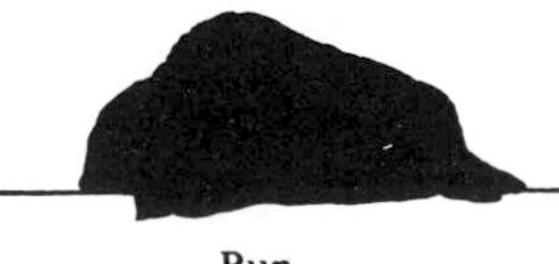

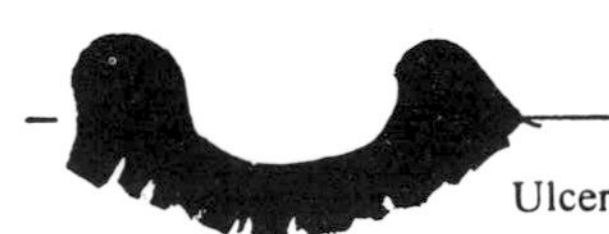

Fig. 17.2. Macroscopic features of bladder cancer.

(a)

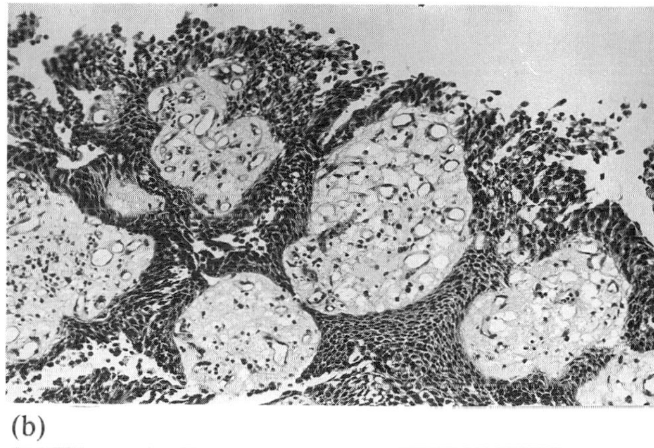

(b)

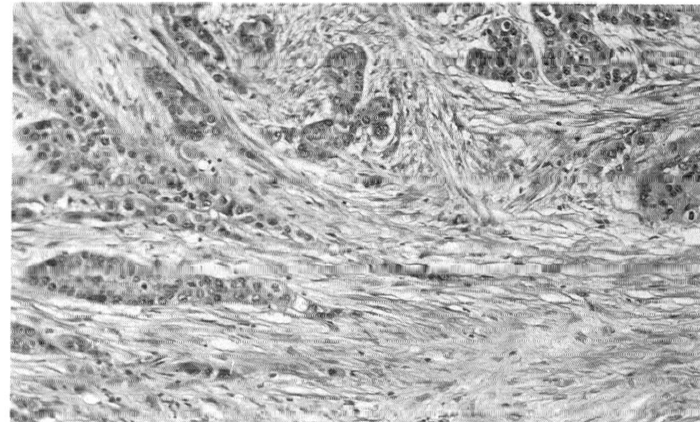

(c)

Fig. 17.3. (a) G1 well-differentiated papillary tumour of bladder. (b) G2 superficial papillar tumour of intermediate differentiation. (c) G3 undifferentiated tumour showing invasion into the muscle.

Adenocarcinoma

Glandular metaplasia occurs in chronic infection (see p. 174) and in time may proceed to the formation of an adenocarcinoma. Other types of adenocarcinoma occur in the vestige of the urachus (which is lined by columnar epithelium).

Spread of bladder cancer

Direct spread

Bladder cancer spreads by direct invasion through the wall of the bladder, through the fat that surrounds it, and into adjacent organs such as the colon, prostate and uterus. Curiously, bladder cancer never crosses Denonvilliers' fascia — the double fold of peritoneum which stands like a fire-resisting door between rectum and bladder, although even more curiously this barrier only works one way — it does not stop a carcinoma that arises in the rectum from invading the bladder.

Implantation

Bladder cancer may be seeded into the urethra, and possibly onto other parts of the bladder by direct contact.

Lymphatic spread

There are few lymphatics immediately under the mucosa of the bladder but its muscular wall has a rich network, and once a bladder cancer has penetrated into the muscle it quickly reaches the local lymph nodes in the pelvis.

Systemic spread

Distant metastases to the lungs, liver or brain are seen from time to time even with apparently early carcinomas of the bladder, but this is very uncommon when compared with direct invasion and lymphatic involvement.

Staging of bladder cancer

The TNM (tumour, nodes, metastases) is an International System of staging which allows different centres to compare their results. The details of the staging system change with better methods of detecting tumour spread. As a rule, when a guess has been made at the depth of invasion, the stage is denoted by the prefix T. Thus a tumour which was thought by palpation to have just begun to invade the bladder muscle would be T2 (see Fig. 17.4). If this clinical suspicion was supported by a deep biopsy the added prefix would be p, i.e. pT2. If the entire bladder had been removed, and the pathologist was provided with the cystectomy specimen, the prefix is P, i.e. P2.

To assign an N stage (lymph nodes) is difficult unless the lymph nodes have all been removed by radical cystectomy: but today the CT scan may reveal lymph nodes and these can be sampled by fine needle biopsy.

One pitfall to beware of is comparing the result of treatment of series that have been staged by cystectomy (P2, P3 etc.) with those staged only by biopsy (pT2, pT3). Very often this simple precaution is forgotten.

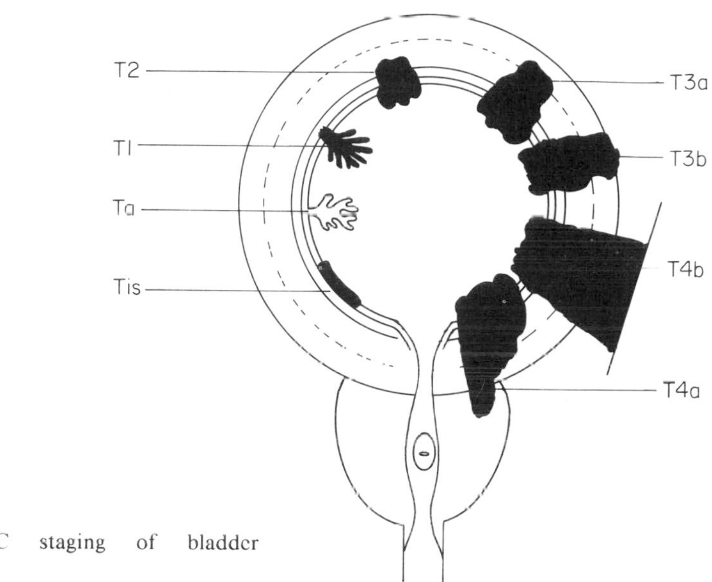

Fig. 17.4. UICC staging of bladder cancers.

Screening of symptomless patients

Patients thought to be at risk (e.g. in the chemical industry) can be screened by searching their urine for malignant cells using the Papanicolaou method (see p. 13). It is difficult to identify malignant cells when they are autolysed, so it is important not to use early morning urine which may have been in the bladder for 8 hours, and to fix all specimens at once by adding a roughly equal volume of 10% formalin solution. The specimen is then sent to the laboratory to be centrifuged, fixed and stained (Fig. 17.5). The diagnosis of cancer depends on the recognition of a huge nucleus in the cell and relatively little cytoplasm, so cells from a well-differentiated (G1) tumour are not distinguishable from normal transitional epithelium unless by chance an entire broken-off frond is found in the smear. *Flow cytometry* is a more sophisticated mechanized method (Fig. 17.6) of measuring the nuclear/cytoplasm ratio in large numbers of cells and avoiding the observer error which so easily arises from boredom when large numbers of urine samples have to be screened, most of which will be normal.

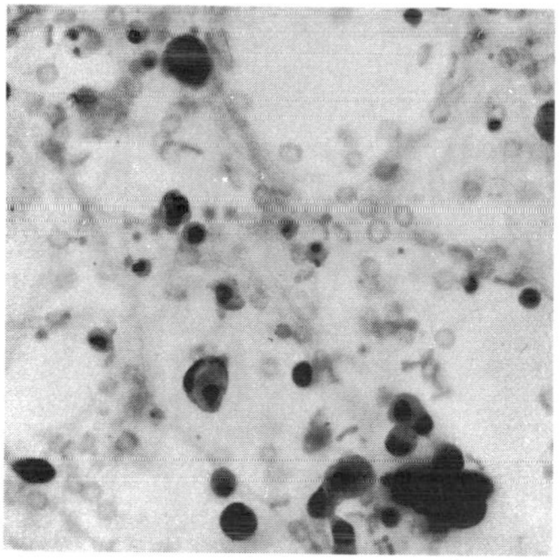

Fig. 17.5. Malignant cells found in the centrifuged urine.

Symptoms

Haematuria is noticed by 80% of patients with bladder cancer (Fig. 17.7) and this is the cardinal reason why every patient with haematuria must be cystoscoped. Equally important is to note that 20% of people with

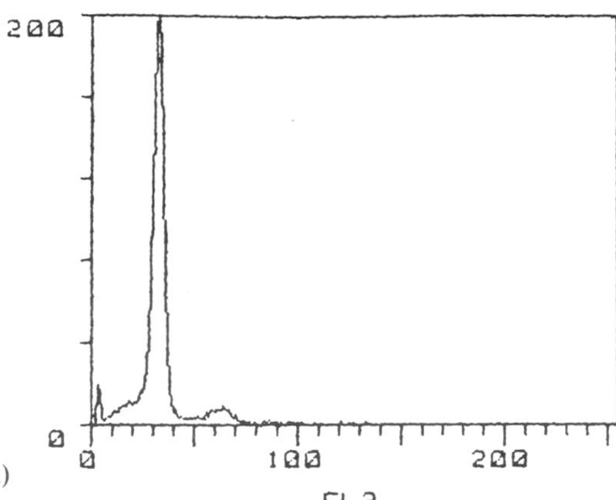

Fig. 17.6. Flow cytometry. DNA histogram of mainly diploid tumour (main peak) with smaller tetraploid peak on the right.

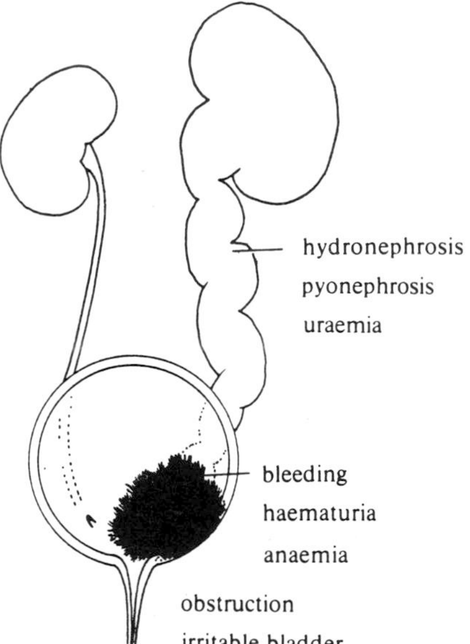

Fig. 17.7. Clinical features of bladder carcinoma.

bladder cancer have *not* had haematuria: in a way their symptoms are even more important.

A bladder cancer irritates the surrounding urothelium making it red and oedematous: the afferent limb of the micturition reflex is overstimulated and the patient has *frequency*, and sometimes also *pain* on voiding. It is easy to jump to the conclusion that they have cystitis. The give-away is the absence of micro-organisms from the urine combined with many cells (cancer cells look very like pus under the ordinary microscope). *Sterile pyuria = cancer or tuberculosis until proved otherwise.*

In elderly men in whom most bladder cancers are seen, irritability of the bladder may suggest prostatic outflow obstruction (see p. 219). To avoid this error the urine is always carefully tested for blood and sent for Papanicolaou staining, and before any operation on the prostate the bladder is always meticulously inspected with the cystoscope.

Other symptoms may bring the patient with a bladder cancer to the doctor — but they are late. *Pain* — a boring, unremitting pain radiating to the perineum and sacrum, signifies extension of cancer outside the bladder. *Anaemia* out of all proportion to the size of the tumour, from long continued loss of blood in haematuria, may drastically reduce the haemoglobin and even bring the patient to hospital with angina pectoris. Finally, any *urinary infection* occurring for no obvious reason in an elderly man should be regarded with suspicion: infection often starts in the necrotic superficial part of a solid tumour.

Physical signs

These are usually absent, but in tumours arising from the urachus there is nearly always an obvious hard mass between the umbilicus and the

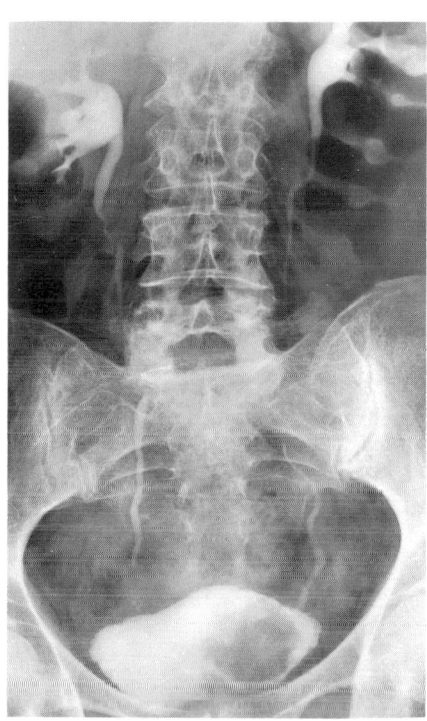

Fig. 17.8. Excretion urogram from a 68 year old man with a three month history of haematuria. Note the large filling defect in the left half of the bladder. The ureter is not obstructed. This was found to be a G2pT1 carcinoma and was treated by transurethral resection.

symphysis, and a similar mass is all too common in advanced cases, particularly those found with schistosomiasis. Rectal examination may detect a mass that cannot be felt in the abdomen.

Investigations

Haematuria = IVU + cystoscopy. This is the first equation every urologist must learn: to it one may add a measurement of the plasma creatinine, haemoglobin, a urine culture and urinary cytology.

The IVU often shows a filling defect in the bladder (Fig. 17.8). If a ureter is obstructed it means the muscle near the ureteric orifice has been invaded and hence the growth is T2 or worse.

Cystoscopy

Today the flexible cystoscope is used in the routine diagnosis of patients with haematuria because it is painless and does not require admission to hospital even for a day. However, if a tumour has been seen in the urogram, or is found on flexible cystoscopy, the next stage is to carry out a cystoscopy under general anaesthesia in order to establish the TNM Grade and Stage of the tumour.

Grade requires a biopsy using the resectoscope (Fig. 17.9) or cup forceps (Fig. 17.10). To establish the pT stage the biopsy must include

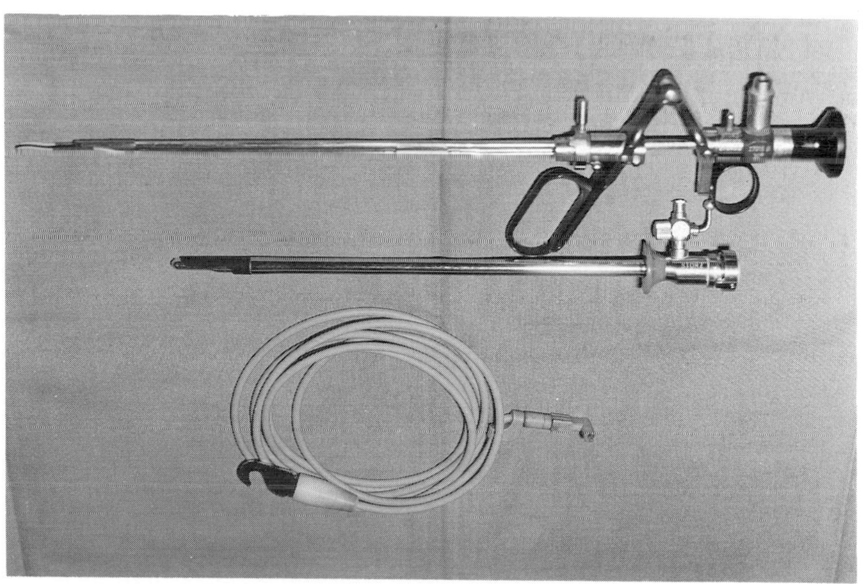

Fig. 17.9. Resectoscope.

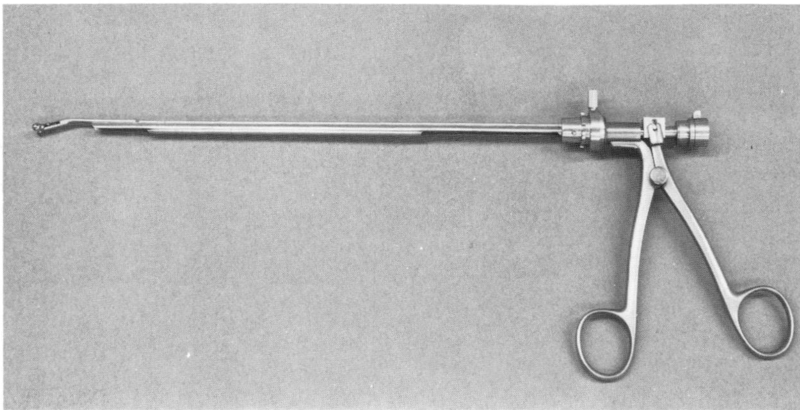

Fig. 17.10. Cup forceps.

muscle from the wall of the bladder (Fig. 17.11). This is supplemented by bimanual palpation after the resection of the tumour, to try and guess whether there is still induration remaining in the bladder wall which would suggest deep invasion, i.e. T3.

Treatment of bladder cancer

Carcinoma in situ (G3 pTIS)

This is fortunately a rare entity which presents as 'cystitis' in middle-aged men, usually heavy smokers, and usually without haematuria. Anaplastic cells are found in the urine on Papanicolaou staining. The bladder looks normal or slightly inflamed on cystoscopy (Fig. 17.12). A biopsy shows that the urothelium has become jumbled up, and many mitoses are visible. This condition responds to several intravesical agents notably BCG (see below) and mitomycin. It also responds to a single course of intravenous cyclophosphamide, but if missed, it is likely to develop into lethal invasive cancer within months.

Ta and T1

The majority of these tumours arise as pretty little pink raspberries, often multiple (Fig. 17.13). Most of them are G1 — well differentiated, and for many years they were all called *papilloma* and treated by diathermy as if they were really benign. They are not: they have to be treated with great respect. If the basement membrane is broken through (i.e. T1) invasion, spread, and distant metastases are all possible and every patient is

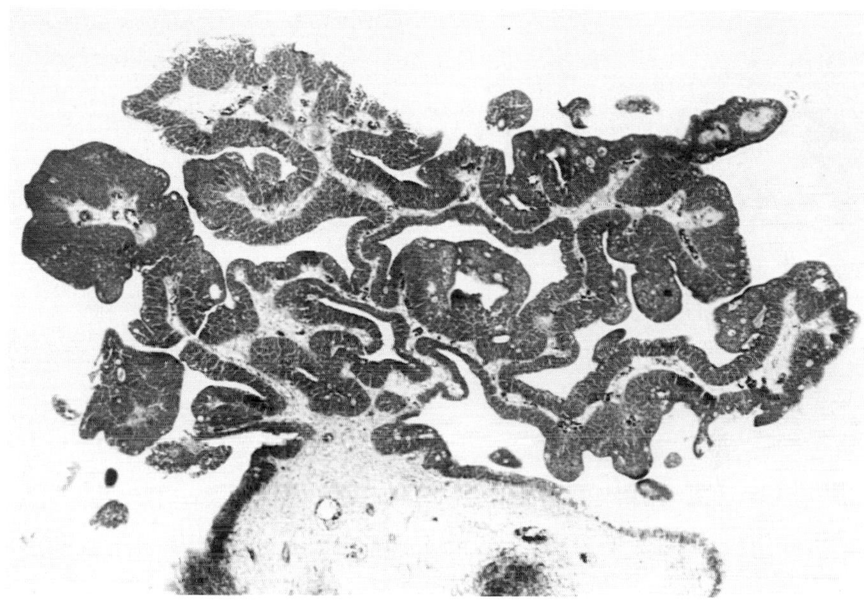

Fig. 17.11. Biopsy taken with cup forceps showing muscle in base of biopsy.

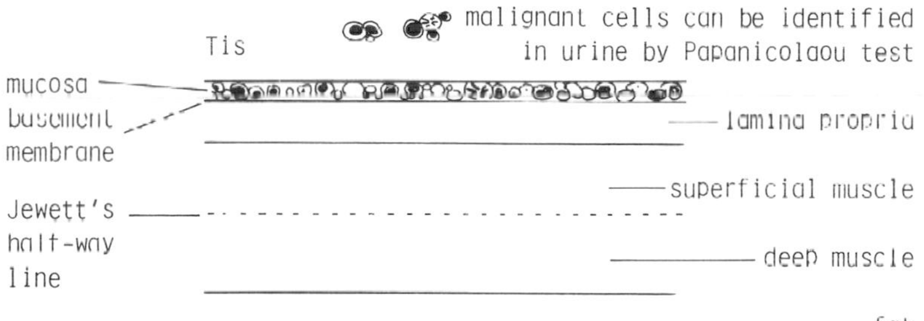

Fig. 17.12. Tis carcinoma of the bladder—'flat *in situ*' or 'malignant cystitis'.

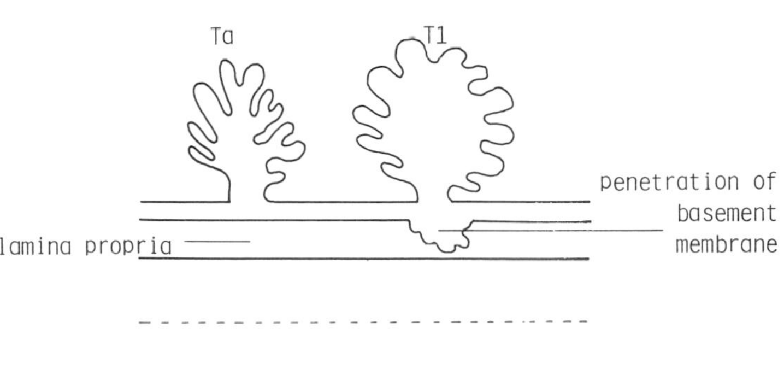

Fig. 17.13. Ta and Tl carcinoma of the bladder. In Ta there is no break-through of the basement membrane into the lamina propria. Unfortunately this is a very rare tumour and Tl is more common.

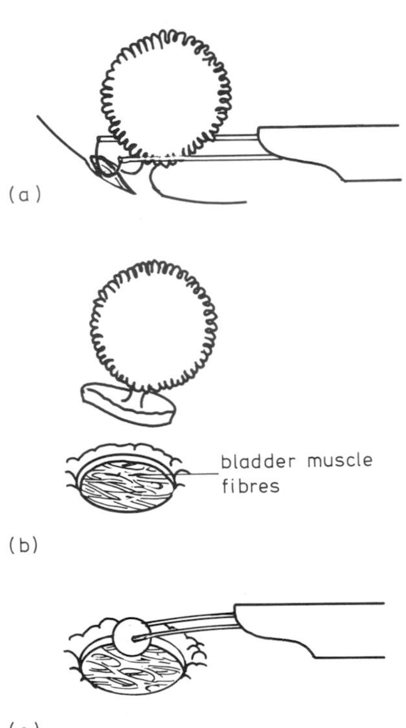

Fig. 17.14. Transurethral resection of a small bladder tumour.

followed up by regular cystoscopy. The initial treatment is by *transurethral resection* using the resectoscope.

Transurethral Resection of a Bladder Tumour (TURBT). When a large tumour has been seen on the IVU or flexible cystoscope it is necessary to be prepared for a considerable loss of blood and these patients must have their blood group determined and blood ready at short notice. These tumours look like a stumpy bush, whose trunk cannot at first be seen. The resectoscope is used to cut away enough of the protruding bush of the tumour to afford a view of the base (Fig. 17.14). This can often be very bloody because it is only when the base has been exposed, that the large feeding vessels can be thoroughly coagulated in the stalk of the tumour. Once this is achieved the resection of the rest of the bush is relatively bloodless (Fig. 17.15). In bulky tumours the pieces resected from the bush are sent to the laboratory in a separate pot from the stalk, so that the pathologist can determine its stage — i.e. how far the growth has penetrated the muscle of the bladder wall. Resecting these bladder tumours can be very time-consuming and difficult, and calls for more skill and experience than is needed for resection of a prostate (see p. 226). The postoperative management and complications are very similar.

Once the larger tumours have been resected, smaller ones are coagulated with the diathermy ball (Fig. 17.16), or the neodymium YAG laser (Fig. 17.17).

Adjuvant chemotherapy. In patients whose tumours keep on recurring, intravesical chemotherapy is given using thiotepa, mitomycin, or adriamycin, which all have the very definite beneficial effect of reducing the

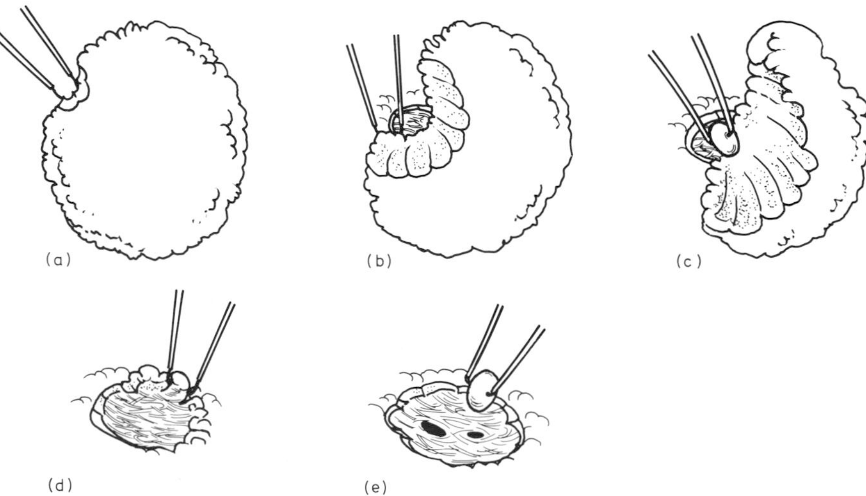

Fig. 17.15. Transurethral resection of a larger tumour: the 'bush' is taken in the first stage (a,b,c) and the 'stalk' in the second (d). The stalk is then coagulated with the rolyball electrode (e).

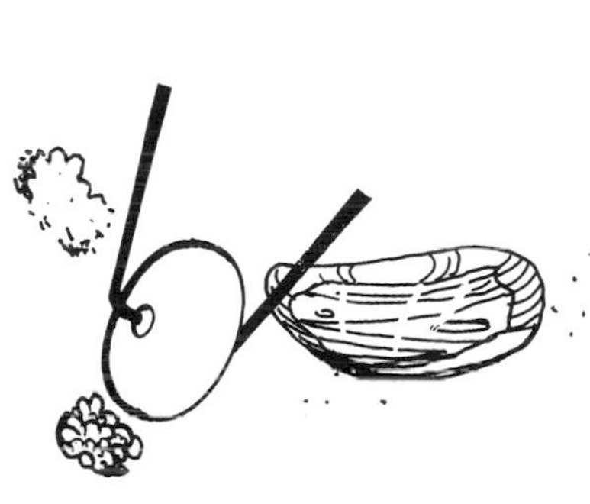

Fig. 17.16. A very small papillary tumour is coagulated with the roly-ball electrode of the resectoscope. The coagulation extends into the wall of the bladder around the stalk of the tumour.

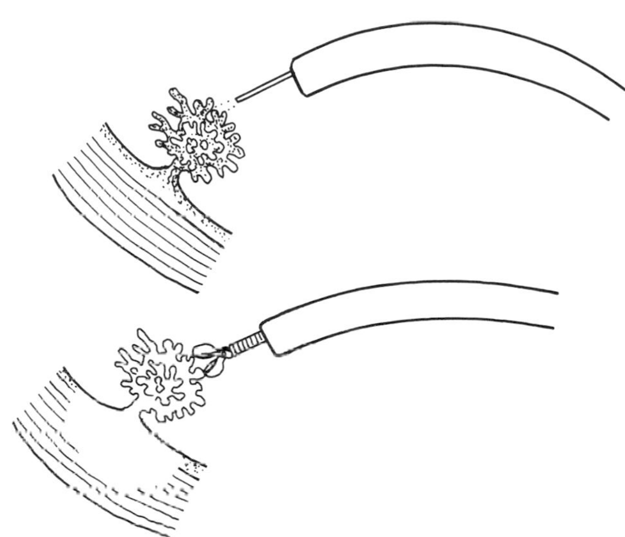

Fig. 17.17. Small papillary tumours may be coagulated with the Neodymium YAG laser passed down a flexible quartz fibre using a flexible cystoscope. A similar depth of coagulation is reached. The tumour turns white but does not disintegrate as it does with diathermy coagulation and its histological features remain virtually unchanged so that a biopsy can be taken after coagulation.

numbers of recurrences, but all have their own side-effects. More recently, *immunotherapy* has been introduced, using various strains of BCG. The effect of this is of great interest: it can produce a complete and apparently permanent clearance of the bladder tumours which endures for several years, but it does cause painful cystitis, which is occasionally so severe as to call for treatment with antituberculous drugs, and may lead to such contraction of the bladder that cystectomy and urinary diversion is necessary.

Although most of these superficial tumours are G1, a small number are G3, and these are very dangerous. Treated by cystoscopic treatment in the usual way, they soon recur and spread deeply into the muscle. Today these are treated (in the writer's department) as if they had already invaded the muscle, i.e. by radical radiotherapy.

T2 and T3 tumours

Nearly all of these are G3, a few being G2. The distinction between T2 (Fig. 17.18) and T3 (Fig. 17.19) is somewhat artificial, being based on the concept of a half-way in the bladder muscle. This half-way line is difficult to find in the cystectomy specimen and impossible to guess at from a biopsy specimen, but by convention the stage pT2 is assigned to

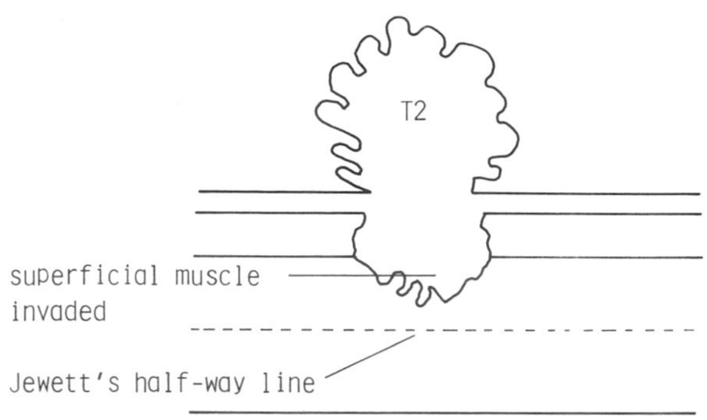

Fig. 17.18. T2 tumour of bladder, where there is invasion of the muscle but not more than half-way through the bladder wall.

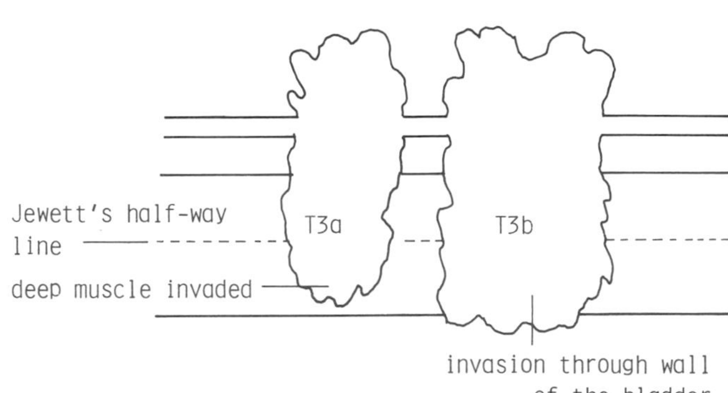

Fig. 17.19. T3 tumours of the bladder. In T3a the tumour is into the deep muscle; in T3b it has reached the outside of the bladder wall.

those in whom no induration can be felt after the surgeon has finished resecting the tumour. The subsequent survival of the patients does in fact suggest that the T3 tumours do slightly less well than the T2 — but the distinction is unimportant compared with the huge worsening in survival that follows invasion of muscle.

There are three main methods of treatment of invasive bladder cancer, and nobody knows which is the best, or how best to combine them: *total cystectomy, radiotherapy, and combination chemotherapy.*

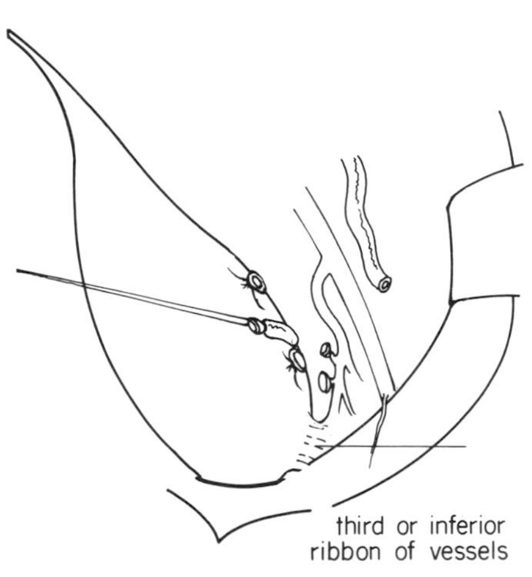

Fig. 17.20. Total cystectomy: three main vascular pedicles must be divided in order to liberate the bladdder.

Total cystectomy. In patients who are relatively fit, the operation of total cystectomy has certain advantages. It gives true P staging, and if combined with radical node dissection, an exact measure of N status. Most surgeons exclude cases with positive lymph nodes (N1) from their results. If no radiotherapy has been used, it is possible to fashion a continent reservoir (see below) for the patient, and in certain well-selected cases it is possible to preserve the nerve supply to the penis so that the patient retains his potency (Fig. 17.20).

Radiotherapy. In almost exactly 50% of patients with these G3 muscle-invasive tumours, the cancer will disappear completely after a course of 5500 cGray delivered with the linear accelerator. Until recently there was no way of discovering which tumour was radiosensitive and which was not: recent observations suggest that the presence of squamous metaplasia and of beta-HCG in the biopsy means that the tumour will be insensitive to radiotherapy — findings awaiting confirmation at the time of writing. It has therefore been customary in most UK hospitals to try radiotherapy first, and to remove the bladder only when the tumour persists or fails to go away completely. This policy, of *radiation* and *salvage cystectomy* has been much criticized by the advocates of early radical cystectomy, and in the debate it has become customary to ignore the important differences in staging — pT (without knowledge of N) versus cystectomy P and N.

Combination chemotherapy. By using various combinations of chemotherapy, details of which change almost monthly — it is possible to get 'complete remission' in from 40 to 60% of cases. These combinations of chemotherapeutic agents are all very toxic, and involve the patient in loss of hair and some risk of sepsis because of bone marrow suppression. So far most centres have been cautious in their use of these regimens, reserving them for patients who refuse, or are refused cystectomy, or as an adjuvant designed to destroy distant micrometastases before or after removing the bladder.

Total cystectomy

Preoperative preparations

The bowel is prepared by a high fluid intake and antibiotics. Anaemia is corrected by appropriate transfusion and smoking is forbidden for as long as possible to minimize chest infection. Six units of blood should be set aside. The site for the ileal conduit is carefully selected and marked before the patient goes to the operating theatre.

Incision

With the patient supine or in the cystoscopy position giving access to the perineum, a long midline incision is made, and the caecum and terminal ileum are mobilized to display the bifurcation of the aorta. The lymph nodes are then dissected off the aorta, common and internal iliac vessels and swept medially, first on one side and then on the other. The bladder is supplied by a series of vessels springing off the internal iliac artery and these are divided between clips or ligatures one after the other. The ureters are divided about 5 cm away from the bladder.

When there have been multiple tumours, the urethra is removed in continuity with the bladder and prostate to prevent urethral recurrences (Fig. 17.21).

Urinary diversion after cystectomy

Ureterosigmoidostomy was for many years the standard urinary diversion (Fig. 17.22). The ureters were led through a long submucosal tunnel in the wall of the sigmoid to prevent leakage of urine and reflux of urine and faeces from the sigmoid back up to the kidneys (Fig. 17.23). This was not always successful, and recurrent urinary infections led to scarring and renal failure. The absorption of urine from the bowel also led to renal tubular failure and hyperchloraemic acidosis. It was and still is a useful technique in parts of the world where adhesive appliances are either unavailable, or cannot be made to stick onto the skin because of tropical heat. It has been given up in the United Kingdom largely because the ureters so often failed to heal onto the bowel after irradiation.

In most patients, and always when preoperative irradiation has been given, the ureters are anastomosed to one end of an isolated loop of ileum (Fig. 17.24) to form an *ileal conduit* — Bricker's operation (Fig. 17.25). The other end is led onto the skin where the urine is collected into an adhesive appliance (Fig. 17.26). Great care is taken to choose the site for this urinary stoma: it must not rub against the belt, or lie in a scar or skin crease, or else the adhesive will not stick.

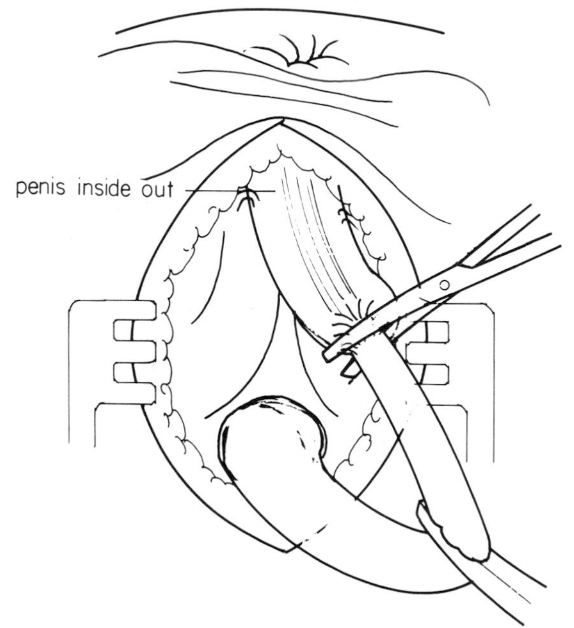

Fig. 17.21. Urethrectomy in continuity with the bladder through a midline incision in the perineum.

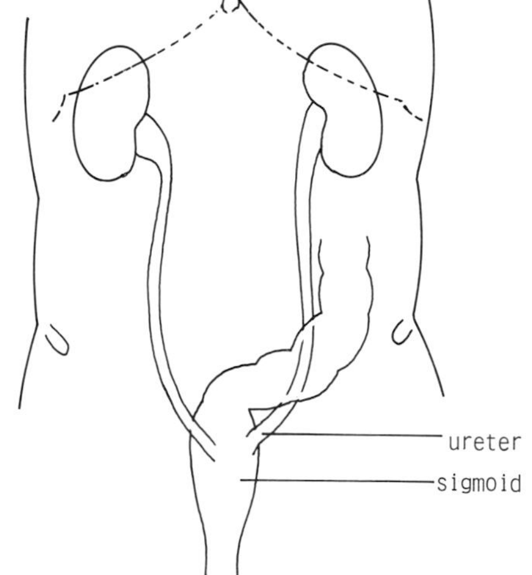

Fig. 17.22. Ureterosigmoidostomy.

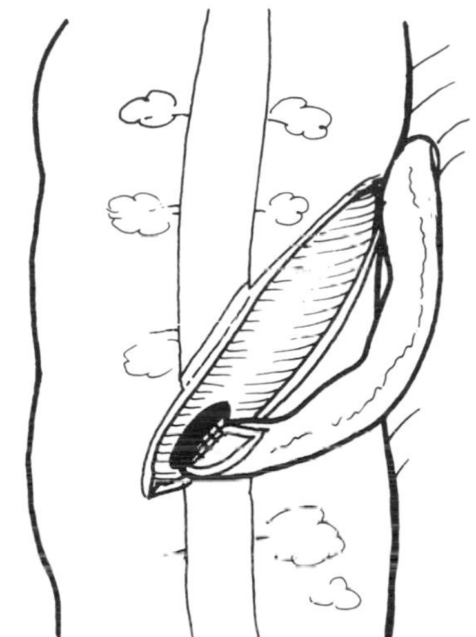

Fig. 17.23. Ureterosigmoidostomy.

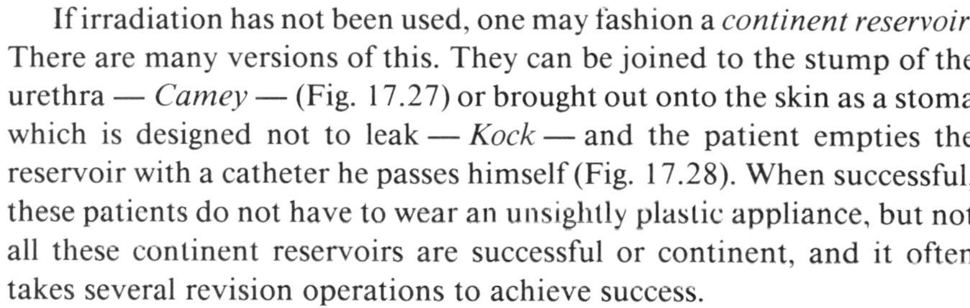

If irradiation has not been used, one may fashion a *continent reservoir*. There are many versions of this. They can be joined to the stump of the urethra — *Camey* — (Fig. 17.27) or brought out onto the skin as a stoma which is designed not to leak — *Kock* — and the patient empties the reservoir with a catheter he passes himself (Fig. 17.28). When successful, these patients do not have to wear an unsightly plastic appliance, but not all these continent reservoirs are successful or continent, and it often takes several revision operations to achieve success.

One of the most interesting forms of diversion has been devised for the special problem of the squamous cell cancer that occurs after bilharziasis where the ureters are dilated, and the poor patient is unable to obtain or to wear adhesive appliances. In this *Ghoneim* and *Kock* reservoir (Fig. 17.29) the sigmoid is invaginated like an intussusceptum and the ureters led down the gap which forms a valve that not only prevents reflux of urine up the ureters to the kidneys but also to the rest of the colon (and so limits the surface area across which urine can be absorbed and prevents acidosis). But this intussuscepted sigmoid is too small to act as an effective reservoir, so a large patch made from terminal ileum is added onto it. The patient is continent because of his anal sphincter, and the early results suggest that he avoids the well-documented disadvantages of ureterosigmoidostomy.

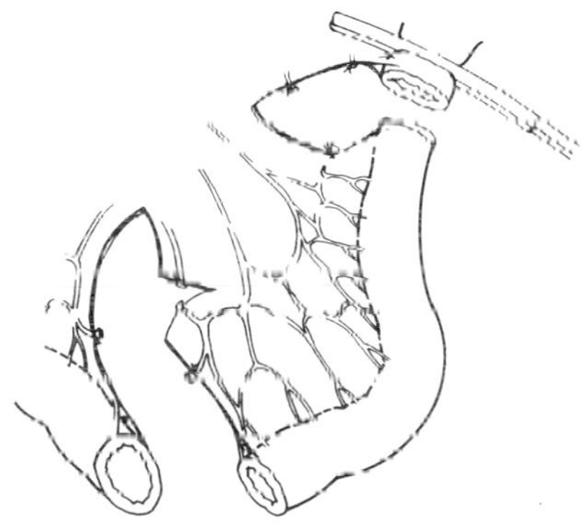

Fig. 17.24. Preparation of an isolated ileal loop. The small bowel continuity is restored by end-to-end anastomosis.

Complications of total cystectomy

This is a very severe and dangerous operation, and the patient needs the utmost in postoperative nursing and medical care. Ileus persists for up to 10 days, during which time the bowel must be kept deflated by a nasogastric tube, or preferably a gastrostomy. Especially after radiotherapy there is a risk of dehiscence of the anastomosis at the site where the isolated segment of ileum was removed to make a conduit, and for the

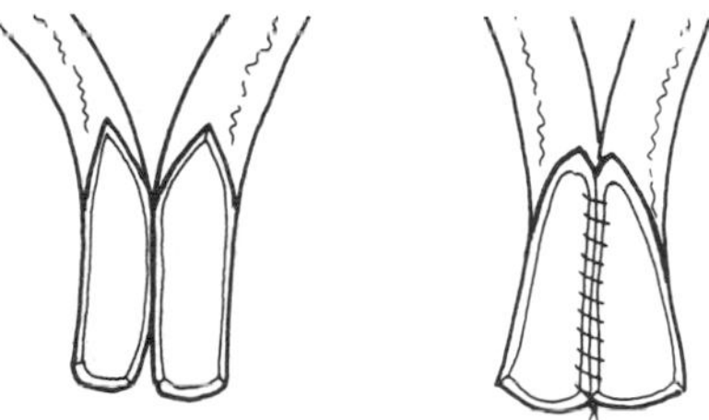

Fig. 17.25. The ureters are spatulated, sewn side to side, and both joined on to the open end of the ileal loop by Wallace's method over suitable splints.

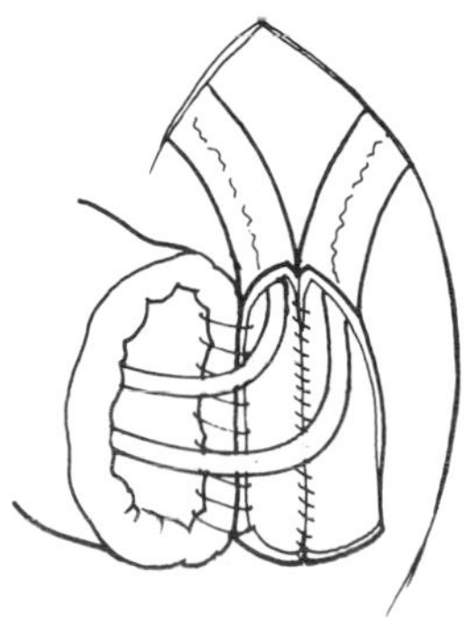

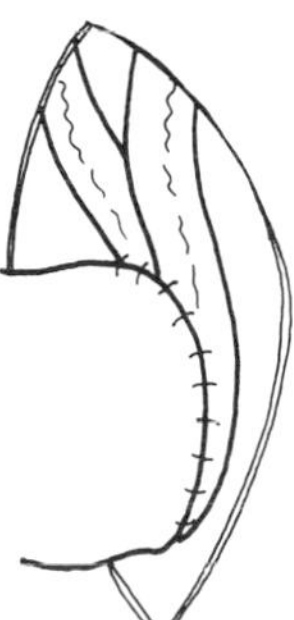

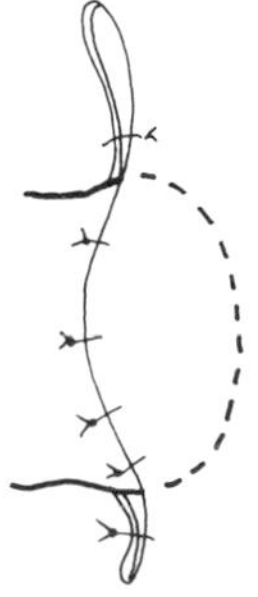

same reason there may be urinary leakage from the anastomosis between ureters and bowel. Wound infection, pulmonary complications, and deep venous thrombosis all add to the hazards of this operation.

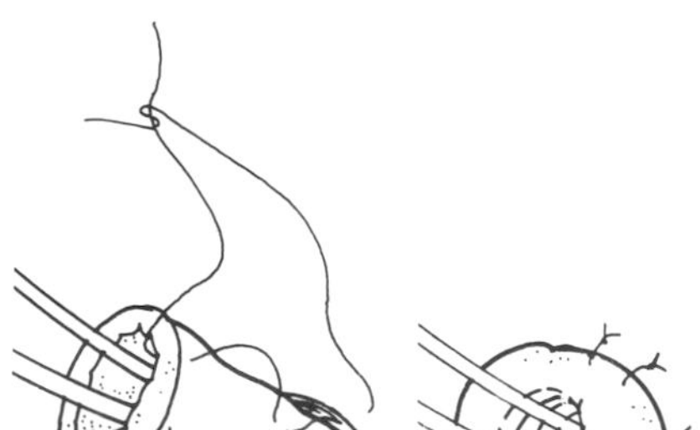

Fig. 17.26. Formation of the urinary ileal stoma. This may be flush, or everted.

Palliative treatment for bladder cancer

All too often treatment fails and we are confronted with an elderly patient, voiding blood-stained urine, with pain and difficulty every few minutes day and night. Sleeplessness worsens his misery and the necrotic tumour in the bladder is often irremediably infected. Since this is essentially a tumour which spreads locally, there is no prospect of a merciful end from metastases. But the surgery can offer much — not for cure — but for relief of suffering. A palliative urinary diversion with a ureteroureterostomy (Fig. 17.30) or an ileal conduit may give considerable relief from the discomfort of painful frequency. A short course of radiotherapy or chemotherapy stops bleeding and relieves pain. The patient should be allowed to have pain-relieving medicines when he needs them — and this is not necessarily regularly — for pain knows no clock. In the end, the surgeon can still give something of value merely by being there from time to time, not because he has anything to offer, but to show that he is still the patient's friend, and that he cares.

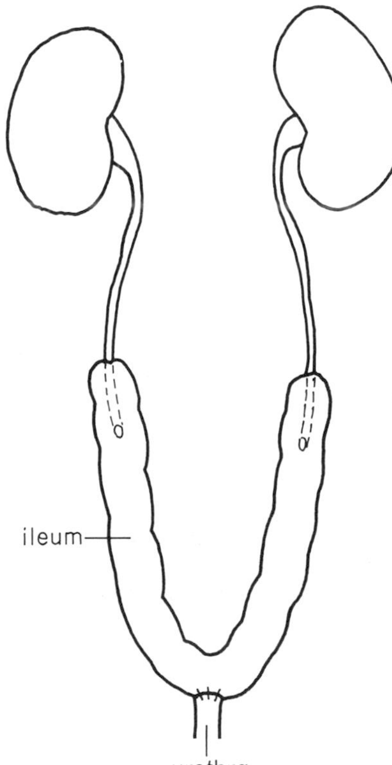

Fig. 17.27. Camey néovessie. The ureters are anastomosed to each end of a length of ileum which is joined to the urethra.

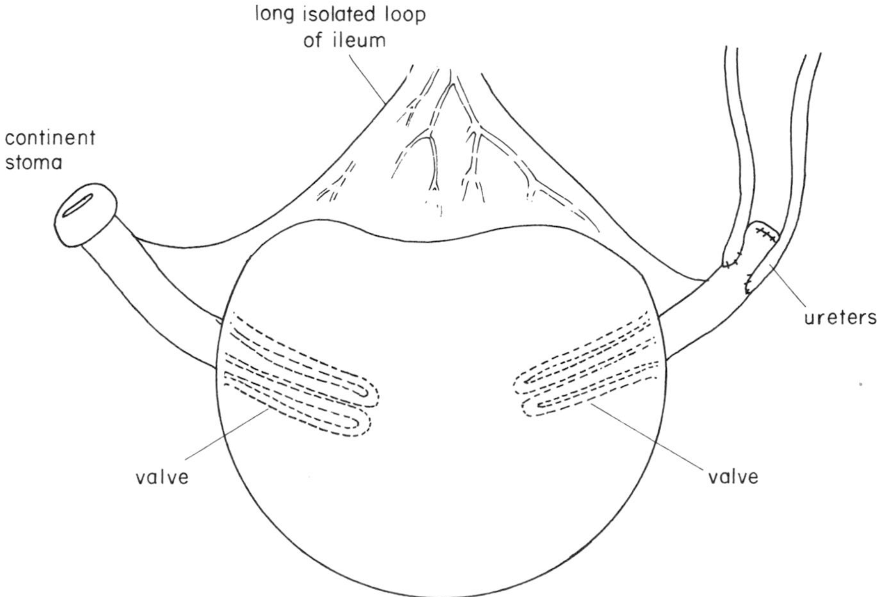

Fig. 17.28. Kock's pouch provides a valved stome which can be catheterized, and a second valve to prevent reflux of urine up the ureters.

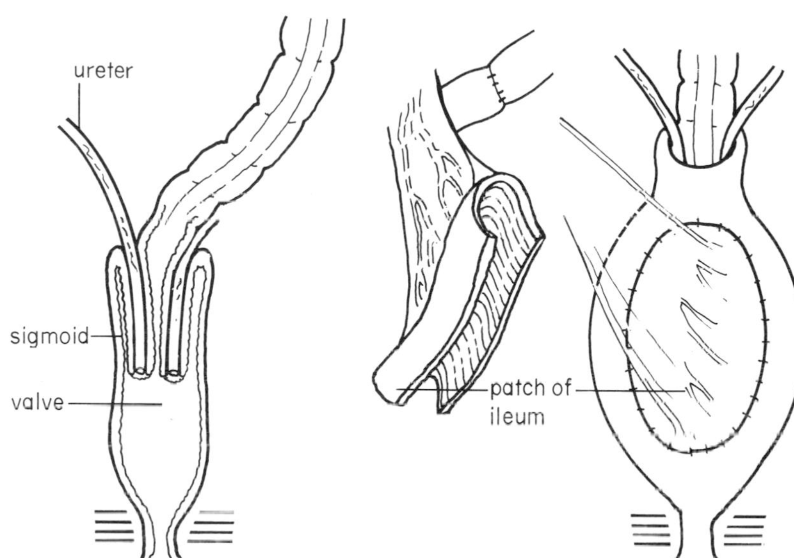

Fig. 17.29. Ghoneim's continent diversion.

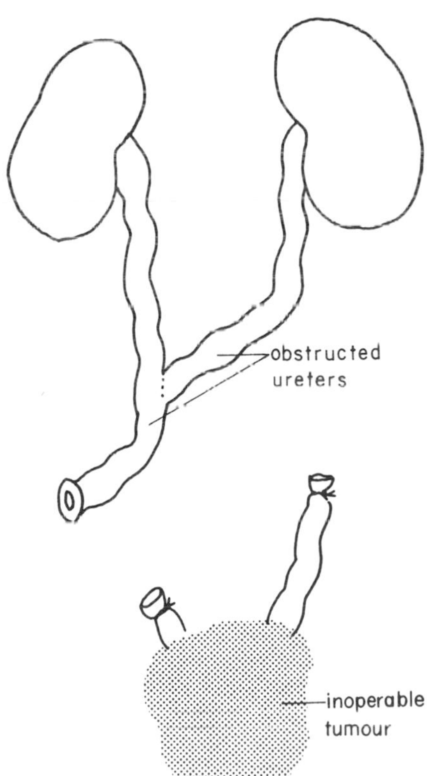

Fig. 17.30. Palliative uretero-ureteric anastomosis with single stoma.

FURTHER READING

BAUS Committee on Industrial Bladder Cancer (1988) Occupational bladder cancer: a guide for clinicians. *British Journal of Urology* **61**, 183–91.

Catalona WJ, Dresner SM & Haaff EO (1988) Management of superficial bladder cancer. In: Skinner DG & Lieskovsky G (Eds) *Diagnosis and Management of Genitourinary Cancer.* WB Saunders, Philadelphia. pp. 281–94.

Daniels JR, Skinner DG & Lieskovsky G (1988) Chemotherapy of carcinoma of bladder. In: Skinner DG & Lieskovsky G (Eds) *Diagnosis and Management of Genitourinary Cancer.* WB Saunders, Philadelphia. pp. 313–22.

Jenkins BJ, Caulfield MJ, Fowler CG, Badenoch DF, Tiptaft RC, Paris AMI, Hope-Stone HF, Oliver RTD & Blandy JP (1988) Reappraisal of the role of radical radiotherapy and salvage cystectomy in the treatment of invasive (T2/T3) bladder cancer. *British Journal of Urology* **62**, 343–6.

Jenkins BJ, England HR, Fowler CG, Tiptaft RC, Badenoch DF, Paris AMI, Oliver RTD & Blandy JP (1988) Chemotherapy for carcinoma *in situ* of the bladder. *British Journal of Urology* **61**, 326–9.

Skinner GC & Lieskovsky G (1988) Management of invasive and high-grade bladder cancer. In: Skinner DG & Lieskovsky G (Eds) *Diagnosis and Management of Genitourinary Cancer.* WB Saunders, Philadelphia. pp. 295–312.

Smith PH & Pavone-Macaluso M (Eds) (1988) *Management of Advanced Cancer of Prostate and Bladder.* Alan Liss, New York.

18 The Bladder — Incontinence and Functional Disturbances of Micturition

COMMON DISORDERS OF MICTURITION

Disorders of the bladder reflex arc

Afferent overstimulation

Anything which makes the lining of the bladder more sensitive or stimulates it unusually may set off a detrusor reflex contraction before the bladder has filled to its normal capacity (Fig. 18.1). Common causes of this are bacterial cystitis, a stone or carcinoma. The main symptom is frequency of micturition with an intense desire to void, and sometimes 'urge incontinence' if the patient cannot reach the toilet in time. Detrusor contractions appear in the static and voiding cystometrogram long before the bladder has filled completely but the detrusor pressure is normal during these contractions and the flow rate is normal though the volume which is passed is only small. The performance of the external sphincter and the bladder neck is normal.

Excess central facilitation

Everyone who has faced an important examination will know how facilitation from higher centres (Fig. 18.2) may sensitize the bladder, and frequency is a common feature of many anxiety states. To distinguish this from the frequency caused by something irritating the bladder is not always easy. With anxiety the frequency occurs only in the daytime and — once the patient is asleep — he is not wakened. Urodynamics show a bladder which empties long before it is full: the flow rate is normal. Under anaesthesia the bladder is seen to be normal and easily holds 400 to 500 ml.

Lack of central inhibition (Fig. 18.3)

Bed-wetting. At some time, early in their descent from the trees, our primate ancestors learned that, to live together, it was necessary to

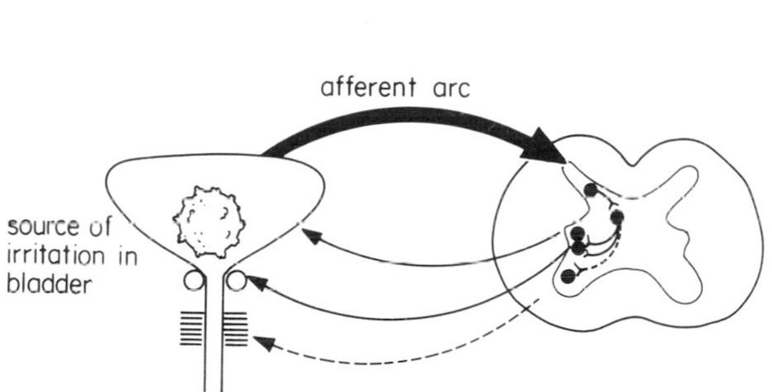

Fig. 18.1. Overstimulation of the afferent side of the reflex arc sets off the detrusor reflex before the bladder is really full.

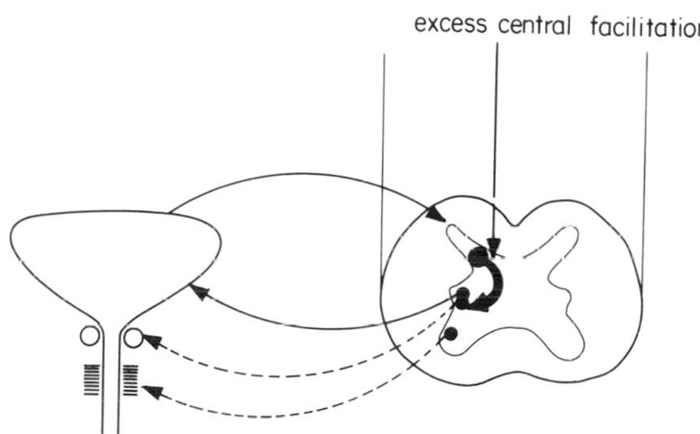

Fig. 18.2. Excessive central facilitation of the reflex arc triggers it to empty before it is really full.

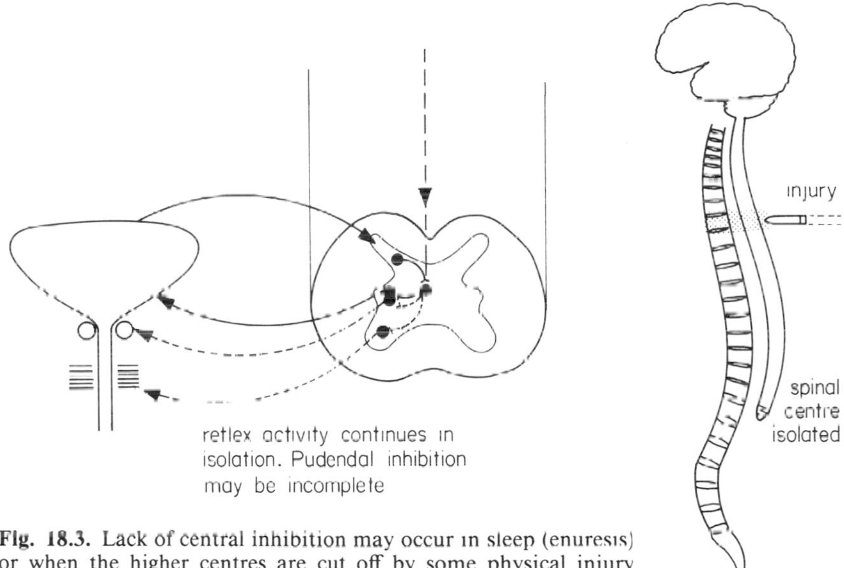

Fig. 18.3. Lack of central inhibition may occur in sleep (enuresis) or when the higher centres are cut off by some physical injury (paraplegia). In paraplegia, the co-ordinated inhibition of the pudendal and internal sphincter innervation is disturbed.

urinate and defaecate outside the cave. This inhibition of the reflex activity of the bladder and the bowel is conditioned in childhood. It may fail, and only very seldom is it possible to discover what has gone wrong. Often these children sleep unusually deeply: parents find them almost impossible to wake suggesting that the night-watchman who is supposed to stay awake to inhibit reflex emptying of the bladder succumbs to sleep in some unlucky children.

But there may also be other reasons for bed-wetting, e.g. anything which makes the reflex more sensitive:

(a) Urinary infection.

(b) Threadworms — which can be seen to wriggle from the anus to the urethra.

(c) Vaginitis usually without an obvious cause in little girls.

(d) Balanitis from infection behind a tight prepuce in little boys.

It is more difficult to evaluate minor disorders of the innervation of the bladder. These may be associated with *spina bifida occulta* but it is seldom possible, with the techniques available today, to pinpoint any definite neurological disorder, let alone put it right.

Because of all these uncertainties it is difficult to know when to begin to investigate this tiresome condition: children develop the sleeping inhibition at different ages. Many perfectly normal children are not reliably dry at night until they are 8 or 9 years old. In some otherwise normal adults the reflex remains unreliable — *adult enuresis.*

Anything which facilitates the reflex may make it worse: urinary infection adds an element of afferent stimulation to the reflex arc, and many investigators claim to find some minor abnormality of the nervous system. As a rule there is nothing wrong and it is doubtful if more than simple testing for infection is needed in the majority of cases. In older children one must be extremely cautious before starting on a full series of urodynamic investigations which are, for the child, demeaning, uncomfortable and sometimes terrifying.

Treatment of bed-wetting uses three principles:

1 *Reinforcement of central inhibition.* The child is encouraged to pass urine by the clock in the daytime. This allows him to learn what it feels like to have a full bladder and to practise how to inhibit the detrusor contractions until the minute hand reaches the hour. It is obviously impossible to train the cortex to inhibit urination during sleep, but it can be useful to practise during the day.

2 *Medication to lighten sleep.* Most of these children sleep very deeply indeed: a variety of drugs are used and one should use the most simple and most safe. Phenylpropanolamine and other alpha-stimulators have been used with good effect.

3 *Building up a conditional reflex.* One may treat the child like a Pavlov dog. He sleeps on two thin sheets which separate two perforated layers of tin-foil connected to a battery and a buzzer which is arranged so that it goes off when the sheet between the tin-foil becomes soaked in urine.

When using this system it is essential that the child is fully awakened and made to urinate. Before long his sleeping inhibitory centre associates the sensation of a full bladder with waking up and urinating. It is futile to misuse the buzzer alarm: letting it sound, waking the rest of the family, making the mother change the wet sheets while all the time the child sleeps on in blissful oblivion. Used intelligently these three arms of treatment usually work.

PARAPLEGIA

High injuries of the spinal cord

In high spinal cord injury inhibitory influences are cut off from the S2 and S3 segments. As a result the detrusor reflex works automatically when the bladder is more or less full but this ideal state of affairs is seldom seen in high spinal cord injuries. For reasons that are ill-understood, the isolated spinal cord centre for the bladder does not behave in the same co-ordinated way as a normal one and the sphincters are not inhibited when the detrusor contracts. The effect is to force the detrusor to work against resistance at the outlet of the bladder: the pressure inside the bladder rises but the bladder does not empty. Before long there is a combination of infection and obstruction to the ureters, and the kidneys develop obstructive uropathy. It is now known that there is a critical pressure in the bladder above which this obstructive uropathy will occur — 40 cmH_2O.

Urodynamic investigations soon show what pressure is developing inside the bladder. In many instances very high pressures occur at the internal and external sphincters and the videocystogram shows how poorly the contraction of the detrusor is co-ordinated with relaxation of the sphincter. There is often reflux up the ureters.

In the early days after the injury the bladder is emptied by frequent intermittent catheterization. Later there are several options: one can make the bladder atonic by dividing or injecting alcohol into the S2 and S3 efferent nerves, so lowering its pressure, and empty it by intermittent catheterization or a patch can be added formed into the shape of a 'clam' from bowel in such a way that it does not contract and the pressure inside the bowel remains low. Also — in men — one can divide the internal and external sphincters transurethrally — *sphincterotomy.* Urine is then collected by means of a condom urinal stuck to the penis.

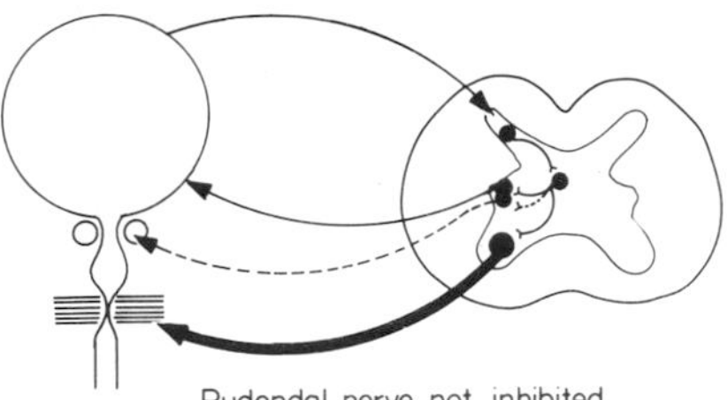

Fig. 18.4. External sphincter dyssynergia: when the detrusor contracts the external sphincter does not relax.

External sphincter dyssynergia

There is an uncommon disorder in which the detrusor and internal sphincter work together harmoniously, but the external sphincter does not relax (Fig. 18.4). This can be easily shown by means of a urodynamic study which records the activity of the external striated sphincter. It may be seen in children and in adults, and there is seldom any detectable organic cause, suggesting that there is some disturbance of behaviour, i.e. a bad habit. There can be a most bizarre picture: a large bladder, a normal detrusor, a bladder neck that opens but an external sphincter that shuts tight. The remedy of this condition is not easy: methods involving biofeedback and retraining are used but are not always effective and in many cases the patient has to be taught intermittent self-catheterization.

Destruction of the spinal centre S2, S3

Unfortunately the bladder centre in the tip of the spinal cord is situated just where the spine is most likely to break. Hyperflexion or dislocation fractures at this level usually destroy the tip of the spinal cord as well as damaging the nerve roots that surround it in the cauda equina (Fig. 18.5). To tell whether the spinal centre is intact or not one can test for the bulbospongiosus reflex by tweaking the glans penis and feeling for a contraction of that muscle. If the spinal centre is completely destroyed the bladder becomes a denervated bag.

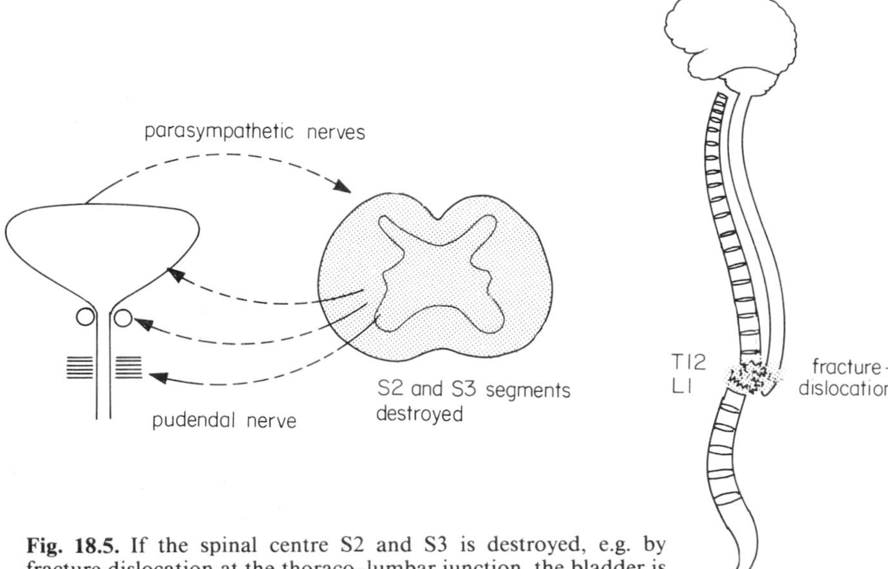

Fig. 18.5. If the spinal centre S2 and S3 is destroyed, e.g. by fracture dislocation at the thoraco–lumbar junction, the bladder is entirely denervated. It behaves like an inert rubber bag.

It may be difficult to be sure of the diagnosis for 4 to 5 weeks after the initial injury. Return of the bulbospongiosus reflex indicates that the spinal centre is intact. Urodynamic studies after this same interval may detect detrusor contractions in response to filling the bladder, especially when using ice-cold water. But when the centre is entirely destroyed, filling the bladder gives a long, flat cystometrogram curve without a flicker of detrusor contraction.

The EMG of the external sphincter shows no action potentials. Such a patient may empty the bladder past the flaccid sphincters by compressing the lower abdomen, but this may raise the pressure inside the bladder, and infection of the residual urine may threaten the kidneys with obstructive uropathy.

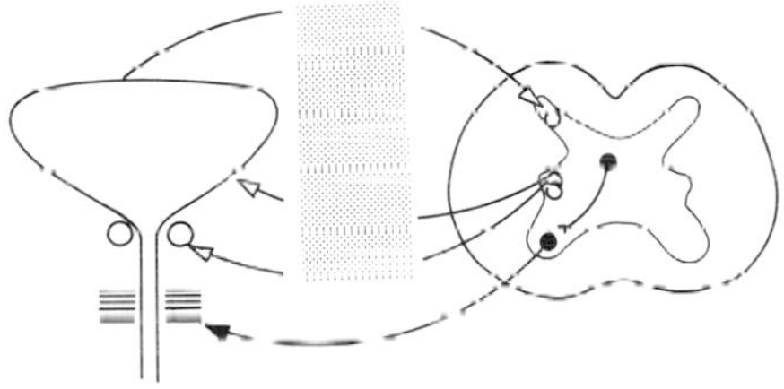

Destruction of the pelvic parasympathetic nerves

Fig. 18.6. If only the pelvic parasympathetic nerves are destroyed, e.g. after surgery, the pudendal nerve and external sphincter continue to work; there may be residual urine and infection.

A similar paralysis of the bladder may follow surgical operations in which the pelvic parasympathetic pathways are cut or removed, e.g. in radical removal of carcinoma of the uterus or rectum when the lymph nodes are removed along the internal and external iliac vessels together with the tissue attached to the side wall of the pelvis. A similar disturbance of function occurs after fractures of the pelvis if the nerves are torn. Clinically and urodynamically there is a big floppy bladder without detrusor contractions, but the somatic motor innervation of the sphincter may be intact and the sphincter may obstruct the outflow from the bladder (Fig. 18.6).

In neuropathy involving the autonomic nervous system, especially in diabetes mellitus, failure of function of the pelvic parasympathetics may give rise to one of two clinical pictures. The bladder may appear to be hypersensitive: it may empty when less than completely full and then empty incompletely. Clinically this may resemble the changes of prostatic outflow obstruction but the symptoms of frequency and urge incontinence will not be relieved by removing the prostate.

The other clinical picture is of a large, overdistended bladder with a big residual urine. Urodynamics show weak detrusor contractions, a large residual urine and a relative obstruction at the neck of the bladder.

Irritation of the spinal reflex arc

One needs care in making this diagnosis which presents clinical and urodynamic features which mimic those of failure of central inhibition or increased sensitivity of the bladder mucosa (Fig. 18.7). Occasionally an irritable bladder is caused by a prolapsed intervertebral disc which juts

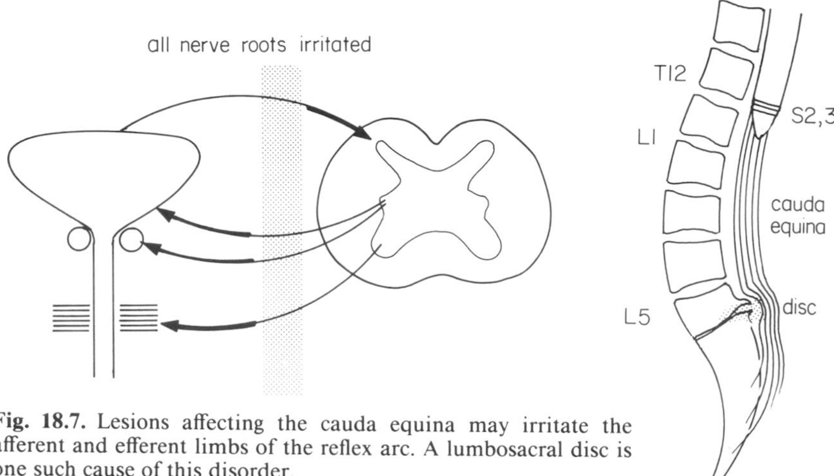

Fig. 18.7. Lesions affecting the cauda equina may irritate the afferent and efferent limbs of the reflex arc. A lumbosacral disc is one such cause of this disorder.

back to irritate the most medial fibres of the cauda equina. Neurosurgical intervention may prevent irreversible damage to the bladder and bring a complete return of bladder and sexual function. Some of the clinical symptoms of frequency and urgency seen in pelvic inflammations may be related to irritation of the pelvic parasympathetic nerves.

There are a larger number of patients in whom no obvious cause can be found for the hyperactive bladder: it is customary to label this condition *detrusor instability* — but this useful term should not be overworked: it is not a diagnosis — it is a name for a condition for which the cause (and indeed the treatment) is unknown.

DISORDERS OF BLADDER FUNCTION CAUSED BY MECHANICAL FACTORS

Diuresis

Diabetes mellitus
Diabetes insipidus
Hydronephrosis
Heart failure
Drinking too much (polydipsia)

It should not be necessary to point out that a patient who has to pass a large volume of urine will have to empty the bladder more often and will therefore have frequency. A very common cause is *diabetes mellitus*: less

Saturday	1·30 am	200	mL
	3 " "	250	"
	4·30 "	250	"
	6 "	250	"
	10 "	150	"
	2 pm	150	"
	5 "	150	"
	8 "	100	"
Sunday	1 am	250	mL
	3·30 "	300	
	5 "	200	

Fig. 18.8. Typical fluid output chart kept by a patient who is unable to concentrate his urine at night.

common are patients with *diabetes insipidus* of pituitary origin or those with a failure of renal tubular function perhaps caused by upper tract obstruction who are unable to concentrate their urine and must perforce produce large volumes of urine.

Many elderly men are referred for prostatectomy because they wake often to pass urine in the night. They have a good flow rate and no residual urine, and study of their fluid chart (Fig. 18.8) shows that they are passing large volumes every 2 to 3 hours throughout the night. They have mild *heart failure* and oedema fluid accumulates during the day and returns to the circulation when they lie down, and is presented as a fluid load which must be got rid of.

Bladder outflow obstruction

There are many reasons for an increased resistance downstream of the bladder: the most important are the enlarged prostate and urethral stricture. If there is an increased resistance at the outflow, the pressure inside the bladder must be increased to get the urine out, and to meet this demand the detrusor responds by *hypertrophy*. The bladder wall becomes thicker and its texture more coarse. In the early phase of this hypertrophic response the detrusor becomes — like the highly tuned muscles of the athlete — more jumpy, more quick to respond to distension. Urodynamic studies show a high pressure in the static and voiding cystometrograms. The flow rate may be normal, but the peak voiding pressure may be very high, and as soon as it exceeds about 40 cmH_2O the upper tracts are threatened. A pressure profile will show a zone of high pressure in the region of the offending prostate (Fig. 18.9).

The patient with these early features of compensatory hypertrophy

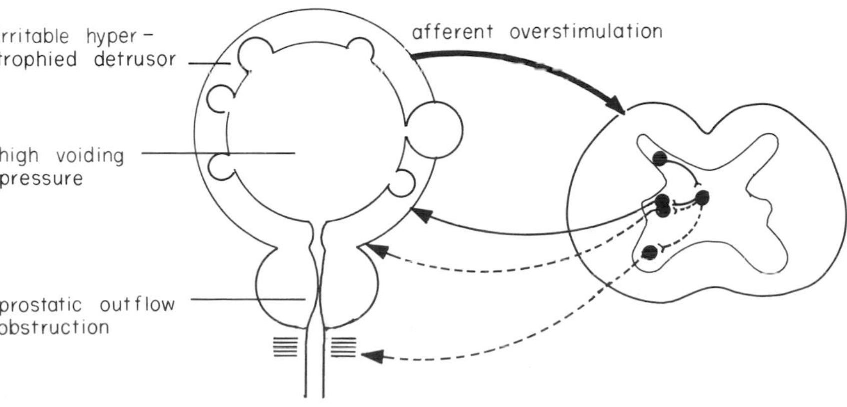

Fig. 18.9. Urodynamic changes in outflow obstruction, e.g. prostate or urethral stricture. The hypertrophied detrusor is also hyper-irritable; its trabeculated and sacculated muscle is abnormally jumpy from afferent overstimulation. There is a high voiding pressure, poor flow, and often abnormal, uninhibited detrusor contractions as the bladder is filled.

from obstruction has frequency and even urge incontinence, symptoms which characteristically vary considerably from time to time. At this stage it can be difficult to distinguish the bladder which is reacting to an increased outflow resistance from one that is irritable from some other cause and before offering any surgical procedure to a patient whose chief complaint is frequency it is necessary to be quite sure that there is an increase in the peak voiding pressure.

In time the clinical and urodynamic picture of detrusor hypertrophy is succeeded by *detrusor failure.* Like any muscle that must continue to work against unusual resistance, the detrusor becomes inefficient, and instead of emptying the bladder completely, it gives up before the bladder is empty and so there begins to be a certain quantity of *residual urine.* As the process continues the detrusor becomes chronically stretched and more and more strands of fibrous tissue appear amongst the coarsened muscle fibres until eventually the hypertrophied detrusor becomes nothing more than an inert, atonic bag with a huge residual urine. A cystometrogram now shows no detrusor contractions: the flow is a mere trickle (Fig. 18.10). By this stage, even if the cause of obstruction is removed, the big floppy sacculated detrusor muscle may not contract and the only way the bladder can be emptied is by abdominal straining. Prolonged drainage with a catheter may enable the bladder to shrink but it seldom restores its original contractility.

Damage to the sphincters

Accidental injury to the external and supramembranous sphincters of the bladder may occur in prostatectomy, and after fractures of the pelvis

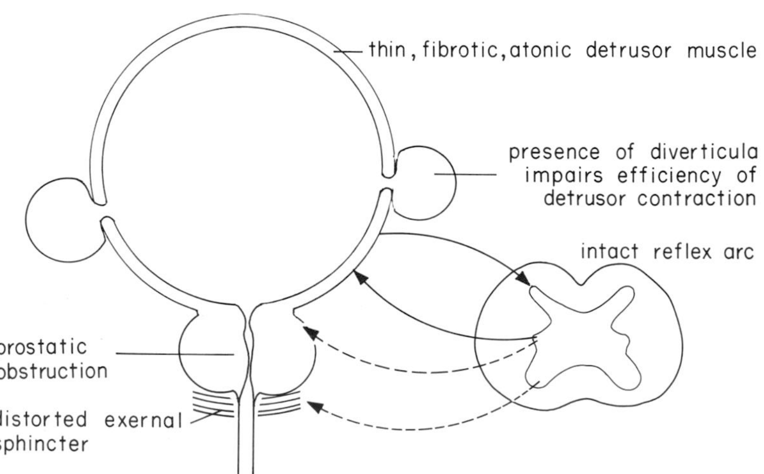

Fig. 18.10. Detrusor failure. After continued, unrelieved outflow obstruction the detrusor finally gives up: its wall becomes inert, floppy, and partly replaced by fibrous tissue. There is chronic retention, a very poor flow-rate, and a low voiding pressure.

complicated by tearing-across of the urethra. If the internal sphincter at the neck of the bladder has also been resected or injured, the patient will be incontinent (Fig. 18.11). A similar change is sometimes seen in carcinoma of the prostate when it invades the sphincters and keeps them stiff and permanently half-open.

Urodynamics will show a detrusor perhaps more jumpy than normal from being always empty and often infected, but the contraction does not produce an excessive voiding pressure. The outflow resistance is negligible. The pressure profile shows no peak at either of the sphincters. The patient may be dry lying down in bed but the urine runs away as soon as he rises. A few patients may be able to interrupt the flow of urine by voluntary contraction of the external sphincter and in some patients exercising this muscle restores continence. Electrical stimulators placed in the rectum or applied to the perineum may help re-educate the external sphincter.

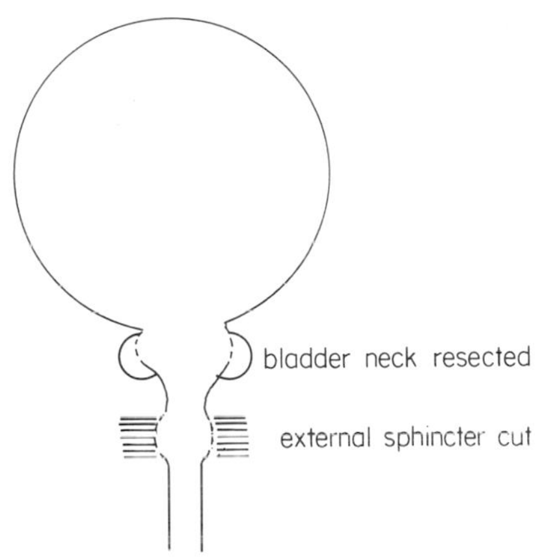

Fig 18.11 Incontinence from surgical division of both the internal and external sphincters.

When, as is so often the case, the patient has lost the use of both sets of sphincters, one may be able to close the urethra by some form of appliance. There are two main types: external appliances such as the Cunningham clip (Fig. 18.12) and implanted gadgets such as the Brantley Scott artificial sphincter (Fig. 18.13). Both suffer from the inherent defect that the pressure needed to keep the urethra closed is greater than the venous pressure in the vessels of the wall of the urethra, so that there is a risk of ischaemic damage to the soft tissues. Pressure necrosis, infection, and mechanical failure are significant complications of all these appliances.

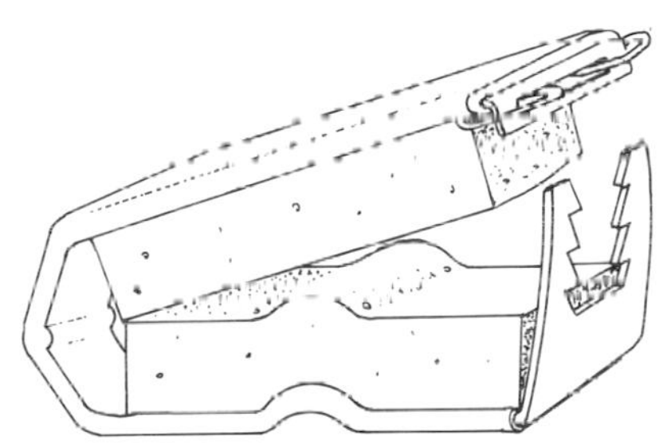

Fig. 18.12. Cunningham's clamp: it is applied across the penis to keep the urethra closed. The pads are made of sponge rubber.

Herniation of the base of the bladder through the pelvic floor

After childbirth many women develop an enlargement of the gap for the vagina in the levator ani shelf (Fig. 18.14) through which the trigone and the anterior wall of the vagina prolapse. As a result the internal sphincter comes to lie outside the levator ani and when the abdominal pressure is raised, this pressure is no longer able to automatically squeeze the urethra above the levator sheet. Patients lose urine when they laugh, cough or strain. This is *stress incontinence.*

Clinically it can be quite difficult to distinguish this from the *urge incontinence* seen in women who cannot get to the toilet quickly enough when their detrusor contracts, especially since a detrusor contraction may be stimulated by a laugh or cough when the detrusor is unstable for whatever reason.

In stress incontinence if two fingers are placed in the vagina on either side of the urethra and are lifted up, this will prevent the escape of urine

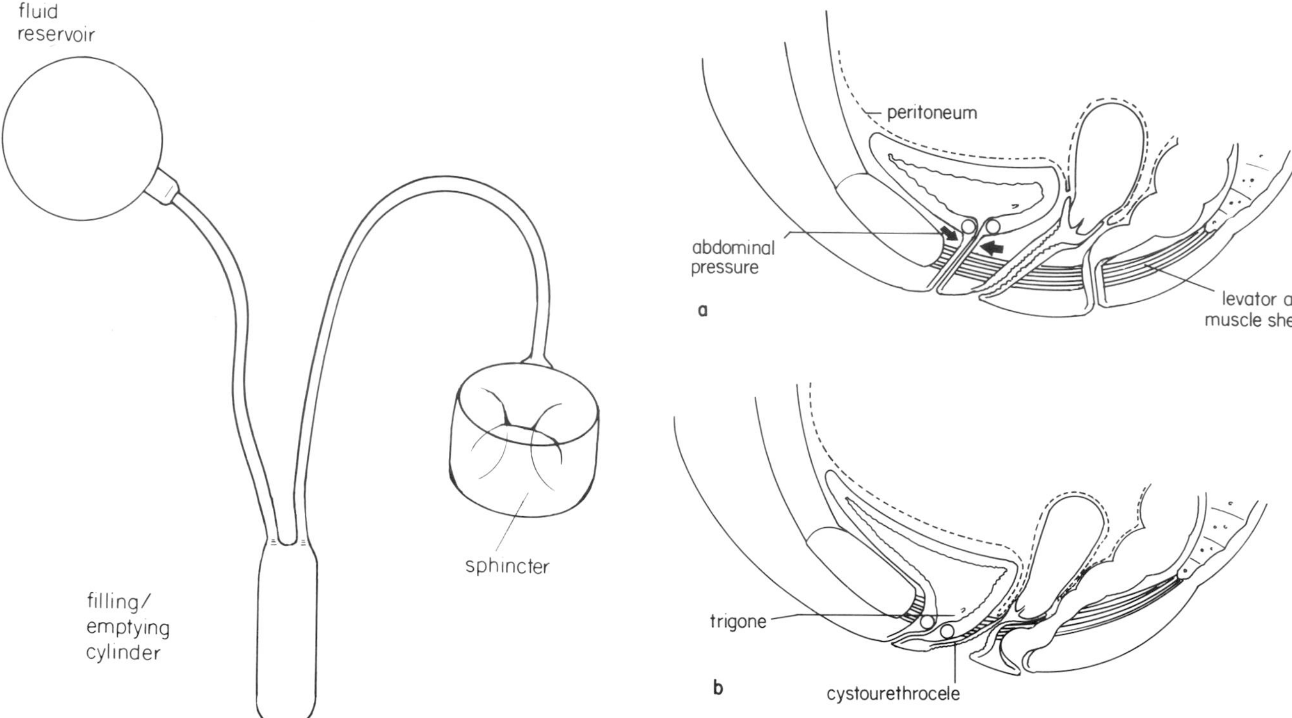

Fig. 18.13. Scott inflatable sphincter. The doughnut-shaped cuff is placed around the urethra and blown up or let down by working a valve which allows fluid to run in or out from the reservoir.

Fig. 18.14. (a) Diagram of the normal perineal floor in a women. When she strains or coughs, the increased intra-abdominal pressure is transmitted to the urethra to compress it and keep the urine in. (b) When there is herniation of the pelvic contents through the levator shelf, the internal sphincter finds itself outside the levator, the intra-abdominal pressure no longer helps keep the urine in and the angle between trigone and urethra is flattened out. The patient is wet at the least exertion. There may be a cystocele.

when the patient coughs — this is the test of Marshall and of Bonney. Today it is usual to check that there is no primary instability of the bladder by a cystometrogram since the chance of effecting a cure by surgery is reduced when the detrusor is at fault.

Operations for stress incontinence

1 *Stamey's sutures.* There are many variations on this theme: two nylon sutures lift the vaginal wall on either side of the urethra, imitating the action of the two fingers in Bonney's test. The sutures are tied over the

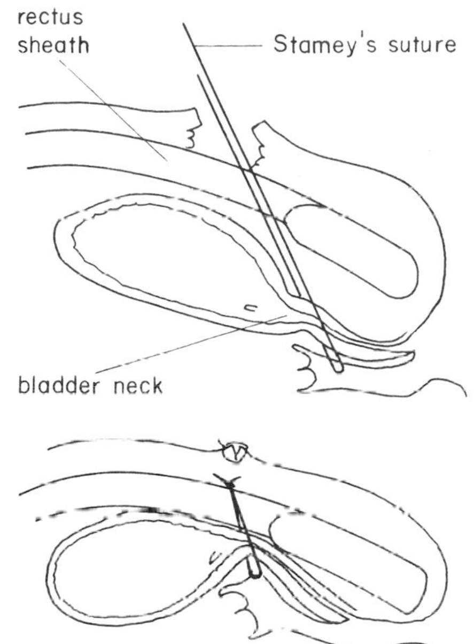

Fig. 18.15. Stamey or Pereira sutures for stress incontinence.

rectus abdominis sheath. Placing these sutures requires care, but the operation is a very minor one, and particularly useful in elderly women (Fig. 18.15).

2 *Vaginal colposuspension.* Through a vaginal approach the ligaments of Mackenrodt are sewn together under the trigone of the bladder to lift it up (Fig. 18.16).

3 *Marshall-Marchetti-Krantz operation.* There are many versions of this, the classical operation for stress incontinence. They have one theme in common — they lift up the trigone and the urethra (Fig. 18.17). A series of sutures are placed (Fig. 18.18) so as to attach the strong tissues of the vagina to the back of the symphysis pubis. Some surgeons pass their stitches through the periosteum of the pubis, others use the so-called ligament of Gimbernat. Many names are attached to what is basically the same operation (not a new phenomenon in surgery).

4 *Millin's sling.* In about 20% of cases, the Marshall operation fails, probably because the tissues fail to unite. Something stronger is needed to hold up the bladder. Various substances are used as a sling or hammock to lift up the bladder neck: the first of these was a strip of the rectus abdominis sheath — the *Millin sling* (Fig. 18.19). Other techniques use foreign materials such as Marlex or Teflon, but the principle is the same

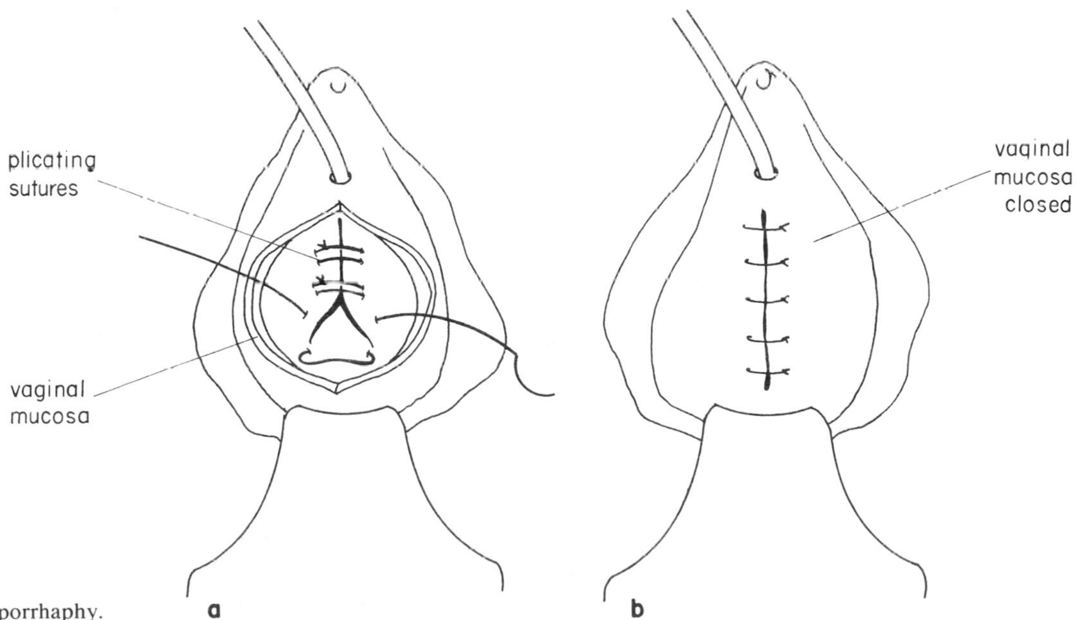

Fig. 18.16. Anterior colporrhaphy.

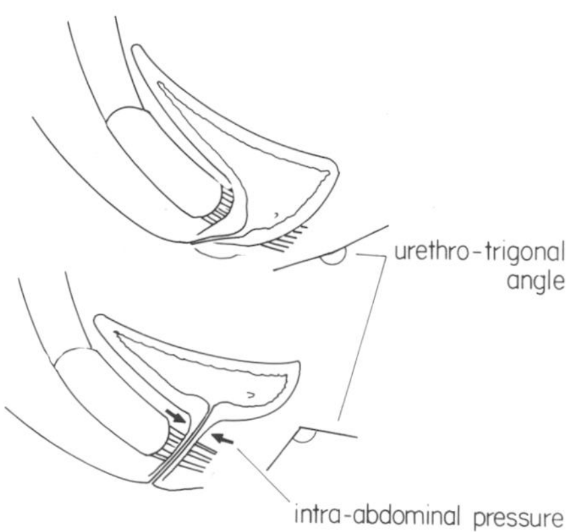

Fig. 18.17. The aim of all operations for 'stress incontinence' is to lift the urethra so that it once more comes within the effect of intra-abdominal pressure to restore the urethrotrigonal angle.

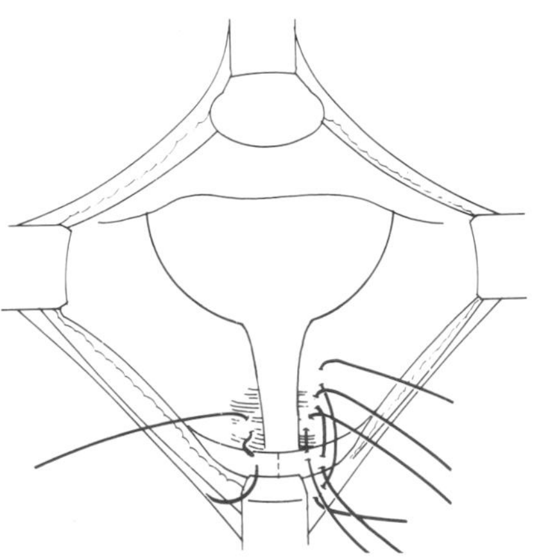

Fig. 18.18. In the Marshall–Marchetti–Krantz operation the urethra is fixed up behind the symphysis in a tunnel made by stitching the vaginal tissues to the back of the symphysis.

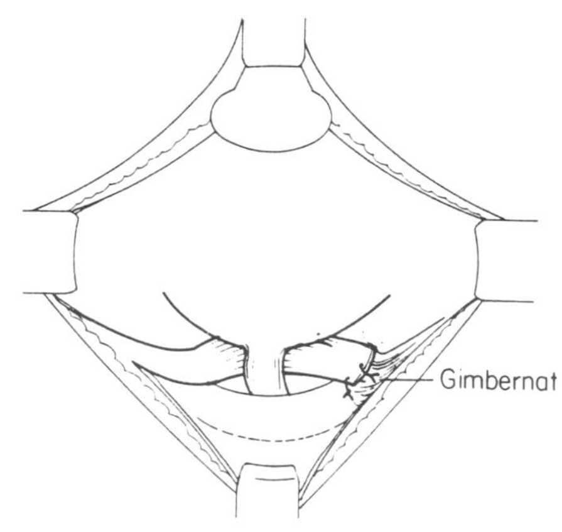

Fig. 18.19. In the Millin and similar sling operations a hammock is made with fascia or synthetic tape to sling up the neck of the bladder. Gimbernat's ligament is a useful anchor for a suture to hold the sling.

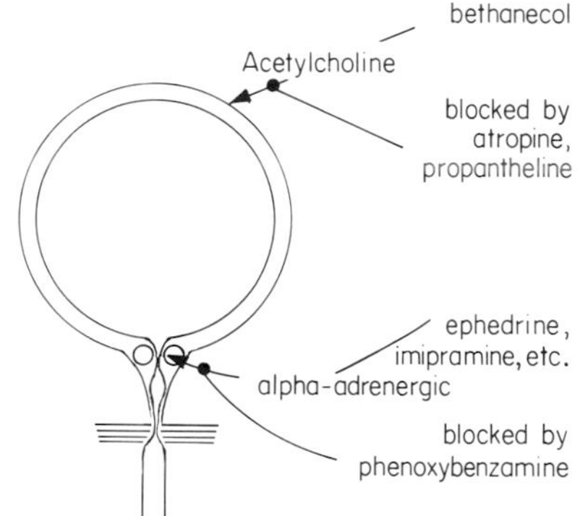

Fig. 18.20. Action of drugs on the bladder.

and as one might expect, many different names are attached to what is essentially the same operation. They all work in about 80% of cases provided the incontinence is really due to the mechanical displacement of the bladder. If in fact the chief reason for the incontinence is not a mechanical displacement of the base of the bladder but a disorder of its reflex activity, then none of these operations work.

PHARMACOLOGICAL TREATMENT FOR DISORDERS OF MICTURITION

Few medications really do good in the common disorders of bladder function. The smooth muscle of the detrusor is usually regarded as cholinergic, that of the sphincter as alpha-adrenergic (Fig. 18.20). To help the bladder empty, one might use bethanecol to release acetylcholine from the postganglionic fibres in the detrusor: but plainly this must be futile in cases of long-standing obstruction where the detrusor muscle is largely replaced by fibrous tissue.

Incontinence from weakness of the internal sphincter may benefit from an alpha-stimulator (ephedrine, imipramine, phenylpropanolamine, mazindol). These are surprisingly effective in adult bed-wetting and minor forms of stress incontinence.

FURTHER READING

Ashken MH, Abrams PH & Lawrence WT (1984) Stamey endoscopic bladder neck suspension for stress incontinence. *British Journal of Urology* **56**, 629–34.

Brocklehurst JC (Ed) (1984) *Urology in the Elderly*. Churchill Livingstone, Edinburgh.

Fidas A, Galloway NTM, McInnes A & Chisholm GD (1985) Neurophysiological measurements in primary adult enuretics. *British Journal of Urology* **57**, 635–40.

Freeman RM & Baxby K (1982) Hypnotherapy for incontinence caused by the unstable detrusor. *British Medical Journal* **284**, 1831–3..

Grundy D & Russell J (1986) ABC of spinal cord injury: urological management. *British Medical Journal* **292**, 249–53.

Heathcote PS, Galloway NTM, Lewis DC & Stephenson TP (1987) An assessment of the complications of the Brantley Scott artificial sphincter. *British Journal of Urology* **60**, 119–21.

King LR, Stone AR & Webster GD (Eds) (1987) *Bladder Reconstruction and Continent Urinary Diversion*. Year Book Medical Publishers Inc., Chicago.

Mundy AR, Stephenson TP & Wein AJ (1984) *Urodynamics, Principles Practice and Application*. Churchill Livingstone, Edinburgh.

Nurse DE & Mundy AR (1988) One hundred artificial sphincters. *British Journal of Urology* **61**, 318–25.

Ryall RL & Marshall VR (1982) Point of view: laws of urodynamics. *Urology* **20**, 106–7.

Sibley CNA (1987) The physiological response of the detrusor muscle to experimental bladder outflow obstruction in the pig. *British Journal of Urology* **60**, 332–6.

Tiptaft RC, Woodhouse CRJ & Badenoch DF (1984) Mazindol for nocturnal enuresis. *British Journal of Urology* **56**, 641–3.

19 The Prostate Gland

COMPARATIVE ANATOMY

In our mammalian ancestors the urethra was supplied with a whole series of accessory glands, most of which seemed to have some function related to procreation, although their exact role is seldom very clear (Fig. 19.1). From what is known of monkeys one can make out a kind of primitive blue-print for the prostate. There are two elements: each shaped like a croissant or a collar not properly buttoned-up in front, and they fit one into the other. The two are separated by the entry of the ejaculatory ducts (Fig. 19.2). The cranial prostate seems to differ from the caudal one: benign enlargement mainly arises in the cranial part, cancer in the caudal.

SURGICAL ANATOMY

The normal adult prostate gland is placed around the urethra like a croissant. It lies behind the symphysis pubis to which it is attached by a tough fascia containing large veins (Fig. 19.3). On either side the pubis and ischium curve around it. Behind it the rectum is separated by

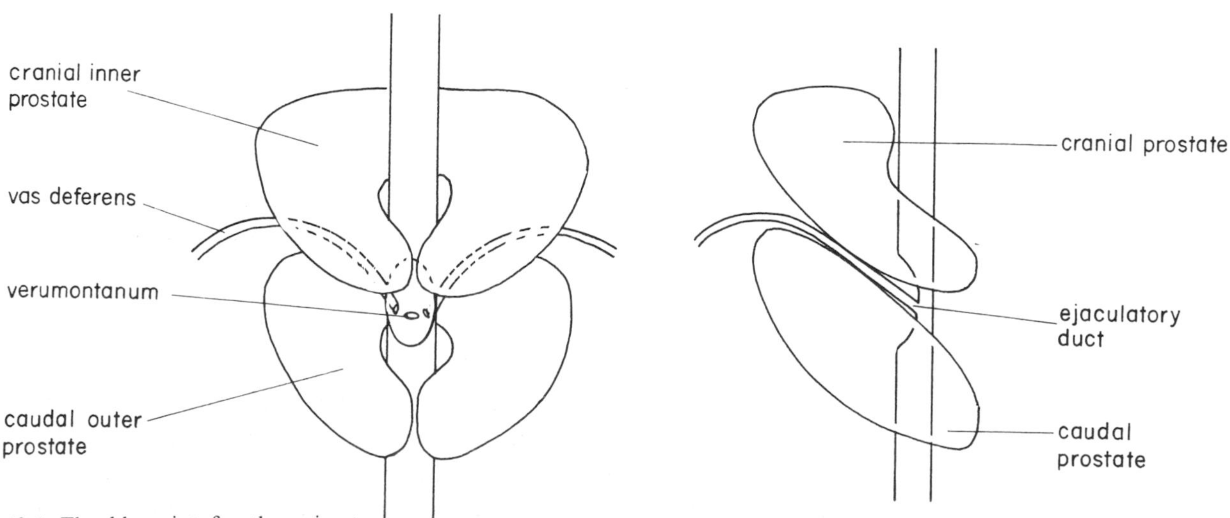

Fig. 19.1. The blueprint for the primate prostate.

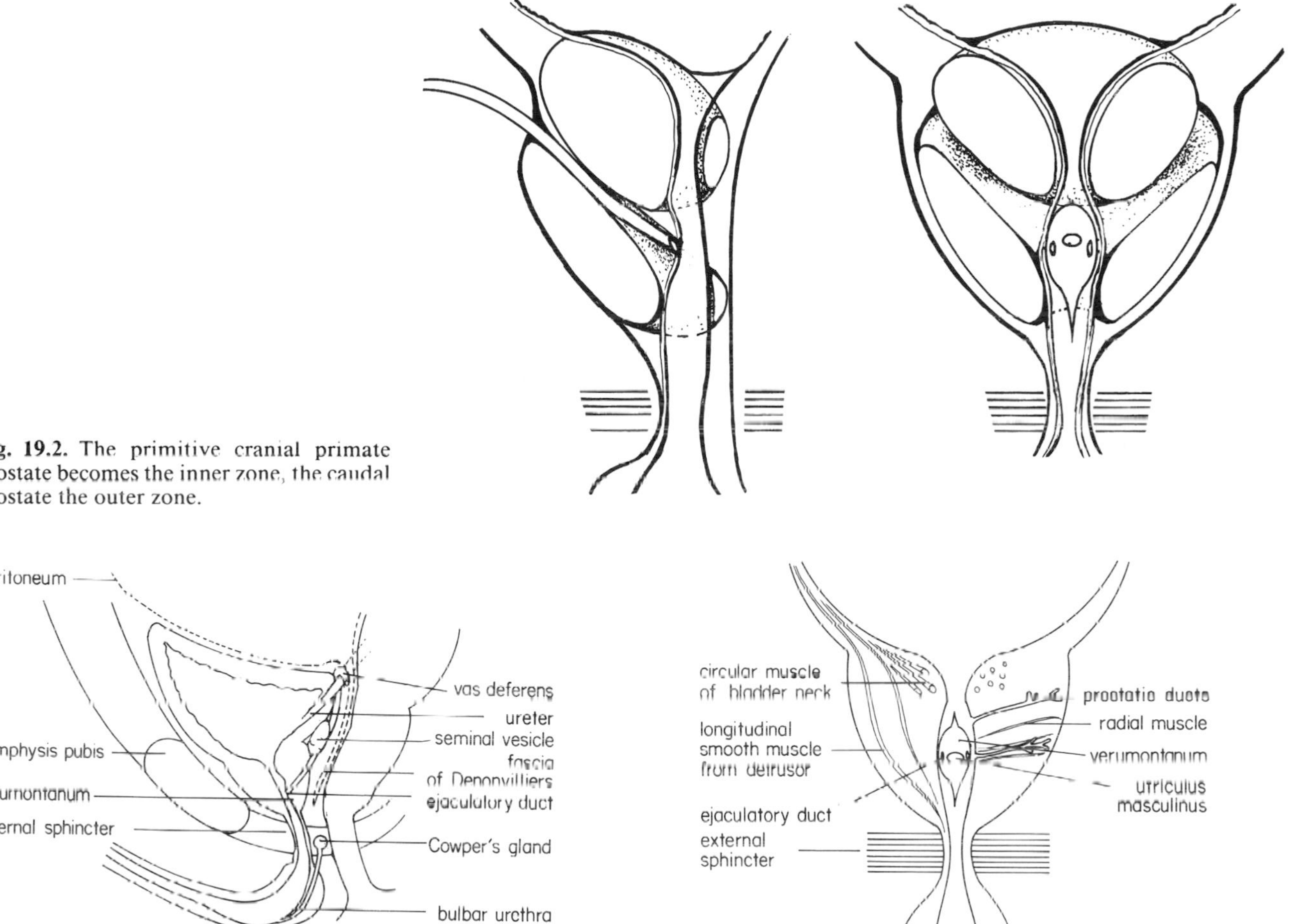

Fig. 19.2. The primitive cranial primate prostate becomes the inner zone, the caudal prostate the outer zone.

Fig. 19.3. Surgical anatomy of the prostate.

Fig. 19.4. Structure of the prostate in coronal section.

Denonvilliers' fascia which is made up of two layers of peritoneum fused together. Between the prostate and the bladder lie the seminal vesicles, vasa, and ureters.

STRUCTURE OF THE PROSTATE

The prostate is a mass of tubes each with a contractile sleeve of muscle and all supported by a stroma of connective tissue (Fig. 19.4). These three elements change with growth and maturity. Glandular and muscular elements are undetectable in the child: they hypertrophy with puberty and in middle age develop the nodules and whorls of benign enlargement.

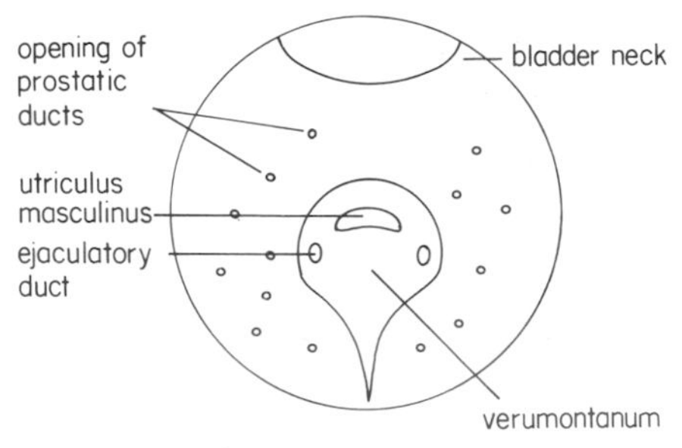

Fig. 19.5. Endoscopic appearance of the prostatic urethra.

The glandular ducts of the prostate run more or less radially out from the prostatic urethra into which they empty. Endoscopy reveals their openings in the prostatic urethra (Fig. 19.5). Half way down the prostatic urethra is the *verumontanum* (Latin: mountainous island), more a volcano than a mountain — its crater the *utriculus masculinus* — vestige of the Müllerian ducts that form the uterus in women. On either side of the verumontanum are the more important ejaculatory ducts.

The normal, healthy young man's prostate has no true lobes. Only as the gland is deformed by benign nodular hypertrophy appear the lateral and middle lobes: hypertrophy must take this form owing to the limitations imposed on the prostate by the symphysis in front and the bladder above. Below the prostate the thinnest part of the urethra passes down through the pelvic diaphragm — the levator ani. The verumontanum lies well above the external sphincter.

FUNCTION OF THE PROSTATE

Nobody knows the normal physiological function of the prostate. It probably contributes a tiny fraction (0.5 ml) to the seminal fluid which may help the sperms swim. The prostate gland probably contracts during sexual intercourse — but this has never been proven.

INFLAMMATION OF THE PROSTATE

Acute prostatitis

The prostate is spongy and contains innumerable channels and ducts which invite infection. If there is obstruction downstream of the prostate, e.g. by a urethral stricture, infected urine may be forced into the prostatic ducts. Acute prostatitis may occur without warning with a systemic illness marked by rigors, fever, and muscular pains. It may follow passage of a catheter or cystoscope, or the accidental injection of phenol in oil in injection for haemorrhoids. Clinically the patient is very uncomfortable and feels aching in the perineum which radiates to the thighs and penis. Passing urine is painful, the stream is thin, there is frequency and often a high fever, palpation reveals a tender swollen gland and the urine may or may not grow pathogens on culture (Fig. 19.6).

If organisms are identified in the urine they should be treated with an antibiotic that really gets into the prostatic tissue in adequate quantities: erythromycin, trimethoprim and cinoxacin give high prostatic tissue antibiotic levels. Antibiotics must be given for up to six weeks.

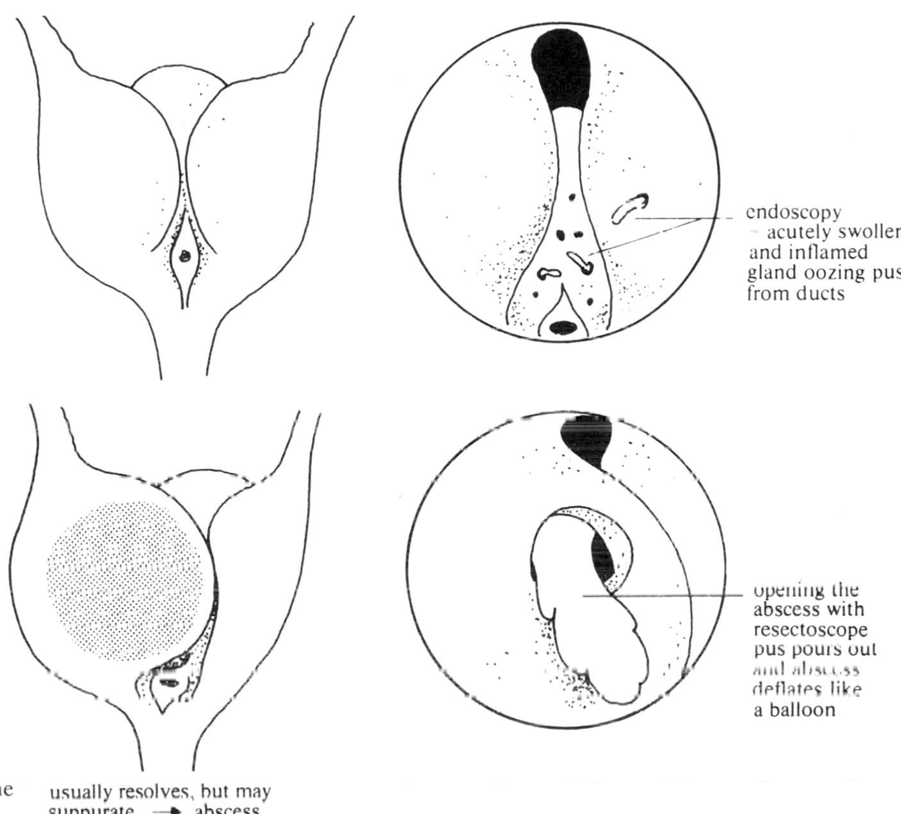

Fig. 19.6. Acute inflammation in the prostate.

Prostatic abscess

Acute inflammation in the prostate, as elsewhere in the body usually heals with resolution but may lead on to suppuration when a fluctuant abscess forms in the prostate, which bulges back towards the rectum as a huge tender mass. It is best for this abscess to be drained *per urethram*. If it is allowed to point though the tough barrier of Denonvilliers' fascia into the rectum it may cause a prostatorectal fistula.

Chronic prostatitis

As with any inflammation, healing is followed by scarring and the prostate is infiltrated with fibrous tissue. Some men have minor exacerbations with discomfort, fever and pain on voiding: organisms may be found in the urine or the fluid expressed by 'massage' of the prostate may grow *Neisseria gonorrhoeae, Chlamydia* or *Trichomonas.*

For each patient with inflammation in the prostate there are dozens

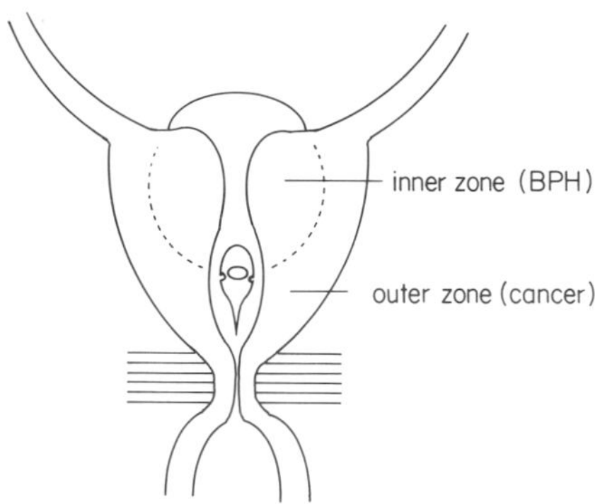

Fig. 19.7. Zones of the prostate.

who complain of pain in the perineum, discomfort on voiding and vague symptoms of sexual inadequacy. Often the trouble is psychosexual, and one must take care not to make the patient worse by treatment that has no justification in pathology or pharmacology. Never commit a patient to a protracted course of 'prostatic massage' without asking yourself candidly whether there is any other chronic inflammation which is better for being deliberately squeezed. Prostatic pain certainly calls for relief. It may be distressing, but it does not necessarily arise in the prostate. May of these men are secretly worried that they may have acquired some loathsome venereal disease. Time, explanation, and the assurance of an expert venereologist may bring profound relief.

BENIGN ENLARGEMENT OF THE PROSTATE

Aetiology

Over the age of 40 all men have some degree of benign nodular hyperplasia of the prostate but only one in ten will get obstruction as a result. The size of the enlargement that occurs in nodular hyperplasia is unrelated to the degree of obstruction: the smallest prostates may cause the worst outflow obstruction and huge glands may cause no obstruction at all.

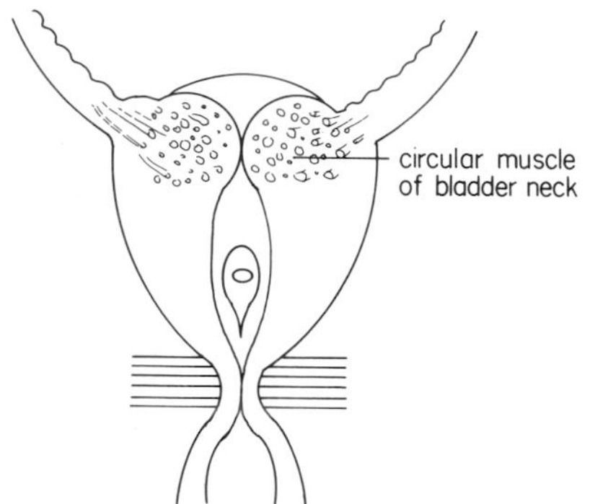

Fig. 19.8. Hypertrophy of the bladder neck.

Pathology

There are two zones in the prostate — reflecting their primate ancestry (Fig. 19.7). The inner cranial zone may be a target for oestrogens and it enlarges for a week or two in the newborn boy, under the supposed influence of maternal oestrogens. The outer caudal zone is thought to be under androgen influences. In the normal, young male, there is no histological or anatomical difference between the zones. The prostate of the 20 year old is made up of acini, muscle fibres and connective tissue. Each of these elements enlarges in benign hypertrophy.

There may be overactivity of the muscle of the neck of the bladder for which no neurological cause can be found (Fig. 19.8). This may give rise to outflow obstruction and the condition occurs at a relatively early age. Later on this overactivity of the bladder neck is confused by nodular hyperplasia (Fig. 19.9) for after the age of 40 all prostates show, here and there, whorls composed of hypertrophied smooth muscle, connective tissue and duct epithelium. As the years go by the whorls become larger, more numerous and confluent. They may become stiff and gristly or form bulky *adenomas* which displace and compress the caudal outer zone of

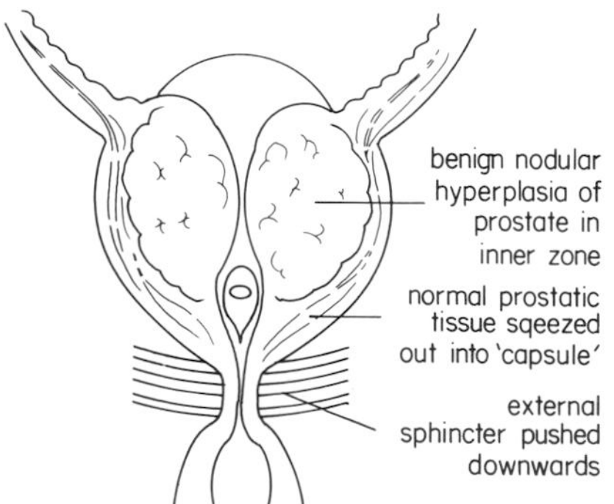

Fig. 19.9. Benign prostatic enlargement.

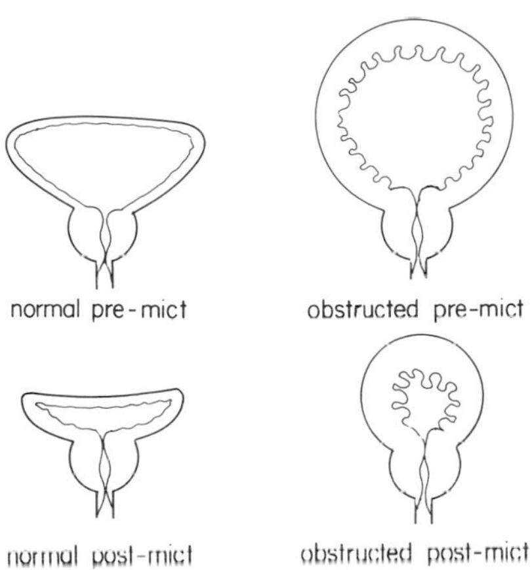

Fig. 19.10. Radiographic appearances of the normal and the obstructed bladder.

prostate into a shell or *capsule.* These bulky adenomas enlarge on either side of the urethra, and grow up through the internal sphincter to form the *lobes* of the prostate. As these adenomas enlarge they displace the verumontanum down towards the external sphincter.

Pathological effects of outflow obstruction

The detrusor responds to outflow obstruction by becoming stronger so as to generate an increased pressure during micturition. At first the wall of the bladder is thickened and becomes spherical as the pressure inside it exceeds that within the abdominal cavity (Fig. 19.10). The hypertrophied detrusor is also more jumpy, and responds to filling with a contraction (sometimes labelled 'instability'). At first this increased power in the destrusor keeps the bladder empty and the flow-rate may be maintained. In this phase of the illness the patient may have a little delay in beginning to pass urine and may notice some frequency and urgency but his stream may not be noticeably impaired.

Even at this stage the peak voiding pressure inside the bladder may begin to exceed the critical level of 40 cmH_2O and the upper tracts begin to be threatened as the ureters become compressed or even frankly obstructed.

Before long the detrusor gives up the struggle and the bladder no longer empties. The volume of residual urine grows (Fig. 19.11) and invites infection. With time, things get worse: the volume of residual urine becomes so large that we speak of *chronic retention.* The bladder,

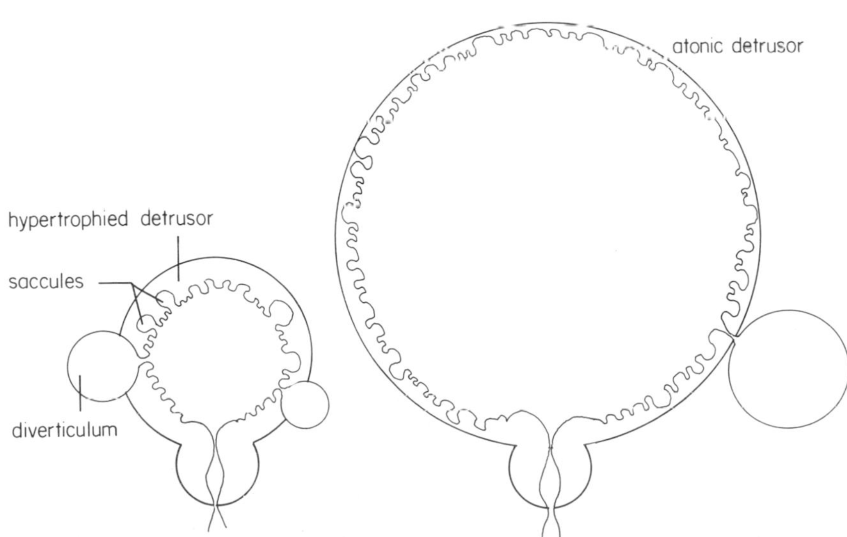

Fig. 19.11. Progressive failure of the detrusor muscle — at first hypertrophy is weakened by development of saccules and diverticula (left); later on, the muscle becomes slack and atonic (right).

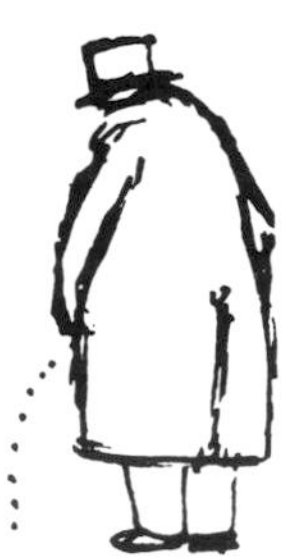

Fig. 19.12.

whose wall is now virtually replaced by fibrous tissue, begins to leak a little urine whenever the intra-abdominal pressure is increased — *retention with overflow*. The ureters are compressed or dilated and the kidneys begin to fail. The patient has now stopped worrying about his urinary frequency. He has lost all sensation in the over-distended bladder. His stream is a mere trickle and he has to spend a long time in the lavatory (Fig. 19.12). Incontinence becomes noticeable, if not to the patient, then certainly to his friends and family.

Changes in the structure of the bladder

The muscle fibres of the bladder are arranged not in neat layers like the gut but in a fine feltwork. In hypertrophy a number of important structural changes take place. The fibrous tissue that creeps in between the muscle strands prevents them from contracting effectively, and at the same time the strands become thick and coarse — resembling the branches of a tree (*trabeculae*) and the mucosa bulges out between them to form *saccules* (Fig. 19.13). Later these saccules enlarge until they form huge balloons — *diverticula* (Fig. 19.14). Once a diverticulum has formed, it never really empties out completely and infection is almost inevitable: worse, the stagnant urine favours squamous metaplasia and the formation of a carcinoma.

Effects on the ureters and kidneys

Increasing the pressure in the bladder above about 40 cmH_2O brings about an increase in pressure in the lumen of the renal pelvis well before the ureter can be seen to become dilated. In time the lower end of the

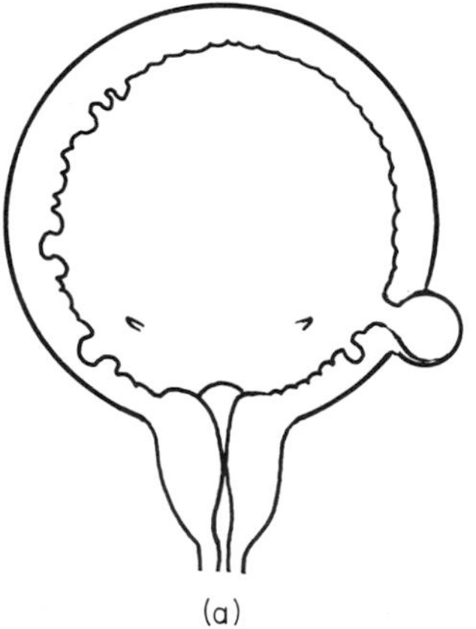

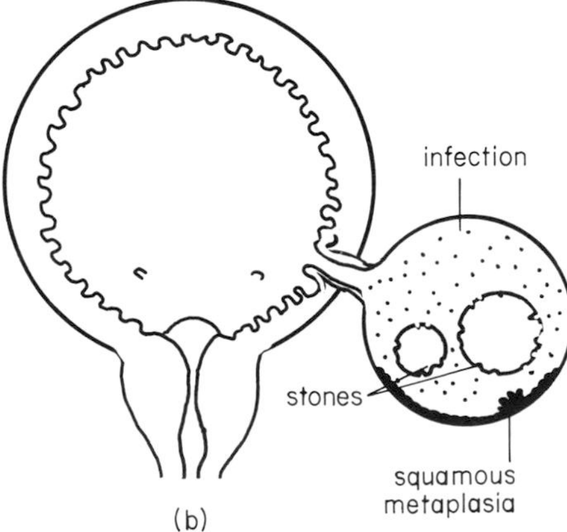

Fig. 19.13. Diverticula predispose to infection, stones, squamous metaplasia and carcinoma.

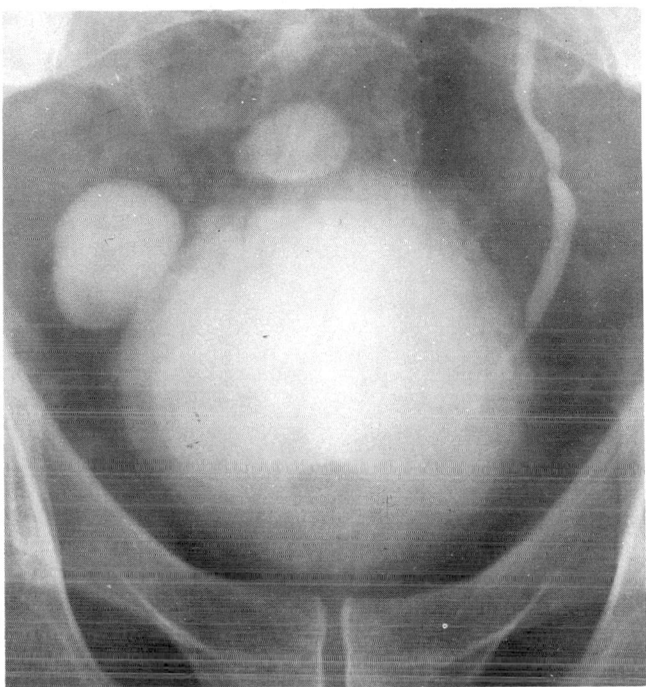

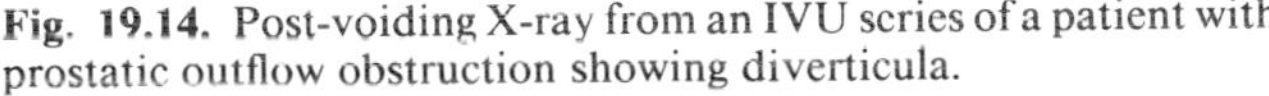

Fig. 19.14. Post-voiding X-ray from an IVU series of a patient with prostatic outflow obstruction showing diverticula.

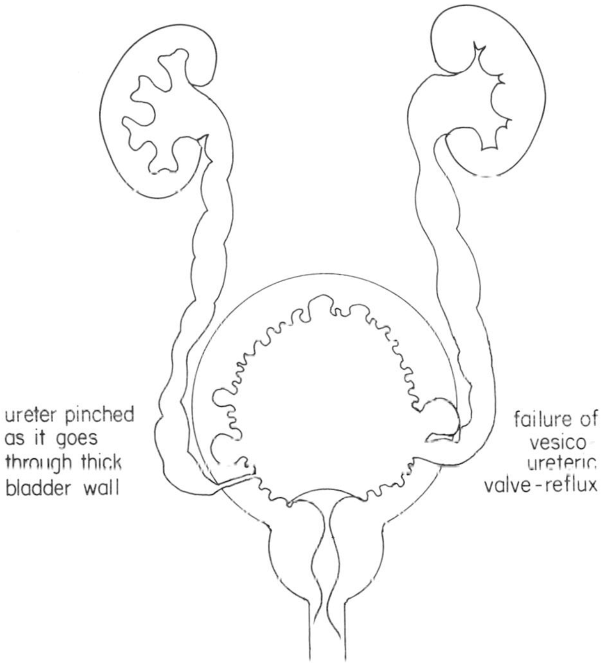

Fig. 19.15. Mechanism of upper tract obstruction in prostatic outflow obstruction: either the ureter is pinched in the thick muscle wall or its valve gives way, allowing reflux.

ureter is nipped by the thickened wall of the bladder (Fig. 19.15) or the valve at its lower end gives way and allows reflux of urine from the bladder to the kidney. The kidney develops obstructive uropathy (see p. 66). At first impairment of tubular function causes hypotonic urine and the need for a diuresis: later there is impairment of glomerular filtration and the creatinine and urea begin to rise. Now begin the symptoms of uraemia — thirst, malaise, confusion, dehydration and anaemia. Prostatectomy at this stage, with dehydration and anaemia uncorrected, is needlessly hazardous. Time spent correcting these abnormalities is well spent.

Infection

If the man with residual urine develops infection it will not go away until the obstruction is corrected, and the first symptoms may be high fever, bacteraemia or acute epididymitis.

Acute retention

The overstrained detrusor may fail suddenly, sometimes associated with some other event such as a myocardial infarction, an accident, a drunken spree or a surgical operation. Often it comes on without any obvious warning. By tradition, acute is distinguished from chronic retention by being painful: in fact it is well to remember that in many patients the acute episode is an exacerbation of a chronic one.

Indications for prostatectomy

The man with outflow obstruction needs an operation before his detrusor is enfeebled by fibrosis and rotten with saccules and diverticula: before his ureters are obstructed and the kidneys affected by obstructive uropathy. Ideally an operation should be considered whenever the peak voiding pressure exceeds 40 cmH_2O but in practice the diagnosis is seldom made at such an early stage.

The symptoms that take the patient to his doctor are usually *frequency* and a *poor flow*: these can of course be imitated by many other conditions. Other bizarre symptoms occur from time to time: patients have been arrested for loitering in public lavatories because they take so long to pass their water.

As things get worse, extreme urgency and frequency lessens as the detrusor gets worn out and insensitive. Later still overflow incontinence with a distended bladder and wet trousers ushers in upper tract obstruction and the symptoms of uraemia: dehydration, indigestion and confusion (Fig. 19.16).

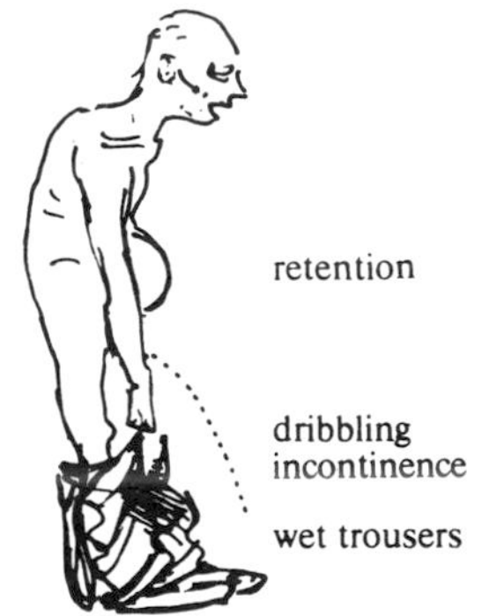

Fig. 19.16.

Physical examination

The size of the prostate is not related to the severity of outflow obstruction, and rectal estimation of its size is inaccurate because urine under pressure in the bladder feels just like an enlarged prostate (Fig. 19.17). Rectal examination is essential to detect carcinoma.

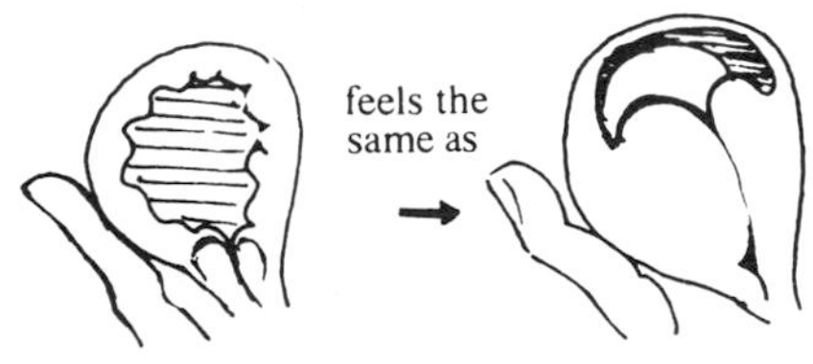

Fig. 19.17. Urine under pressure in the bladder feels just like prostatic adenoma.

Investigations

The urine is examined for malignant cells and sent for microbiological culture. In the blood the creatinine and acid phosphatase are measured and to save an unnecessary needle, it may be wise to request a haemoglobin and blood group.

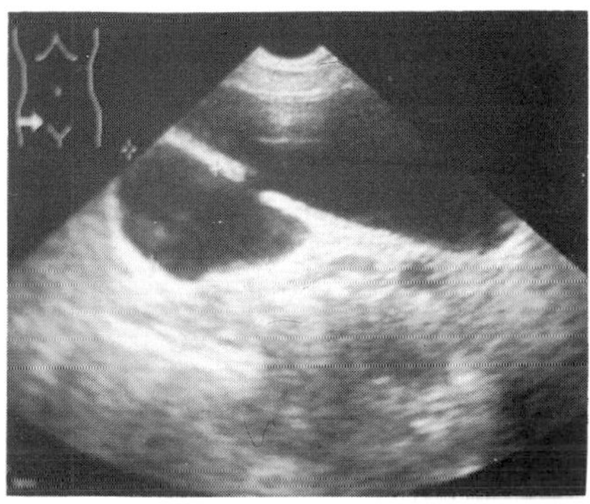

Fig. 19.18. Ultrasound scan after trying to empty the bladder; there is a large volume of residual urine as well as a diverticulum.

An objective measure of the *flow rate* is useful, but watching the patient pass urine may give even more information and an expensive flow-meter is not an absolute necessity. A *plain radiograph* of the urinary tract will detect stones that might be imitating prostatic symptoms, and may call for treatment on their own account. An *ultrasound scan* of the abdomen with views of the bladder before and after voiding is most useful: it shows a large bladder, it shows the thickness of its wall, and depicts the presence of diverticula. Above all, the post-voiding scan shows any residual urine (Fig. 19.18). The scan may show the prostate bulging up in to the base of the bladder. The ultrasound may also reveal widening of the ureters and dilatation of the kidneys signifying severe back-pressure from the outflow obstruction in the bladder.

Intravenous urography was the classical method of investigation for many years and when in doubt, is still a valuable technique, but it is not needed in an ordinary straightforward case of prostatism.

Differential diagnosis

Bladder cancer may mimic prostatism exactly. One in five patients with cancer of the bladder do not have haematuria. Malignant cells may be found in the urine (if the tumour is undifferentiated). Filling defects may be detected in the ultrasound scan or the urogram when the tumours are large, but cystoscopy is the only safe test.

Prostatic cancer may be suspected when the prostate feels hard on rectal examination, but only half the suspiciously hard prostates turn out to be cancer — the rest have calculi or fibrosis. A relatively short history, especially with incontinence should raise the suspicion of cancer. There may, of course, be metastases in the pelvis and a raised acid phosphatase.

Urethral stricture giving symptoms without previous urethritis or injury is uncommon but the diagnosis is sometimes made only when examining the urethra at endoscopy, which is always done before any operation on the prostate.

Neuropathic lesions are the most difficult to diagnose, e.g. central prolapse of a lumbar disc irritating the cauda equina, diabetic neuropathy and multiple sclerosis.

Be wary of the *diuresis* caused by water retention in cardiac failure, *frequency* caused by anxiety, and the *nocturia of depression* — the sad old man who wakes in the small hours of the night because he is lonely and depressed, he passes urine, he cannot get back to sleep, so he makes a cup of tea: he still cannot sleep so he passes urine again. To make these diagnoses you must listen to what the patient is trying to tell you.

Treatment

There is no medical treatment for benign prostatic enlargement: innumerable pills, hormones, injections and other remedies have been advocated, but none of them work. When the obstruction is mainly due to want of relaxation of the neck of the bladder, then an alpha blocker such as prazosin or phenoxybenzamine will allow the bladder neck to open, but this usually requires prostatectomy or bladder neck incision before long. It is a useful diagnostic test.

The elective cold case

A poor flow rate, residual urine, a thickened bladder wall, sacculation and upper tract obstruction are all relatively late features demanding prostatectomy. Men without these features, whose only symptom is frequency, should be treated very warily and need urodynamic evidence of a raised voiding pressure. Even then some time spent in observing the natural course of the disease is often wise. The patient should always be referred to a specialist urological unit where transurethral resection can be offered.

Acute retention of urine

When acute retention of urine comes as the culmination of a crescendo of prostatic symptoms then prostatectomy is almost inevitable: very few patients will be able to resume normal micturition. In those who have had no such symptoms it is reasonable to pass a catheter, empty the bladder, and see if they can pass urine normally later on. The majority of patients need a catheter and their prostatectomy should be arranged with the minimum of delay. Do not catheterize a patient and send him home. When there is likely to be considerable delay — e.g. in transporting him to a hospital — a catheter should be passed and left indwelling.

Chronic retention

The patient with a painless distended bladder without a raised creatinine may undergo prostatectomy on the next convenient operating list: it is seldom necessary to empty his bladder, but if he is *uraemic* the situation is entirely different. He will be dehydrated and his apparently normal haemoglobin level may be falsely high. On decompressing the bladder there may be a profuse *post-obstructive diuresis* to correct which may require more salt and water than he can comfortably drink. An intravenous infusion of saline may be needed over the first few days to keep up with the diuresis and correct the pre-existing dehydration.

During this period, heart failure often calls for treatment: anaemia may need transfusion and thought should be given to the mental condition of the patient who is often sick, frightened, confused, and fuddled by drugs given for his pain. He needs kind voices to talk to, plenty of light, company and stimulation. Do not isolate him: avoid sedation as a substitute for attention. There is no company he desires so much as that of his family and friends. A little alcohol, within reason, may be a great comfort in his time of need and it never did the kidneys any harm (whatever damage it might do to the liver).

Haematuria

Big veins on the surface of the middle lobe may bleed furiously without any warning and bring a man to hospital with clot retention. This is rare, but it demands emergency clot evacuation with the resectoscope sheath and Ellik evacuator, followed by a careful cystoscopy to seek for a carcinoma. *Beware the decoy prostate* — the big adenoma which hides a little carcinoma on the trigone.

Infection

Drain off the urine to empty the bladder: give time for infection to be thoroughly controlled before embarking on resection of the prostate, which will be covered with prophylactic antibiotics. A rushed operation courts the risk of bacteraemia.

Surgical treatment of benign enlargement of the prostate

Preparation for prostatectomy

It is essential that the patient understands that after any form of operation on the bladder neck or prostate there is likely to be retrograde ejaculation of semen afterwards. Much distress arises if this is not explained, and a younger patient who has not developed any of the absolute indications may wish to put off the operation until it becomes unavoidable.

Blood should be grouped and serum saved, for blood loss can be quite unpredictable and is sometimes quite large. Antibiotics are given when a catheter has been in place for more than 24 hours and whenever the urine is known to be infected.

Preliminary cystoscopy

The bladder and urethra are carefully inspected with the cystoscope to detect stones, diverticula and cancers.

Transurethral resection (TURP)

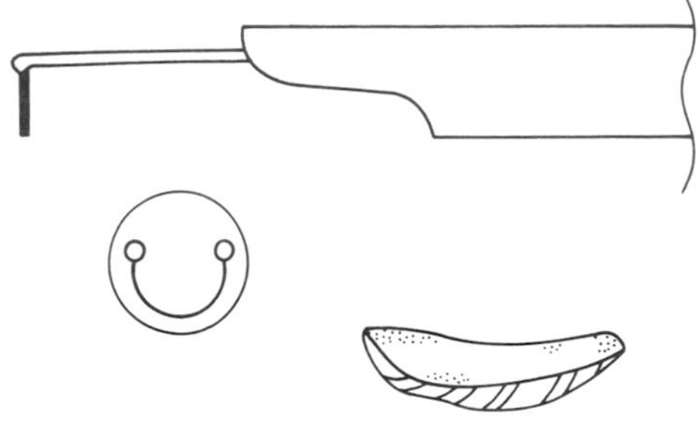

Fig. 19.19. Resectoscope.

A resectoscope is passed, which has a semicircular loop with which long half-cylinders of tissue can be cut out by means of an arc caused by the passage of a very high-frequency cutting current through the tissue (Fig. 19.19). A continuous current of an isotonic non-electrolytic solution (usually 2% glycine) is used to wash the chips into the bladder. The surgeon aims to remove all the obstructing inner benign adenoma that has arisen in the cranial prostate, and to leave behind the compressed outer caudal prostate with the verumontanum and external sphincter (Fig. 19.20). In performing the resection small arteries and veins are cut across which are sealed with the coagulating current.

When all the adenoma has been resected, the inner surface of the compressed outer prostate — the so-called *capsule* — is exposed. The chips are evacuated by means of an Ellik's evacuator (Fig. 19.21) and the bleeding is stopped (as far as possible) with the coagulating current. In fact it is seldom possible to stop the bleeding completely, and small veins may continue to bleed over the next day or two, which may cause clots to form. To prevent this the bladder is kept washed out continually with a slow trickle of saline that runs in and out through a three-way Foley catheter. The catheter is removed after about 48 hours and the patient is usually allowed to go home a day or two later.

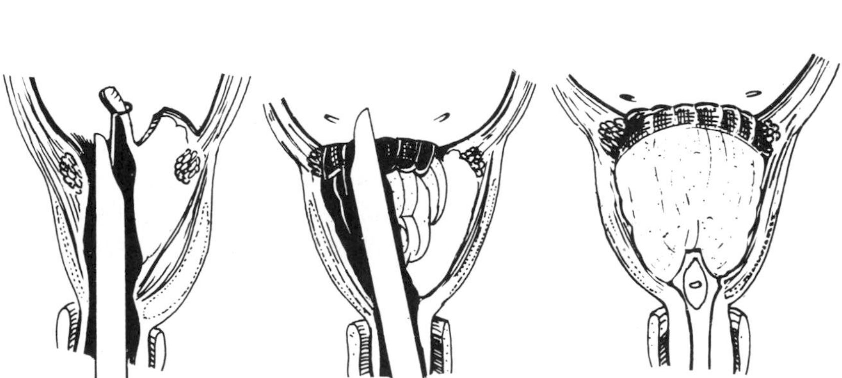

Fig. 19.20. Transurethral resection of the prostate gland. With a series of slices of the resectoscope loop, the adenoma is taken out leaving the 'capsula' intact.

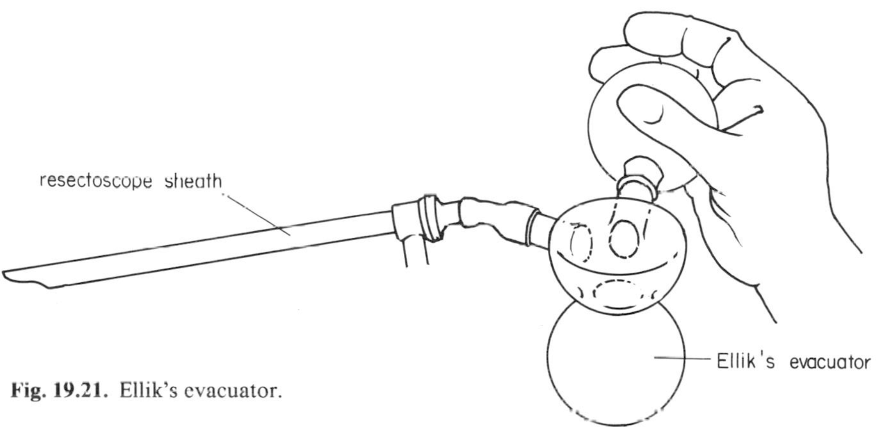

Fig. 19.21. Ellik's evacuator.

Open prostatectomy

The technique of transurethral resection requires specialized training and when the surgeon has not had the opportunity to acquire this skill the gland may have to be removed by an open technique: this is still needed when the gland is very large indeed.

There are several methods of open prostatectomy but the best is that of Millin — the *retropubic prostatectomy*. Through a Pfannenstiel incision the front of the prostate is exposed, and a transverse incision made along it to reveal the outer surface of the adenoma (Fig. 19.22). The adenoma is then shelled out (Fig. 19.23) of the compressed capsule

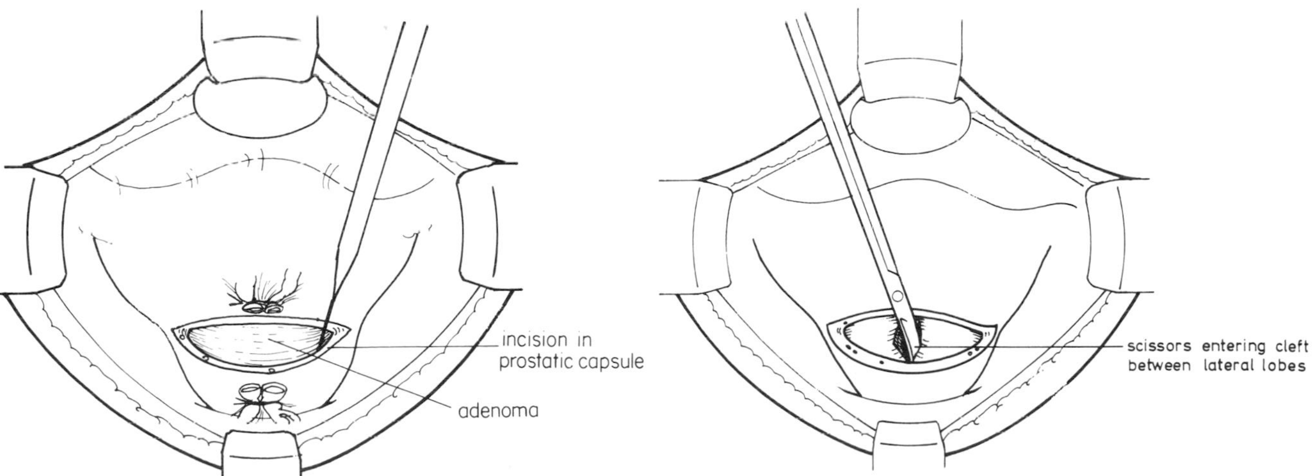

Fig. 19.22. Retropubic prostatectomy.

Fig. 19.23. The plane of the cleavage between the adenoma and capsule is developed, sparing the verumontanum and a strip of mucosa along the back of the prostatic urethra.

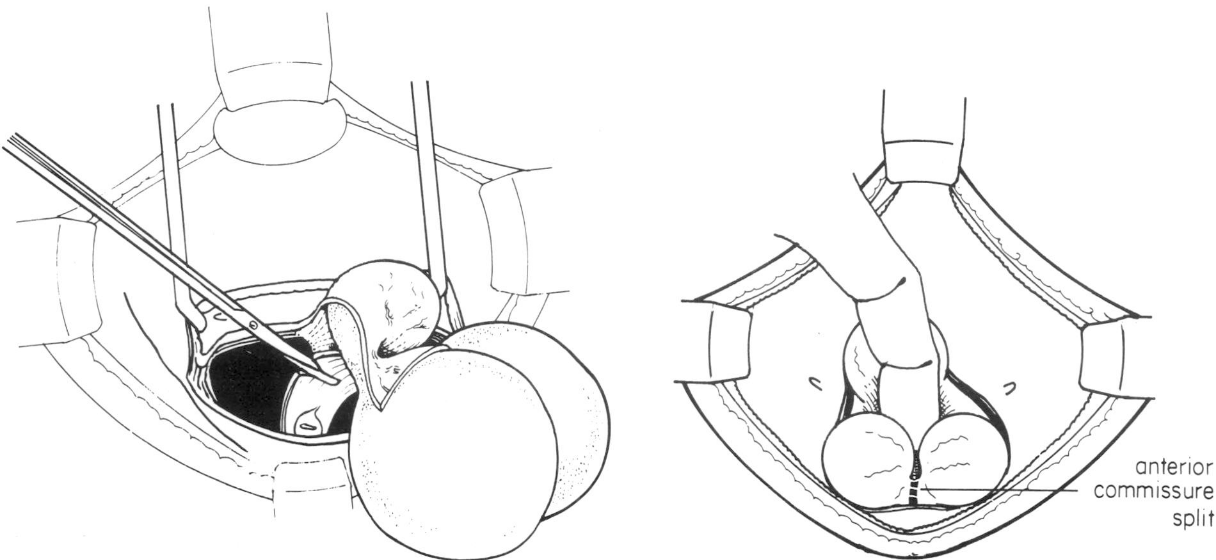

Fig. 19.24. Lateral and middle lobes are removed in one lump by dividing their remaining attachment to the prostatic urethra, preserving the verumontanum.

Fig. 19.25. Transvesical prostatectomy.

(Fig. 19.24). The bleeding is controlled by sutures placed in the corners of the incision in the capsule, and finally it is closed over a catheter.

Transvesical prostatectomy

This is the oldest and easiest of all forms of prostatectomy but seldom indicated today. The bladder is opened. A finger is thrust firmly into the internal meatus until it splits, allowing the finger to enter the plane of cleavage between adenoma and capsule, and so to enucleate it (Fig. 19.25).

There is usually more bleeding at and after all forms of open prostatectomy, and the verumontanum and sphincter cannot be seen as clearly as they can at transurethral resection so that there is a greater risk of causing incontinence.

Perineal prostatectomy

It is possible to remove the adenoma through a perineal approach. This is an exceedingly difficult operation and there is no place for it nowadays.

Postoperative complications

The catheter may be blocked by a fragment of prostate or clot in the eye of the catheter. This may need to be sucked out with a bladder syringe, but if this fails, the catheter may have to be changed. Reactionary bleeding can be severe, filling the bladder with clot, and calling for an immediate return to the operating theatre where the resectoscope sheath is again passed, the clots removed with the Ellik evacuator, and the offending bleeding vessel coagulated. Infection can give rise to bacteraemic shock (see p. 69).

After the patient goes home he should rest quietly around the house for the first week: a good rule is to allow him to do all the things a man can normally do with his carpet slippers on. Thereafter he can gradually resume normal activities. The first week of inactivity is in order to allow the sealed-off vessels to heal strongly. Increasing the intra-abdominal pressure may give rise to secondary haemorrhage: minor loss of blood on about the 10th day is very common, but severe bleeding calling for readmission and clot evacuation occurs in only 1% of cases.

After open prostatectomy the patient usually remains in hospital for about a week to allow the wound to heal, and the catheter usually stays in position for about 4 days.

CARCINOMA OF THE PROSTATE

Aetiology

A different incidence of carcinoma of the prostate is reported in different countries: it is rare in the Japanese and more common in men of African ancestry. It does not appear to be increasing, and it is unrelated to industrial agents, smoking, social status, fertility or previous benign hyperplasia.

Incidence

Small cancers are found in 14% of 50 year-olds and this proportion increases steadily until at the age of 80 nearly 100% of glands can be shown to contain small foci of carcinoma if they are examined by step section. Similar small 'latent' cancers are to be found in other organs, e.g. lungs, adrenals, thyroid, kidney and stomach and it may be that a critical mass is needed before a cancer can spread. In some 10% of prostates resected for retention, and seeming to be benign on rectal examination, cancer is found in the chips, and this proportion increases the more chips are examined and the more sections are taken of each.

Site of origin

Cancer seems to arise as a rule in the periphery — the outer caudal prostate of the primate which in most elderly men forms the so-called capsule that is squeezed flat by benign hyperplasia (Fig. 19.26). As a result, transurethral or open prostatectomy, which leaves this tissue flattened into the *capsule* does not prevent subsequent cancer.

Pathology

Grade

Histologically cancer arises in the glands of the prostate and one of the first changes that can be seen is loss of one of the two layers of cells that normally line an acinus (Fig. 19.27). Thereafter the classification becomes exceedingly confused and unreliable: several systems are in use of which the Gleason (Fig. 19.28) and MD Anderson schemes are most common — but the single most reliable index of future behaviour is provided by *flow cytometry* — a technique which, by measuring the ratio of nucleoprotein to cytoplasm provides an objective measure of what proportion of the cells are (normal) diploid, and how many are polyploid. A cancer that is diploid — whatever its other histological features — has a virtually normal life expectancy. Non-diploid cancers on the other hand have a much worse prognosis.

Stage

TIS — pre-invasive cancer is a difficult entity. It is a histological concept whose natural history is really unknown but believed to be innocent. As a result it is usually regarded as needing no treatment (Fig. 19.29).

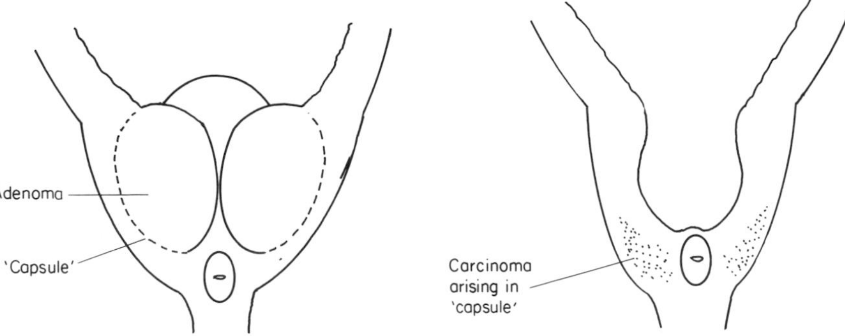

Fig. 19.26. Cancer arises in the caudal or outer prostate, which is left behind as the so-called 'capsule' when an adenoma, which arises in the inner cranial prostate, is removed.

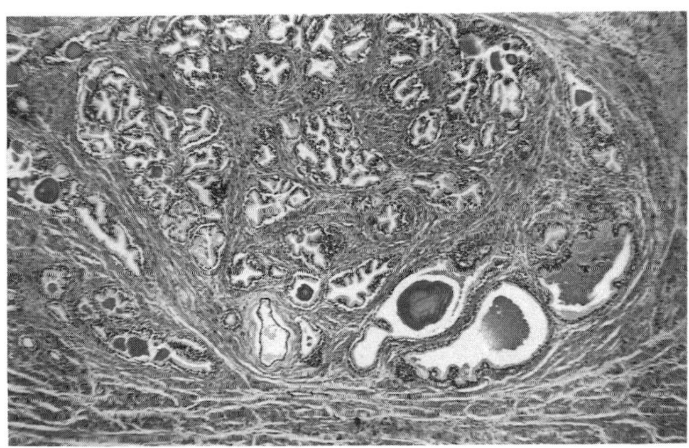

(a)

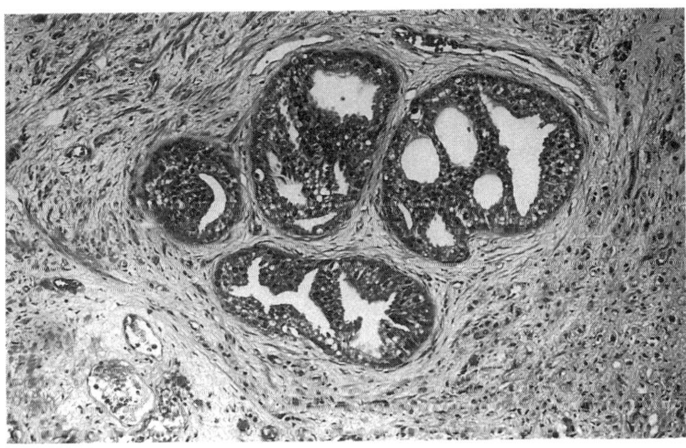

(b)

Fig. 19.27. (a) Benign hyperplasia of the prostate. The acini are lined by two layers of cells. (b) Carcinoma of the prostate: this shows an area of pattern 2 of the Gleason classification surrounded by anaplastic infiltrating tumour of pattern 5.

T0 — no tumour palpable is the common variety, where cancer is unexpectedly found on examining the chips of an adenoma which felt normal and was thought to be benign.

T1 — focal (single or multiple) carcinoma. The tumour is intracapsular and to the finger in the rectum, seems to be surrounded by a normal gland.

T2 — tumour confined to the gland. There is a smooth nodule deforming the contour of the gland but not extending through the lateral sulci or invading the seminal vesicles. Histologically there is diffuse carcinoma with or without extension to the capsule.

T3 — tumour extending beyond the capsule with or without invasion of lateral sulci and seminal vesicles.

T4 — fixed or infiltrating neighbouring structures — the stage at which the diagnosis is made in the majority of cases of prostatic cancer.

This staging system is based upon rectal examination, but in recent years has been supplemented by the increasing use of transrectal ultrasound, which is said to give more accurate images of small confined cancers in the prostate and to detect early breaches in its capsule (Fig. 19.30). The proportion of false positive and false negatives which are found in careful comparisons between ultrasound records and step sections of the specimens provided by total radical prostatectomy has, in recent years, cast grave doubt on the value of transrectal ultrasound. CT scanning has been equally disappointing, and it is too early to evaluate the information provided by NMR.

Spread of cancer of the prostate

Prostatic cancer spreads by direct invasion up into the trigone of the bladder, but its backward invasion into the rectum is prevented by

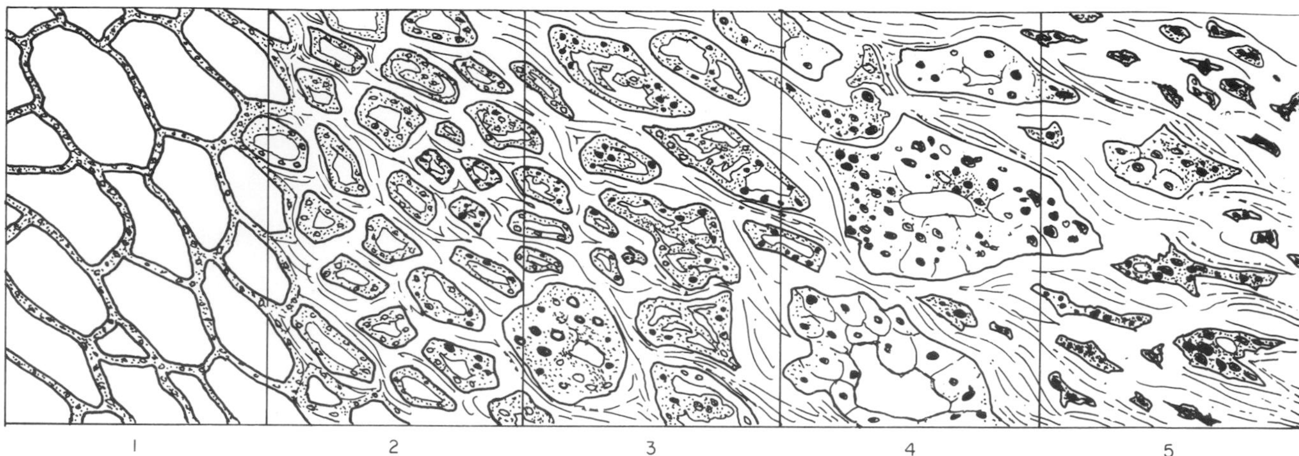

Fig. 19.28. Gleason's system of classification of carcinoma of the prostate. This system is based on the over-all patterns of growth as recognized with the low power. There are five patterns: **1** Well-differentiated uniform single glands, closely packed with relatively circumscribed boundaries. **2** Well-differentiated glands, slightly spaced apart; boundary of tumour less well circumscribed. **3** Moderately differentiated glands, small to large, growing in space infiltrative patterns. **4** Raggedly infiltrating fused-glandular tumour; frequently with pale cells which may resemble hypernephroma of kidney. **5** Anaplastic carcinoma with minimal glandular differentiation diffusely infiltrating the prostatic stroma. Two patterns are recorded for each case, i.e. 2+3, 3+5, etc. so that there is a possible range of scores from 2 to 10. After Gleason D. F., Mellinger G. T. and the VACURG (1974) Prediction of prognosis for prostatic adenocarcinoma by combined histological grading and clinical staging. *Journal of Urology* **111**: 58–64.

Denonvilliers' fascia, so it tends to spread around the rectum and upwards around the ureters, often compressing them.

Lymphatic spread from cancer of the prostate occurs into the internal iliac nodes and then flows upwards along the para-aortic nodes. A direct lymphatic and venous connection from the prostatic system to those in the pelvis, femoral heads and vertebral bodies carries tumour cells directly into these bones.

Markers

Normal prostatic tissue secretes acid phosphatase, and if there is an excess of prostatic cells either in the prostate or in metastases then acid phosphatase spills over into the blood where it can be measured. The method used to measure it is usually an enzymatic one, and the result expressed in *King-Armstrong* units, but the same enzyme can be measured by radioimmunoassay, a method which detects even smaller amounts. The trouble is that in practice the radioimmunoassay appears to be really too sensitive to be of practical value.

The same criticism applies to the *prostatic specific antigen* which is an exceedingly sensitive index of the presence of prostatic tissue.

Clinical features

In about 20% of patients the carcinoma is found by chance when transurethral resection is performed for symptoms of outflow obstruction and has not been suspected on rectal examination (i.e. T0, T1). A short history should make one suspicious that the obstruction may not be

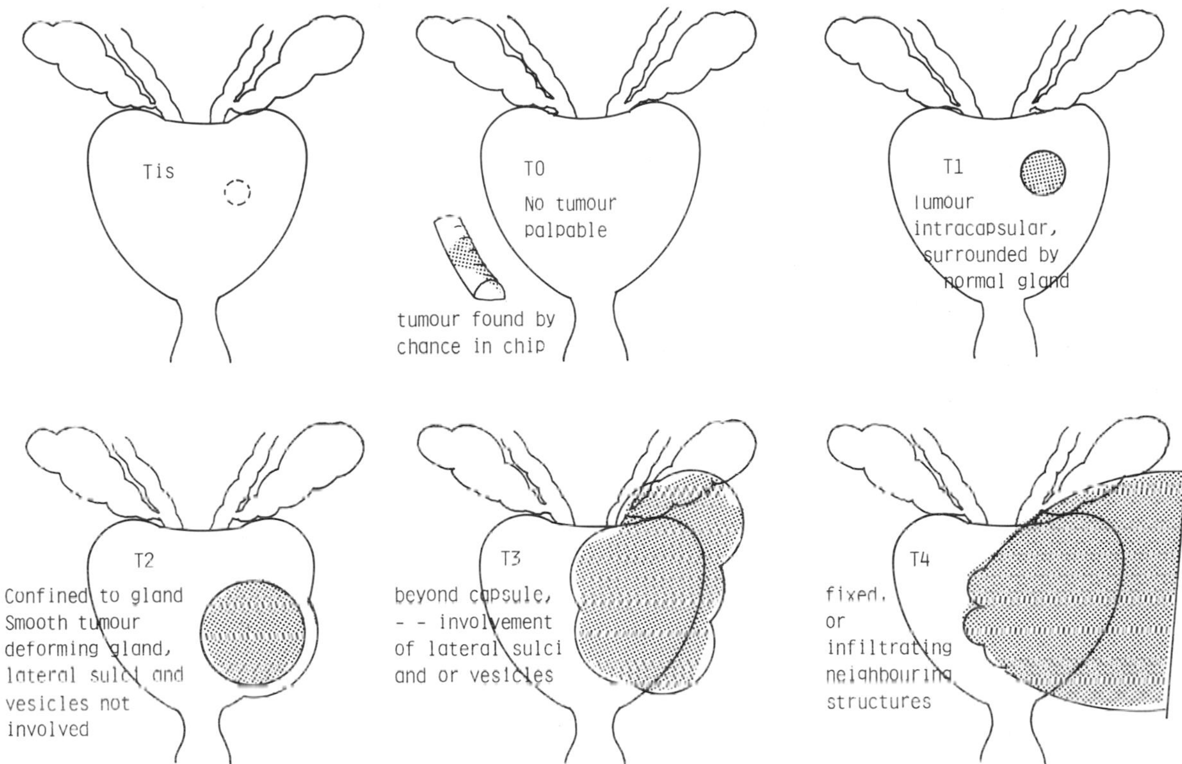

Fig. 19.29. T-staging of carcinoma of the prostate.

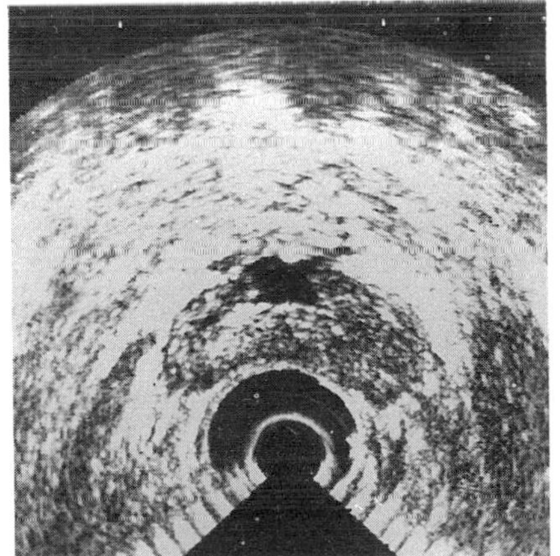

Fig. 19.30. Transrectal ultrasound scan of the prostate showing carcinoma breaching the periphery (capsule) of the gland.

benign. Many present with widespread distant metastases, usually in bones, causing widespread bone pain often and easily mistaken for arthritis. Three unexpected manifestations of carcinoma of the prostate deserve notice, because they are so easily missed:

1 *Intestinal obstruction.* Encircling of the rectum by tumour gives rise to spurious diarrhoea and large bowel obstruction (Fig. 19.31).

2 *Ureteric obstruction.* Uraemia is often caused by carcinoma infiltrating the tissues around the ureters resembling the ureteric obstruction seen in idiopathic retroperitoneal fibrosis (Fig. 19.32).

3 *Haemorrhages and subcutaneous bruising* may occur from the fibrinolysins secreted by the malignant prostatic tissues. If undiagnosed this can give rise to uncontrollable haemorrhage at transurethral resection. It can be corrected with aminocaproic acid. Before setting out to resect a cancer of the prostate when there are widespread metastases it should always be checked by haematological assessment.

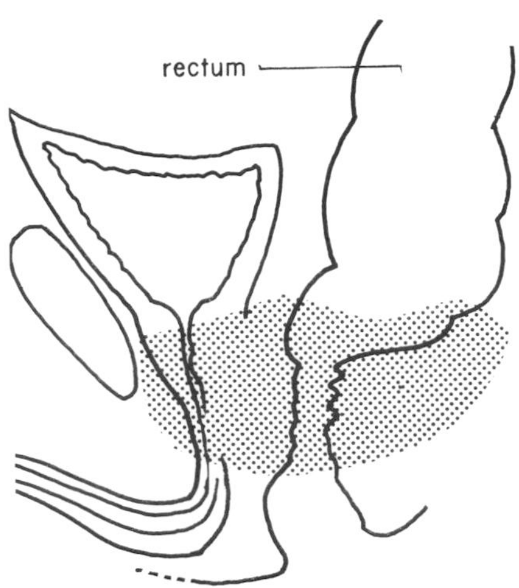

Fig. 19.31. Rarely a carcinoma of the prostate will encircle the rectum and cause intestinal obstruction.

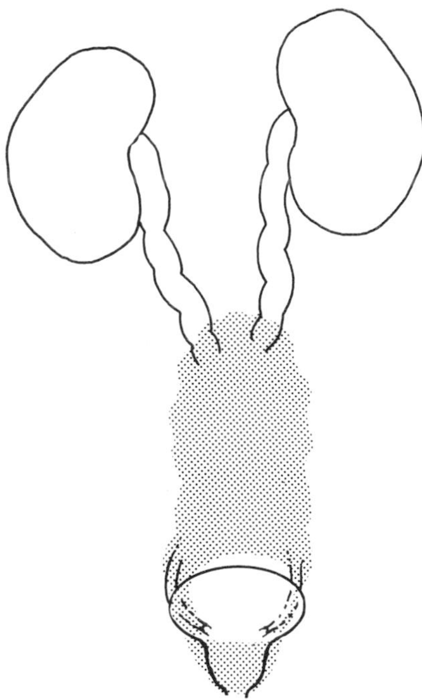

Fig. 19.32. Cancer of the prostate may spread up in the retroperitoneal tissues and provoke intense fibrosis which may obstruct the ureters and mimic retroperitoneal fibrosis.

Investigations

In the routine work-up of a known or suspected cancer of the prostate the histological diagnosis is usually obtained by transurethral resection for outflow obstruction. When a hard nodule is found in the prostate by the finger, or an unusually light or unusually dark area is revealed by transrectal ultrasound scanning (Fig. 19.33) a biopsy is taken by means of the Franzen needle (Fig. 19.34) which provides cytological material or the Trucut and similar automatic biopsy needles which obtain a core of tissue from the prostate (Fig. 19.35).

Biopsy of the prostate

This little investigation is very commonly performed but is not without its dangers. The patient is placed in whatever position is customary for rectal examination.

1 For *cytology*, the needle is passed along a special guide housed in a glove inserted into the rectum. The finger-tip feels the nodule: the needle is advanced into it, and powerful suction applied to the syringe. The drop of blood-stained fluid obtained by this means is spread on a slide, fixed, and examined by Papanicolaou stain.

2 For *histology*, the Trucut or similar needle is passed either through the rectum or via the perineum (Fig. 19.35). A core of tissue is obtained, fixed in formalin, or sent for frozen section. With the newer automatic spring-loaded instruments 10 or 20 cores can be obtained at a single sitting (Fig. 19.36).

When these instruments are introduced through the rectum, antibiotic cover is essential, otherwise there is a risk of faecal organisms being introduced into the bloodstream.

Staging of prostatic cancer

Lymphangiography has been shown to be useless in evaluating spread into the lymph nodes from carcinoma of the prostate, and the only reliable method has been to carry out a dissection of the nodes along the obturator vessels and the internal iliac artery at open operation. This is a formidable operation on its own account, often followed by oedema of the penis and scrotum. If these nodes are seen to be enlarged in a CT scan, they can be aspirated by means of a fine needle introduced under CT control. None of these methods are justified for the usual patient with cancer of the prostate.

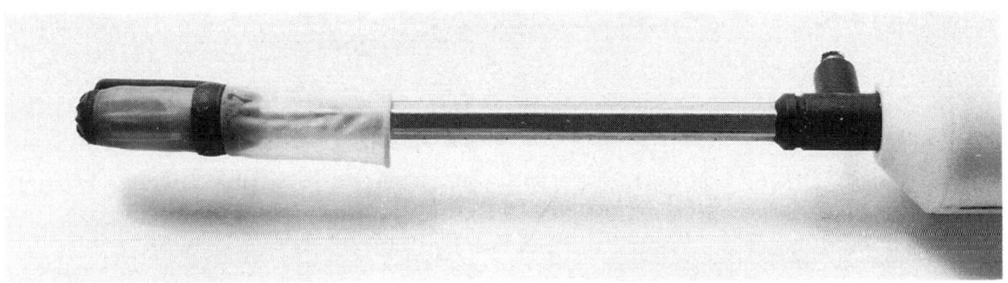

Fig. 19.33. Transrectal ultrasound may detect cancer either because of increased echoes (more calcium deposited) or less echoes (less calcium). There is a wide margin of false positives and false negatives.

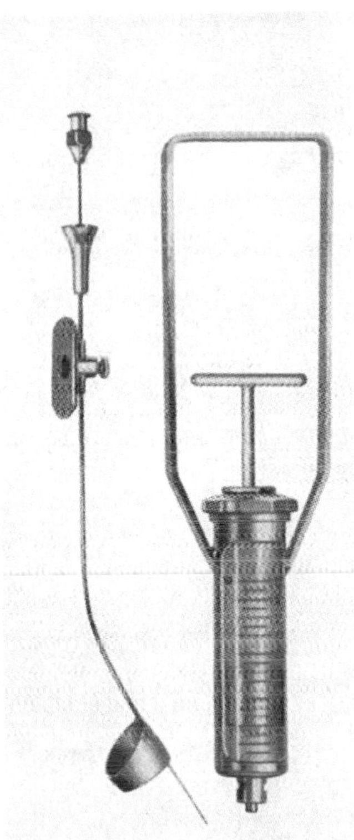

Fig. 19.34. Franzen needle for obtaining cytology from the prostate.

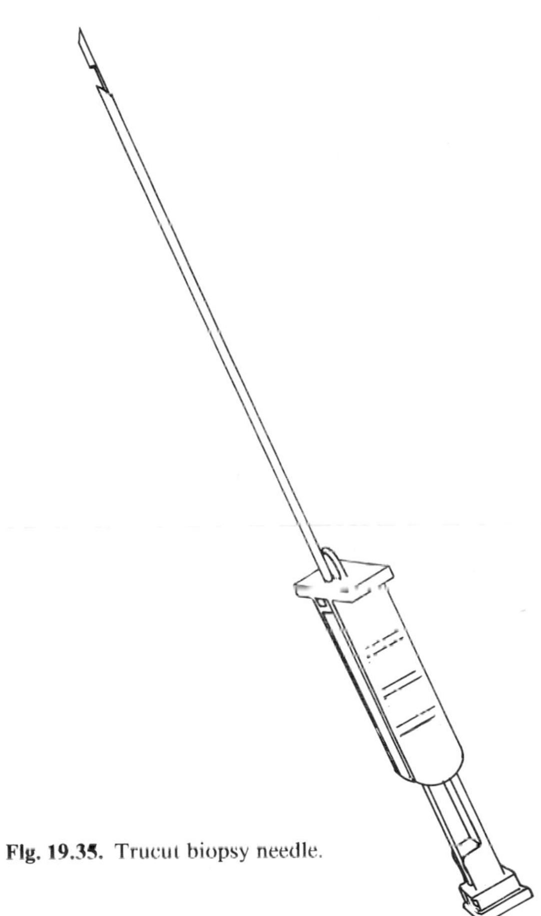

Fig. 19.35. Trucut biopsy needle.

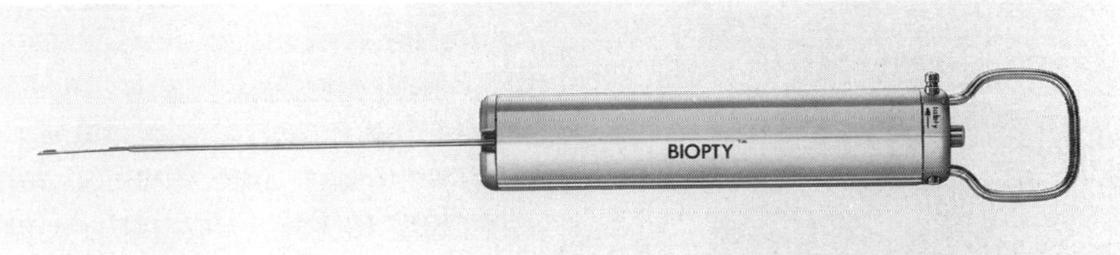

Fig. 19.36. Spring-loaded BIOPTY needle for obtaining many biopsies from the prostate.

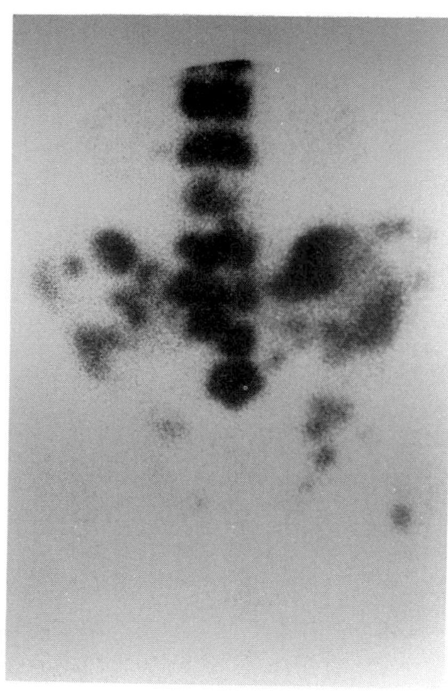

Fig. 19.37. Bone scan showing multiple 'hot spots' of cancer in the pelvis and vertebrae.

Bone scanning

When carcinoma has been confirmed in the prostate, a bone scan is performed. Phosphate (MDP) labelled with radioactive ^{99m}Tc is taken up by bones according to their blood supply. The radioactivity is measured with a gamma camera. Wherever there is an increased blood supply the gamma camera shows a 'hot spot', but it does not tell you whether the hot spot is from cancer or arthritis, or even a recent fracture (Fig. 19.37). Whenever there is any doubt the bone scan must be checked by an appropriate radiograph.

Superscan

If every bone in the body is riddled with prostatic cancer, it will take up the isotope-labelled phosphate, giving a 'superscan' which at first glance, may seem normal.

Treatment of carcinoma of the prostate

No subject in the whole field of urology is more controversial than the treatment of carcinoma of the prostate.

Stage T1

In the incidentally found cancer, whether detected by chance in what was thought to be a chip from a benign gland, or found by biopsy of a tiny nodule in the gland, there are three possible methods of management:

1 Defer treatment;

2 Remove the entire prostate by radical prostatectomy;

3 Treat with radiotherapy.

If all the published results all over the world are critically reviewed, it would appear that there is no difference in the survival rate between either of these three forms of treatment. However, until very recently little account has been taken of the variation in the inherent malignancy of the cancers that were detected in this way. When careful attention is paid either to their histological criteria (using the Gleason or the MD Anderson systems of classification) a very obvious difference emerges: the more anaplastic and undifferentiated tumours do much worse. Evaluating these histological criteria is a process that is fraught with observer error, but when a cohort of cells are examined with the technique of *flow-cytometry* — an entirely objective machine-method of comparing the size of the nucleus with the cytoplasm — it appears that cells with the normal *diploid* complement of nucleoprotein have a normal life expectancy, and those with anything more, do badly (Fig. 19.38).

To date, the various alternative methods of treatment, which at first glance seem to offer the same kind of survival for the patient with confined T1 disease, have not been critically evaluated with respect to careful histological assessment, let alone flow cytometry.

The message (at the time of writing) is clear — in incidentally-found cancer of the prostate, nothing needs to be done, except when the histological features (or the flow cytometry) are bad.

In those 'bad' cases, what should be done? There are two alternatives.

Radical prostatectomy. Radical extirpation of the prostate is a form of treatment widely advocated in the United States. Nowadays the operation is performed through the retropubic approach. The lymph nodes in the obturator group are removed and examined by frozen section. If negative, the veins in front of the prostate are suture ligated (Fig. 19.39), and the tissues on either side of the prostate which contain the nerves responsible for erection are swept aside (Fig. 19.40). The entire prostate is removed together with the vesicles. The trigone is reconstructed and sutured to the urethra over a catheter (Fig. 19.41).

Radiotherapy. Two techniques are commonly used: the most usual is by means of the linear accelerator, but equally good results are claimed from

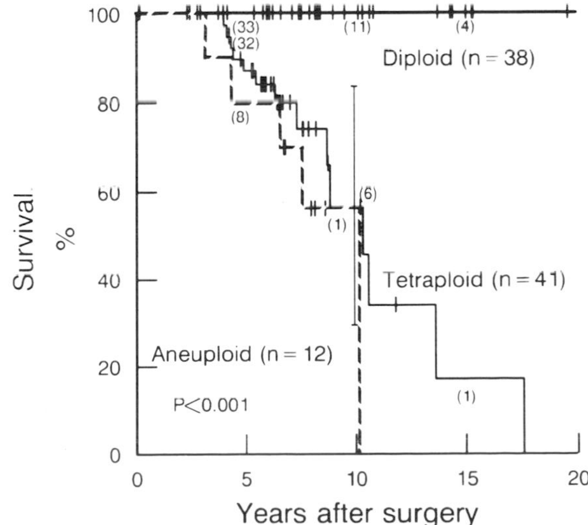

Fig. 19.38. Probability of survival after radical retropubic prostatectomy for patients with Stage D1 (i.e. with positive lymph nodes at operation) prostatic adenocarcinoma shown by various DNA ploidy patterns. Cause-specific survival for normal versus abnormal DNA patterns. From Winkler H. Z., Rainwater L. M., Myers R. P., Farrow G. M., Therneau T. M., Zincke H., and Liever M. M. (1988) *Mayo Clinic Proceedings* **63**: 103–112, courtesy of Dr M. M. Lieber.

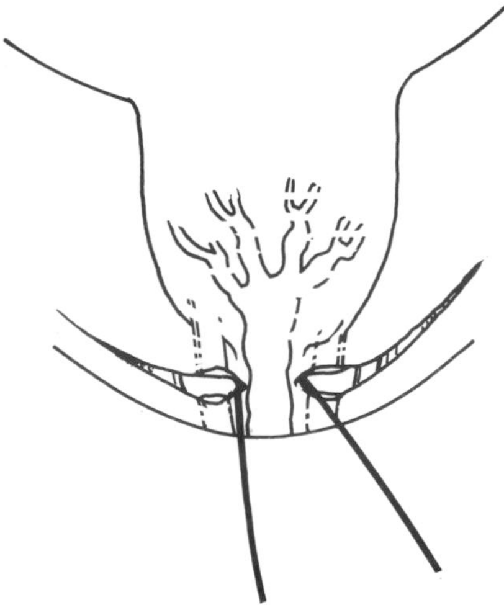

Fig. 19.39. Walsh's radical nerve-sparing prostatectomy: through a retropubic approach the dorsal vein of the penis is divided between ligatures.

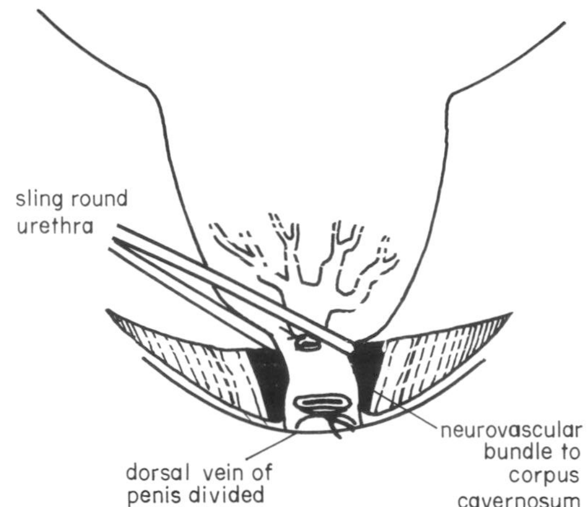

Fig. 19.40. Walsh's operation: a sling is placed around the urethra. The neurovascular bundles to the corpora cavernosa are preserved.

the implantation of radioactive seeds of iodine or gold. These may be implanted through a Pfannenstiel incision (which allows the lymph nodes to be sampled) or through the perineum, under the control of transrectal ultrasound.

Treatment of metastases from carcinoma of the prostate

About 80% of prostatic cancers depend upon a continuing supply of testosterone in order to survive. If the inner part of the testicles which secrete testosterone is removed (*subcapsular orchidectomy*), metastases shrink away and pain is dramatically relieved (Fig. 19.42). The same end can be achieved by giving the patient natural or synthetic oestrogens, of which the cheapest, safest and most effective is *diethyl-stilboestrol*, but it has the disadvantage of causing coronary and cerebral vascular thrombosis.

After orchidectomy there remains a tiny source of testosterone from the adrenals, and for a time adrenalectomy was used to relieve pain from metastases. Today one may give *LHRH agonists* — chemicals which imitate the action of the natural messenger which causes the anterior pituitary to release the gonadotrophins which result in the secretion of testosterone by the testis and the adrenal. These are often combined with

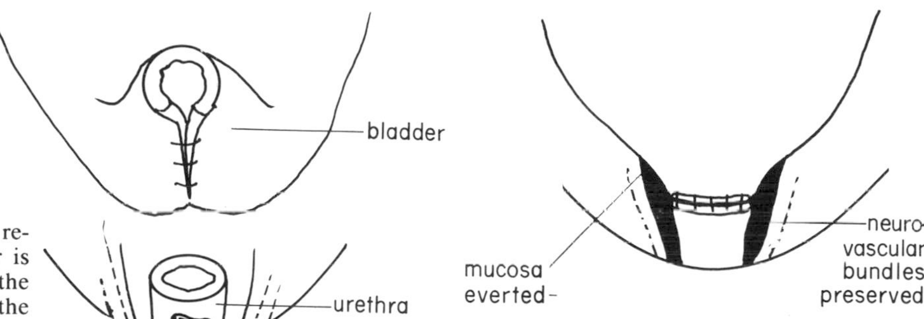

Fig. 19.41. Walsh's operation: after removing the entire prostate the bladder is formed into a tube and anastomosed to the urethra. The neurovascular bundles to the corpora cavernosa are still preserved.

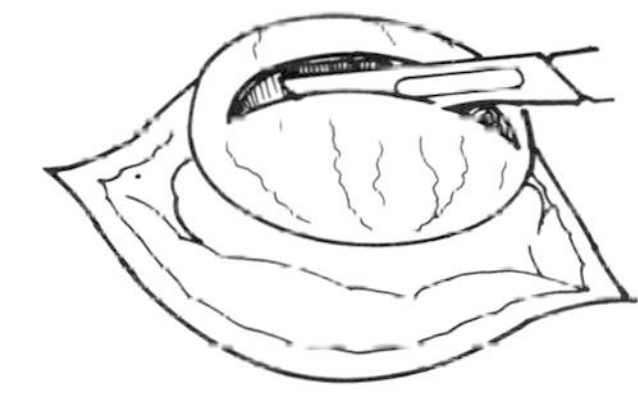

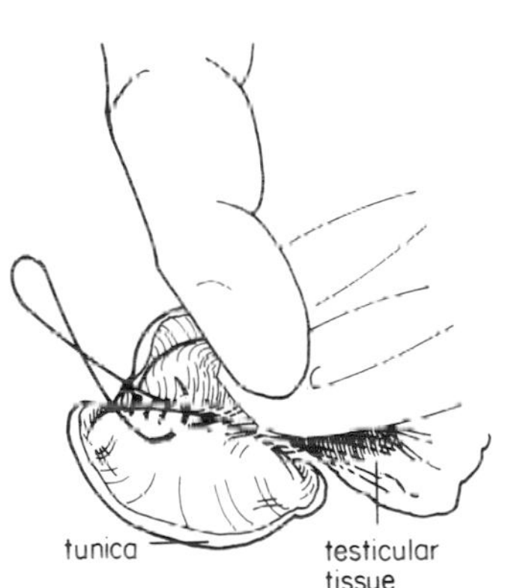

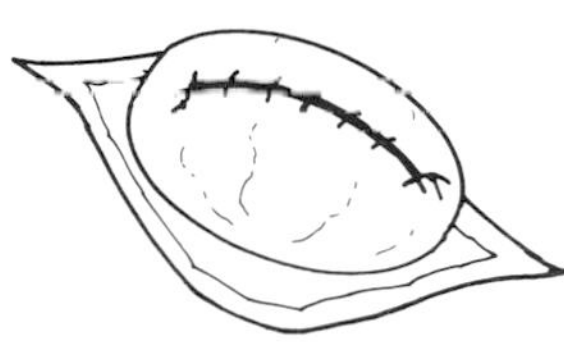

Fig. 19.42. Subcapsular orchidectomy for cancer of the prostate.

substances such as *cyproterone* and *flutamide* which block the action of testosterone on the prostate cells. These chemicals are exceedingly expensive, and controlled studies comparing them with stilboestrol or orchidectomy show negligible difference.

Survival does not seem to be prolonged by hormone therapy and today it is usual to withhold hormone treatment until patients develop metastases that are likely to give rise to a pathological fracture, or are causing pain.

Very often a patient does very well for several years after the cancer has been accidentally discovered in the prostate. Eventually his metastases begin to hurt, and then for another prolonged period of time — often 10 to 15 years — he remains untroubled by any symptoms after orchidectomy or a small dose of stilboestrol. Finally, symptoms return: increasing the dose of stilboestrol, or offering any of the other hormone manipulations, now makes no difference. The usual explanation is that a clone of prostatic cancer cells that are insensitive to any hormones has outgrown the rest.

Until very recently there was little that could be offered to such patients. However, combination chemotherapy based on platinum now promises relief in more than 70% of patients: so far there is no evidence that it can prolong life, and it is too toxic to be used when the patient has no symptoms. By the time this edition is printed new and more useful chemotherapy will certainly have been introduced.

FURTHER READING

Blandy JP & Lytton B (Eds) (1986) *The Prostate*. Butterworth, London.
Blandy JP (1978) *Transurethral Resection*. 2nd Ed. Pitman Medical, Tunbridge Wells.
Blandy JP (1986) *Operative Urology*. 2nd Ed. Blackwell Scientific Publications, Oxford. pp. 168–72.

Chilton CP, Morgan RJ, England HR, Paris AMI & Blandy JP (1978) A critical evaluation of the results of transurethral resection of the prostate. *British Journal of Urology* **50**, 542–6.

Hinman F jr (Ed) (1983) *Benign Prostatic Hypertrophy*. Springer-Verlag, New York.

McCullough DL (1988) Diagnosis and staging of prostatic cancer. In: Skinner DG & Lieskovsky G (Eds) *Diagnosis and Management of Genitourinary Cancer*. WB Saunders, Philadelphia. pp. 405–16.

McGuire EJ (1986) Functional changes in prostatic obstruction. In: Blandy JP & Lytton B (Eds) *The Prostate*. Butterworth, London. pp. 23–32.

Murdoch DA, Badenoch DF & Gatchalian ER (1987) Oral ciprofloxacin as prophylaxis in transurethral resection of the prostate. *British Journal of Urology* **60**,153–6.

Paulson DF (1988) Surgical therapy for cancer of the prostate. In: Skinner DG & Lieskovsky G (Eds) *Diagnosis and Management of Genitourinary Cancer*. WB Saunders, Philadephia. pp. 417–24.

20 The Urethra

The urethra is lined with epithelium, transitional near the bladder, skin near the external meatus, and modified columnar epithelium in between. It receives many 'paraurethral' glands whose ducts lie in the corpus spongiosum around the tube.

In the male, two of these ducts are particularly large — *Cowper's ducts* which drain a pair of *Cowper's glands* lying in the levator ani sheet (Fig. 20.1). The corpus spongiosum is continuous with the glans penis: it is joined firmly to the other two erectile bodies — the *corpora cavernosa* (Fig. 20.2).

Attachments of the corpora

The two corpora cavernosa in the male are firmly attached to the medial aspect of the ischiopubic rami, and the corpus spongiosum is in turn firmly bound to the corpora cavernosa right back to the bulb (Fig. 20.3). Above the bulb, the prostate is firmly bound to the symphysis pubis. The

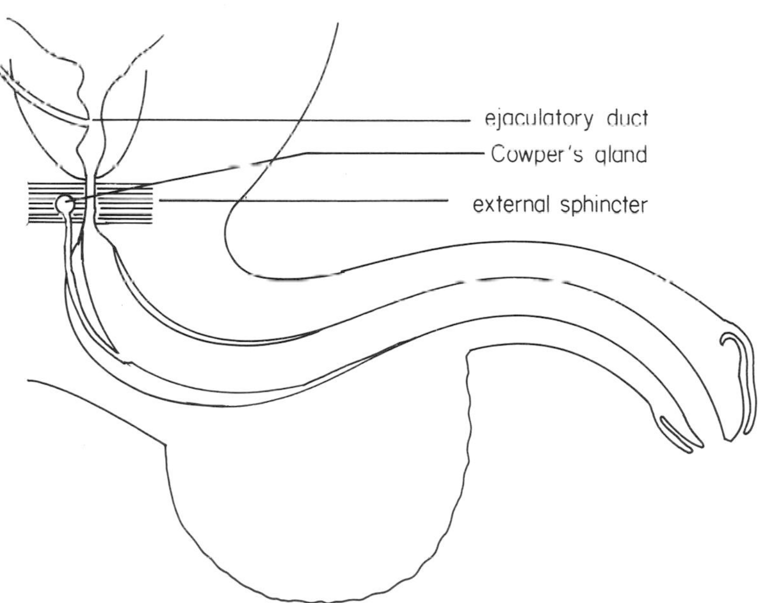

Fig. 20.1. Diagram of the anatomy of the normal male urethra.

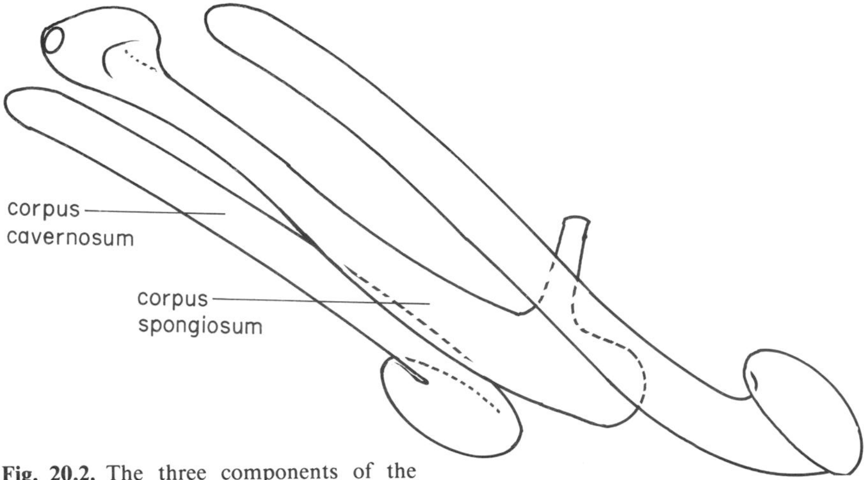

Fig. 20.2. The three components of the penis.

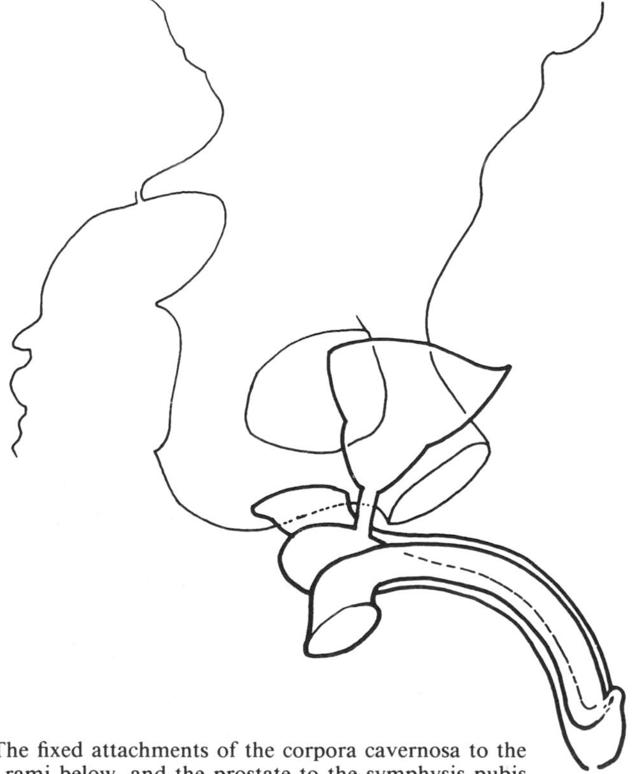

Fig. 20.3. The fixed attachments of the corpora cavernosa to the ischiopubic rami below, and the prostate to the symphysis pubis above: the membranous urethra is the weak link.

membranous urethra, which is thin and weak, bridges the gap between the prostate and the bulb.

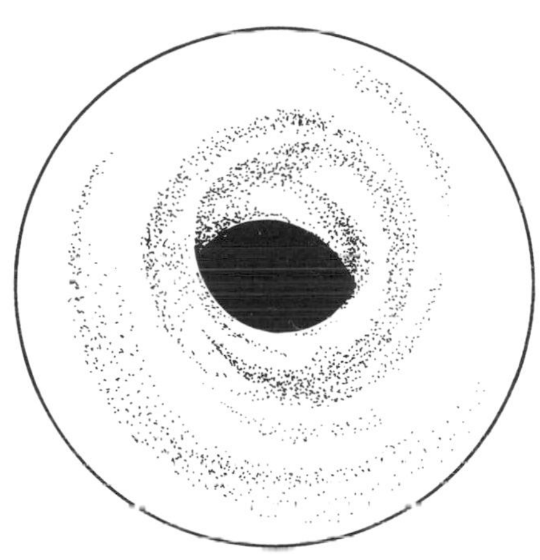

Fig. 20.4. The mucosa of the bulbar urethra is rifled like a gun-barrel.

Investigations

Endoscopy. The urethra is examined with the 0° telescope, and nowadays forms a routine preliminary to any cystoscopy. In addition to the openings of the paraurethral glands, a number of crescentic ridges are to be seen in the bulbar urethra resembling the rifling of a gun-barrel — these are normal, but may be mistaken for strictures (Fig. 20.4).

Urethrography. Ascending urethrography is made by injecting contrast medium through a Knutsson's syringe or a narrow Foley catheter, and oblique views are taken which depict the whole length of the urethra (Fig. 20.5). In females, a double balloon catheter may be used to fill out the urethra.

Descending urethrography is obtained by taking X-rays as the patient is passing urine.

Female urethra

In the female the tube is shorter: where it leaves the bladder it is surrounded by a thick roll of internal sphincter, often thrown into folds

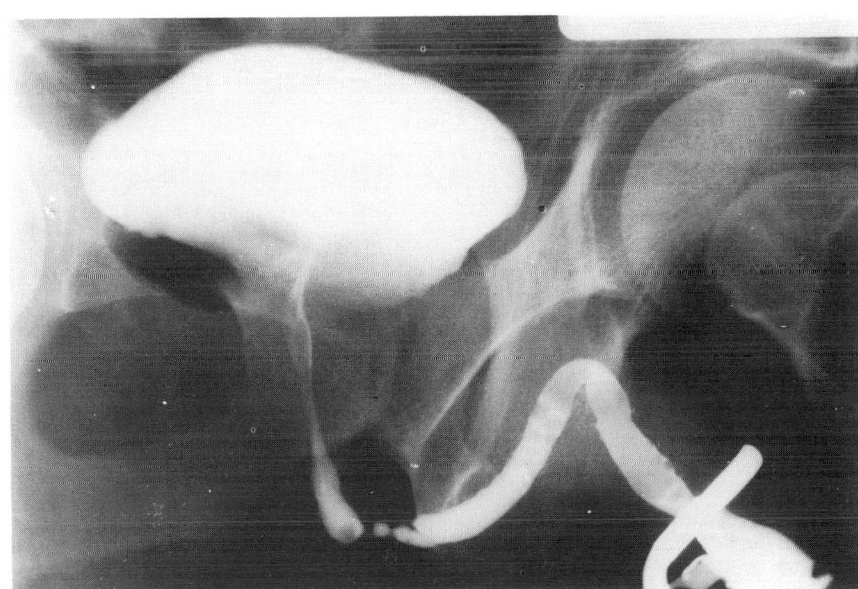

Fig. 20.5. Urethrogram: on the right can be seen the Knutsson's syringe. There is a stricture in the bulbar urethra.

and oedematous frills. The lower third of the urethra is lined by squamous epithelium like that of the vagina and in about 30% of women this extends onto the trigone where it is easily recognized as a thin whitish film of so-called vaginal metaplasia — in fact a normal variation which requires no treatment (Fig. 20.6).

The female urethra is surrounded by erectile spongy tissue continuing down to the glans of the clitoris. The whole tube is provided with mucus secreting glands which may become infected, and occasionally form a distinct abscess.

Sphincters of the urethra

Male

There are three components to the sphincter apparatus of the male (Fig. 20.7). There is the ring of alpha-adrenergic smooth muscle at the neck of the bladder, which forms part of the prostate. There is the shelf of the levator ani, striated muscle, which is slung from the pubis and surrounds the urethra except for a gap in front for the dorsal vessels of the penis, and in between, the *external sphincter* which is so crucial a landmark in transurethral surgery. This is a ring of muscle which can be seen to contract and relax, rather like an anus, through the endoscope. It lies just downstream of the verumontanum, and just upstream, and distinct from, the levator ani sheet. This ring of muscle is of the utmost importance in preserving urinary continence: it contains both smooth and striated elements, and if it is injured (e.g. during transurethral resection) there will be total incontinence, impossible to correct.

Female

One can identify the same three elements in the female (Fig. 20.8): above is the circle of smooth muscle of the bladder neck, and most

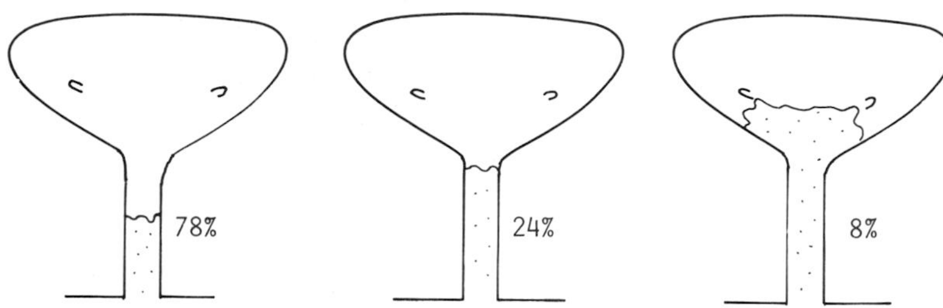

Fig. 20.6. Variations in the junction between the squamous (vaginal) epithelium and the transitional (urothelium) of the bladder.

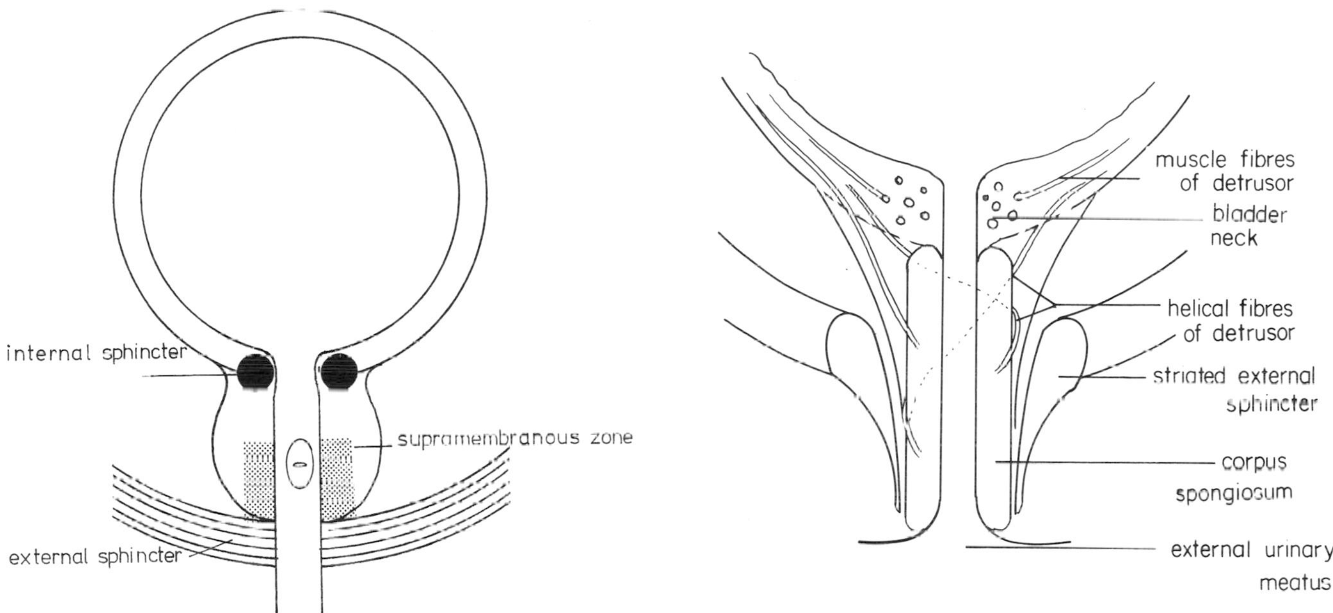

Fig. 20.7. Relationship of prostatic urethra to the sphincters.

Fig. 20.8. Muscle structure of the female urethra.

inferiorly, the sheet of levator ani. In between is a very important component, partly striated, partly smooth, which corresponds to the *external sphincter* of the male and forms part of the urethral wall.

CONGENITAL DISORDERS OF THE URETHRA

Errors in the genital folds

The genital folds roll in to form the male urethra, and are responsible for forming the corpus spongiosum (Fig. 20.9). If they fail to develop or fuse completely, the distal part of the corpus spongiosum may not form properly, and there may be a defect on the under surface of the urethra giving rise to *hypospadias* (see p. 273).

Sometimes the rolling in of the genital folds gives rise to two urethras, not one, and the accessory urethra may be complete or incomplete (Fig. 20.10). These are very rare anomalies, of which the most common is the *anterior urethral diverticulum* — where urine fills the second barrel of the double barrelled urethra and causes outflow obstruction (Fig. 20.11).

Congenital midbulbar stenosis probably occurs from an error in the

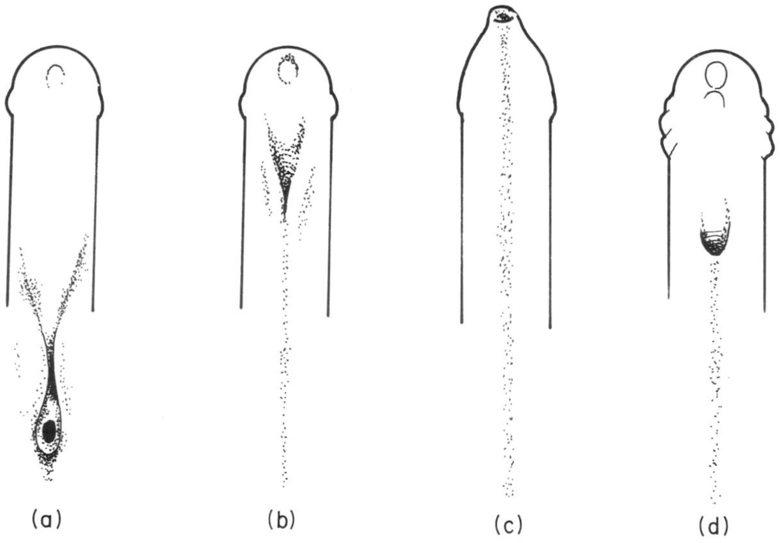

Fig. 20.9 Inrolling of the genital folds proceeds from behind forwards (a,b,c) until the urethra reaches the tip of the glans penis and is closed over by the prepuce. Incomplete inrolling leads to varying degrees of hypospadias (d).

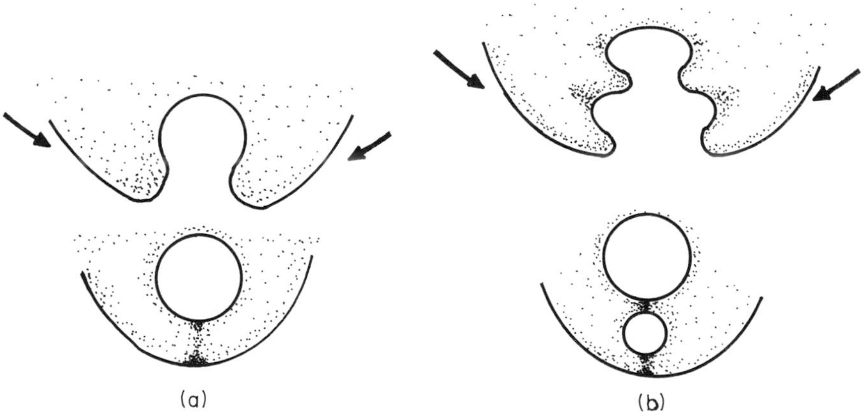

Fig. 20.10. A wrinkle in the inrolling genital fold may give rise to a double urethra.

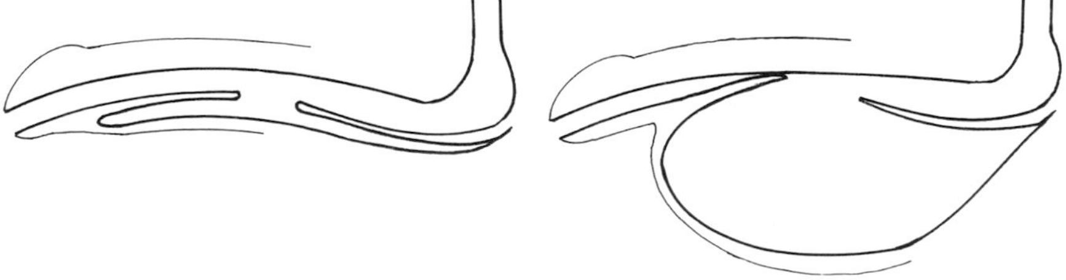

Fig. 20.11. On urination a ventral double urethra fills out: the anterior part of the septum acts as a valve. There is a balloon-like swelling in the perineum and obstructed urination.

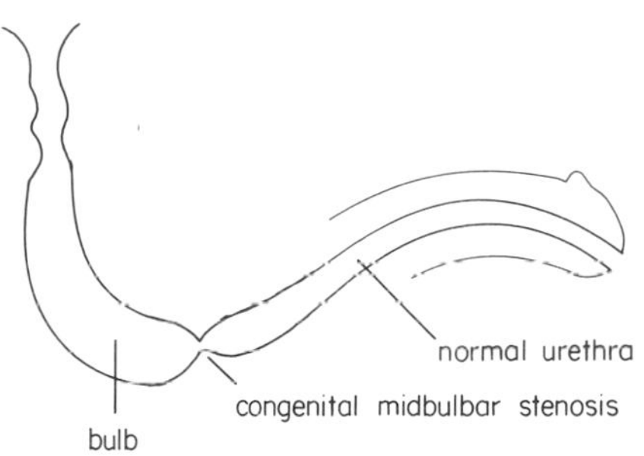

Fig. 20.12. Mid-bulbar stenosis of the urethra: a very similar stricture is caused by perineal trauma.

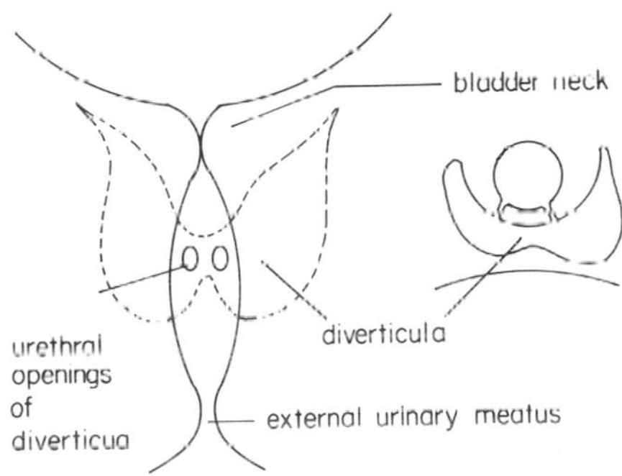

Fig. 20.13. Urethral diverticula in the female—saddle-bag type.

in-rolling of the genital folds. It presents as a narrowing in the bulbar urethra, resembling an exaggeration of the normal rifling that is found there (Fig. 20.12). It is treated as for any other urethral stricture (see below).

In females there can be congenital diverticula in the urethra which arise as a pair of saddle-bag-shaped sacs whose origin is not clear (Fig. 20.13). They sometimes become infected.

Errors in the development of the cloacal membrane

The cloacal membrane may fail to develop correctly, and when it dissolves, there may be large defect in the lower part of the abdominal wall (see p. 166). This is *exstrophy*, and it occurs in varying degrees of severity.

Congenital urethral valves

The embryological cause for this anomaly is still not clear. Just level with the verumontanum there is a thin, tough, membrane with a slit-like hole in it, rather like the spinnaker of a sailing yacht or a parachute (Fig. 20.14). It is sometimes detected before birth by fetal ultrasound, because upstream there is always a greatly obstructed bladder, obstructed ureters and kidneys. It may be associated with failure of muscular development of the abdominal wall and undescended testicles — the

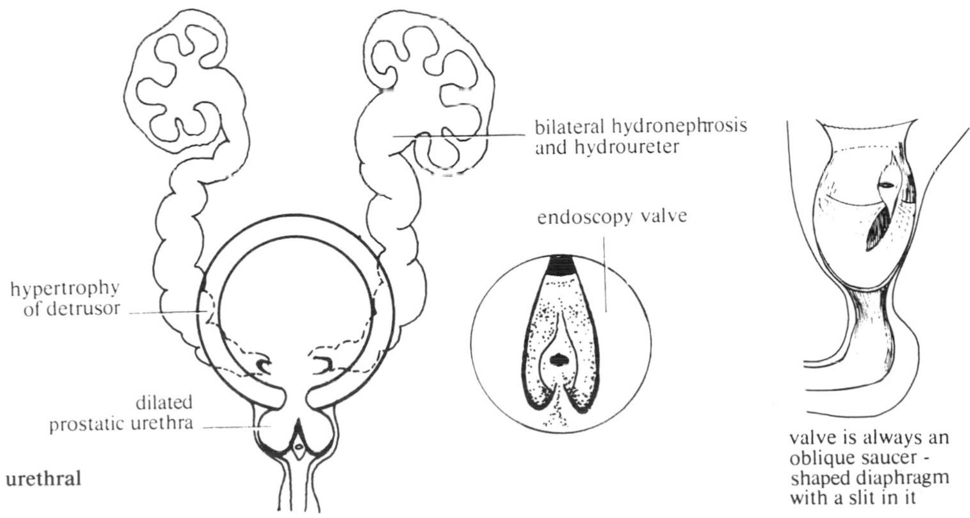

Fig. 20.14. Congenital posterior urethral valves in the male.

prune-belly syndrome. The diagnosis is usually made with a cystogram: the treatment is easy — the little membrane is destroyed with a diathermy or a fine knife.

TRAUMA TO THE URETHRA IN THE MALE

Perineal injury

Fall-astride injury of the urethra has been known from time immemorial — in the days of sail, seamen used to fall from the rigging astride a spar and in the days of coal, Johnny Head-in-Air would fall astride a manhole cover in the street. Today it is an injury of sportsmen and motorcycle riders (Fig. 20.15). A blunt force squashes the perineal urethra up against the sharp inferior margin of the symphysis and tears it, sometimes fracturing the bone at the same time. It is always the bulbar part of the corpus spongiosum which is injured, and because it is firmly held to the corpora cavernosa the two ends cannot retract, but stay close together (Fig. 20.16). Urine and blood may escape from the damaged urethra into the closed space enclosed by the fascial layers of Scarpa and Colles where a swelling consisting of blood and urine will collect (Fig. 20.17). If the urine is concentrated or infected, it may cause necrosis of the overlying skin and in neglected cases the entire skin of the scrotum and penis can slough away.

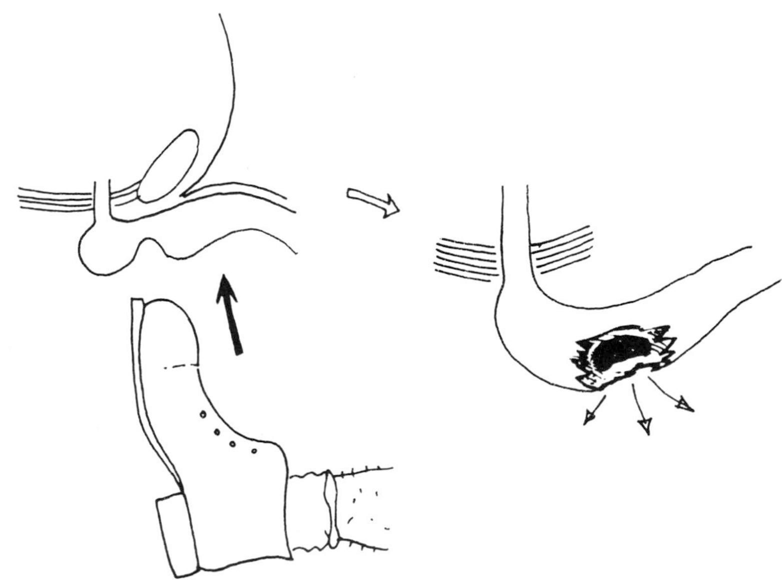

Fig. 20.15. Perineal injury to the urethra.

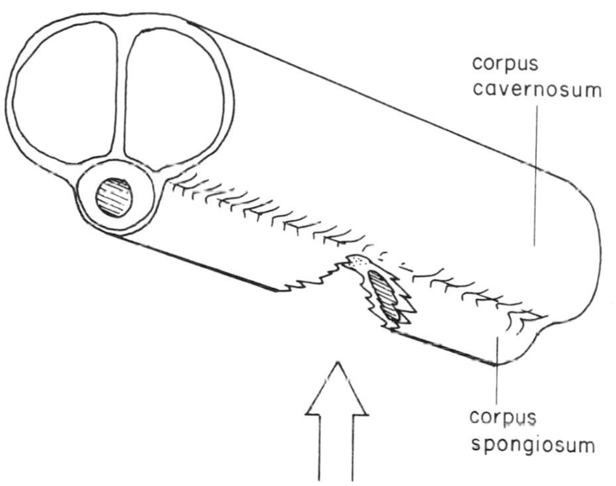

Fig. 20.16. In perineal injury the corpora cavernosa hold the ends of the corpus spongiosum together.

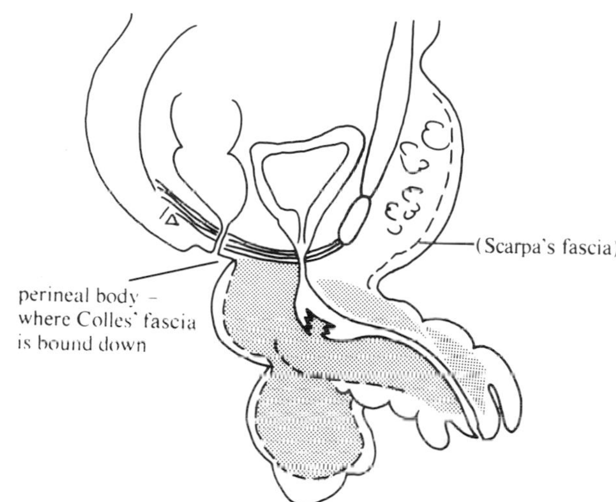

Fig. 20.17. Infected urine may escape into the scrotum and perineum.

Management

There has been a typical injury, a bruised perineum and blood at the external meatus. The most important thing is to prevent the escape of urine into the fascial space, and a suprapubic cystostomy is performed as an emergency, using an appropriate trochar and cannula.

If there has been a delay in getting the patient to hospital and a collection of blood and urine has formed in the perineum it is drained. No attempt is made to explore or suture the lacerated urethra.

After about 10 days the urethra is inspected with a urethroscope. Often the laceration will be found to have healed up completely. Sometimes there is a stricture, which is treated by urethrotomy or dilatation. Only very exceptionally is a urethroplasty needed (see p. 265).

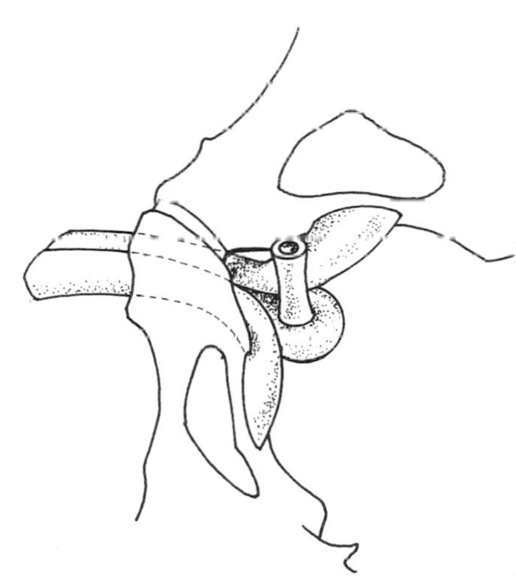

Fig. 20.18. Looking down on the strong attachments of the bulb and the corpora to the ischio-pubic rami. Note how thin and vulnerable is the membranous urethra.

Fractured pelvis with rupture of the urethra

Because the membranous urethra is relatively thin and weak, and bridges the gap between the prostate which is stuck to the symphysis above, and the bulbar urethra which, through its dense attachments to the corpora cavernosa on either side, is held to the ischial tuberosities, any fracture which displaces these bones is apt to tear the membranous urethra (Fig. 20.18).

Orthopaedic surgeons recognize many varieties of fracture of the pelvis, but for the urologist there are essentially three types.

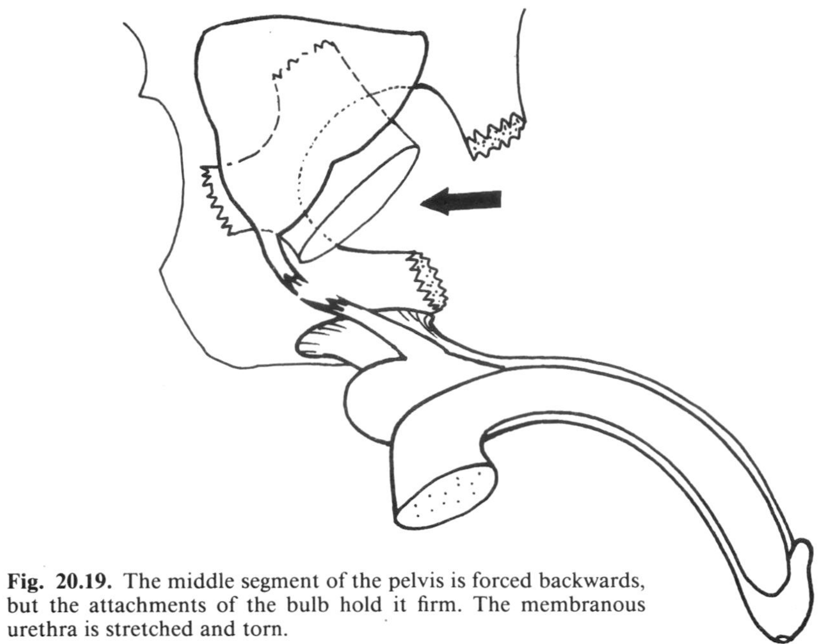

Fig. 20.19. The middle segment of the pelvis is forced backwards, but the attachments of the bulb hold it firm. The membranous urethra is stretched and torn.

1 Minimal displacement injury

The patient is usually compressed from front to back, e.g. when leaning on a wall when a car backs into him — and the pelvic ring is broken where it is most thin — at the pubic and ischial rami on either side of the symphysis pubis, giving a mobile middle segment (Fig. 20.19). As the symphysis is forced backwards, it carries the prostate with it, but the bulbar urethra is held firmly by the corpora cavernosa on either side. The membranous urethra stretches, and finally ruptures either completely or incompletely.

Moments later the pressure is relieved, and the symphysis springs backwards *nearly* to its former position: nearly, but not quite. It usually ends up a little behind its proper place, so that the prostatic end comes to lie just behind the bulbar end, producing either a transverse septum (if the injury has been complete) or an S-shaped bend (Fig. 20.20).

Management. When the patient arrives in the emergency room an X-ray will show the typical fracture. A urethrogram is easily obtained by injecting about 20 ml of sterile contrast medium into the urethra. If the contrast medium extravasates, then there has been some damage to the urethra: if some of it enters the bladder, then the injury is incomplete. If none enters the bladder, there is probably a complete tear.

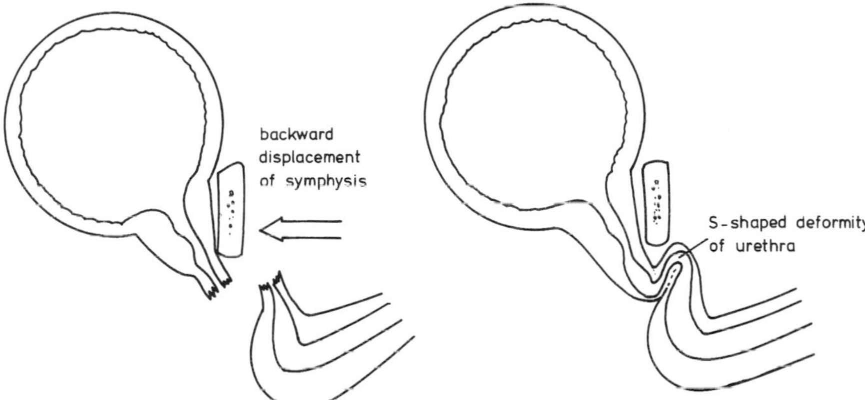

Fig. 20.20. The displaced segment of pelvic ring returns almost to its previous position but the prostatic end of the torn membranous urethra lies a little behind the bulbar end.

A suprapubic tube is inserted as an emergency measure. In many of these patients there are other, important injuries which must be taken care of. It is often 4 to 5 days before the patient has recovered, loss of blood has been replaced, and it is safe to operate. At this time a urethroscopy is performed, using stringent aseptic precautions. If the way can be seen clearly into the bladder, past an incomplete laceration, a fine silicone catheter is inserted and left in position. In such an injury a septum may form as the soft tissues heal, which can easily be divided with a knife later on.

If no way can be seen into the bladder, and the patient is sufficiently fit to undergo an operation, the urethra is approached through a perineal incision. When the corpus spongiosum is dissected off the corpora cavernosa, the bulb is found to have been severed. The soft tissues are separated by recent haematoma. The ends of the urethra are easily found and approximated over a narrow silicone catheter.

Delayed intervention. Sometimes the patient is too sick to allow such an early repair of a ruptured urethra. In such a case the lumen is lost, and a hard layer of scar tissue separates the ends of the divided urethra. The same approach is used as in the recent injury: the ends are freed and anastomosed together, but the operation is very much more difficult than when attempted within a few days of the accident.

2 *Gross displacement of the pelvis*

Here the anatomy of the injury is entirely different. The patient has usually been driving a car and a huge force is carried up his straight leg.

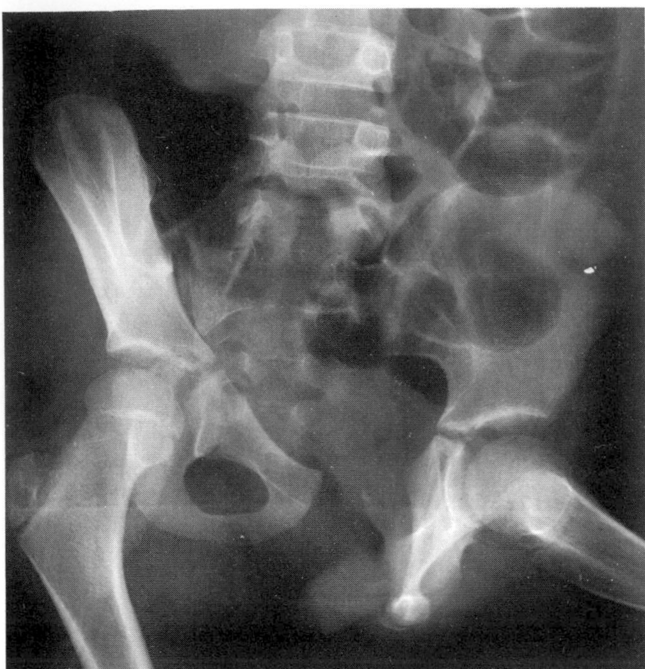

Fig. 20.21. X-ray of a fracture showing gross displacement — the right innominate bone has been forced right up.

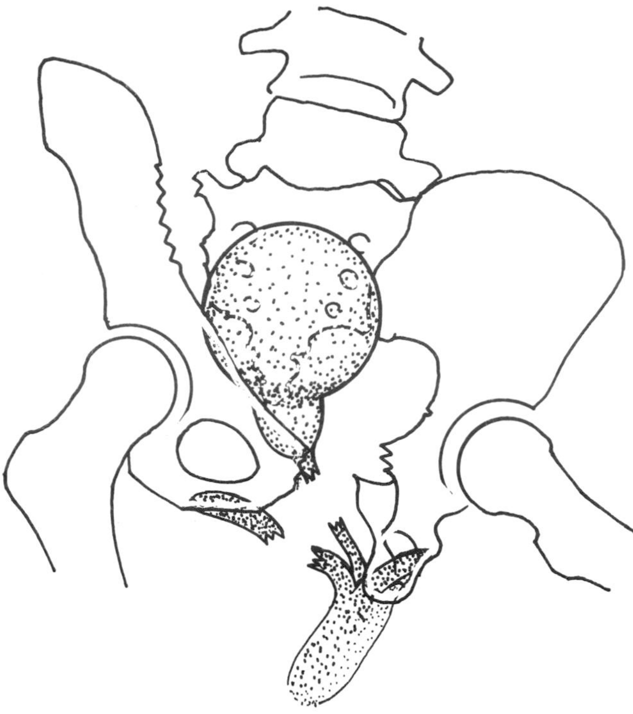

Fig. 20.22. The penis and corpora cavernosa are attached to the left side of the pelvis, the bladder and prostate to the right side; the distance between them is the distance between the bony fragments.

The acetabulum may be smashed and the femur may be fractured but the principal injury (for the urologist) is a fracture dislocation of one half of the pelvis (Fig. 20.21). As a rule the symphysis gives way, or the thin rami are broken to one side of it, and at the same time either the sacroiliac joint or the bone just lateral to it gives way. One half-pelvis is forced upwards, carrying with it the prostate and bladder. The bulbar urethra may be torn up with the prostate and bladder, in which case the membranous urethra is not damaged, but more often it remains attached to the ischiopubic ramus on the other side and the membranous urethra gives way.

In this pattern of injury the bones do not spring back to their normal position afterwards. The innominate bone remains displaced, and the distance between the bones is a measure of the gap between the torn ends of the urethra (Fig. 20.22).

In this type of injury the force that has been applied is far greater than in the antero-posterior injury: large veins have nearly always been torn and the loss of blood into the pelvis is very large indeed. Other injuries to the head, chest, liver and spleen are common. The first 48 hours after admission are preoccupied with controlling haemorrhage and saving life. This is no time to be worrying about a nice reconstruction of the displaced urethra.

On the other hand, the sooner the ruptured urethra is sewn together, the better the result. If possible, the displaced bones should be repositioned. Sometimes this can be effected by external mechanical fixation, using an external device with steel pins placed in the innominate bones. Once the soft tissues have been repositioned, the gap between the ends of the urethra is minimized, and it is not difficult to sew them together.

If for some reason it has not been possible to reduce the displaced fracture of the pelvic ring, and the bones are left permanently dislocated, then a long gap has to be bridged between the prostatic and bulbar urethra.

Management. Resuscitation and the emergency treatment of other major injuries occupies the first few days of the care of this patient, during which time a suprapubic catheter is inserted early on. As soon as is convenient an ascending urethrogram is performed to show whether or not the urethra has been damaged: if the contrast runs into the bladder freely, then the urethra is intact and nothing more needs to be done.

If, as is more usual, there is extravasation of the contrast medium, then the urethra is damaged, and the first objective is to attempt to get the soft tissues back into position by replacing the dislocated innominate bone. This can be done by external fixation (Fig. 20.23). If this is feasible, all that remains is to bring the ends of the urethra together. Through a Pfannenstiel incision the upper prostatic end is mobilized by dividing the attachments of the prostate on one or other side, and brought down without any tension to the bulbar urethra (Fig. 20.24).

If it has been impossible to reduce the dislocation, it is still desirable to join the severed ends together, but this requires more extensive mobilization of the prostate and bulbar urethra.

All too often the opportunity to effect this early reconstruction has been lost and the pelvis has healed in a malunited position, with the severed ends of the urethra widely separated, and a deep malunited callus around the fractured symphysis between the upper and lower ends.

This difficulty is solved by a perineal approach. The bulbar urethra is dissected from the corpora cavernosa, which are parted in the midline, exposing the inferior edge of the symphysis. A semicircular window of

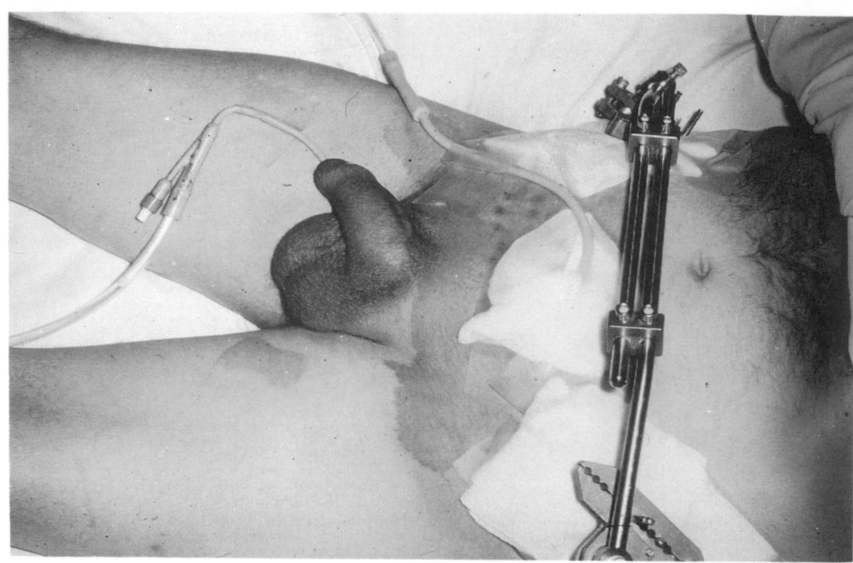

Fig. 20.23. External fixation for displaced pelvic fractures.

bone is now removed from the symphysis, just large enough to allow the bulbar urethra to be brought up to the prostate and the ends to be sewn together (Fig. 20.25).

3 *Gross displacement of the pelvis combined with rectal injury*

This is an even more severe injury, caused by massive crushing and rolling injuries, e.g. being run over by a tank-transporter. Skin and muscles are torn down from the pelvic bones which are crushed and

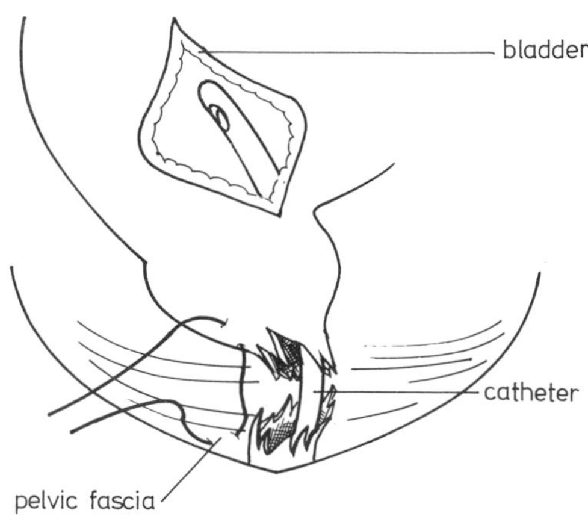

Fig. 20.24. When the patient has recovered from the initial injury and shock the prostate has to be separated by sharp dissection from the pubis and approximated to the urethra over a suitable splint.

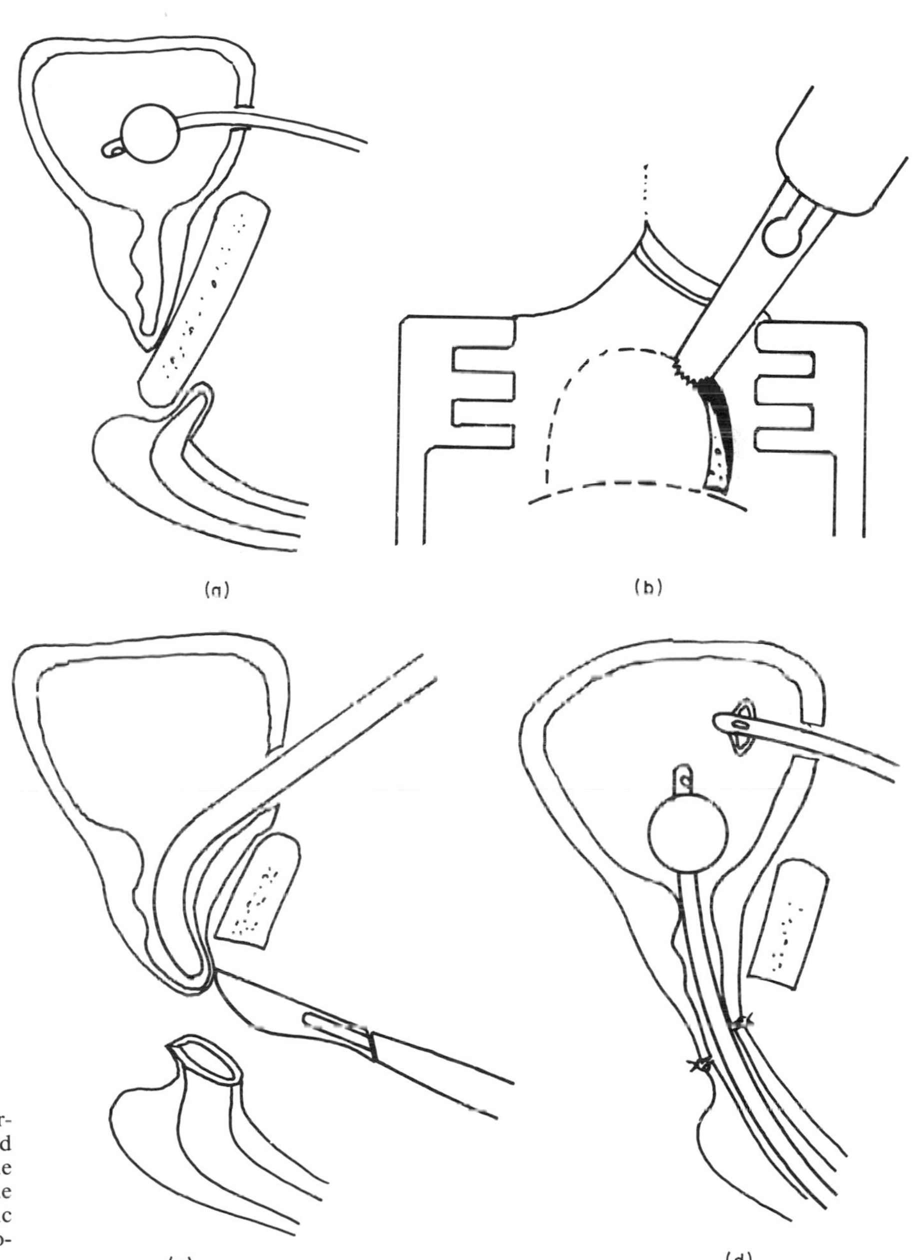

Fig. 20.25. The prostatic urethra is separated from the bulb by a barrier of malunited callus. (a) A window is cut out from the inferior edge of this callus (b) revealing the periosteum behind which (c) is the prostatic urethra to which the bulb is easily anastomosed.

broken in many places. The front of the rectum is split and the tear in the urethra runs up into the bladder (Fig. 20.26). There is tremendous loss of blood and inevitably severe multiple injuries to other organs such as the liver and spleen.

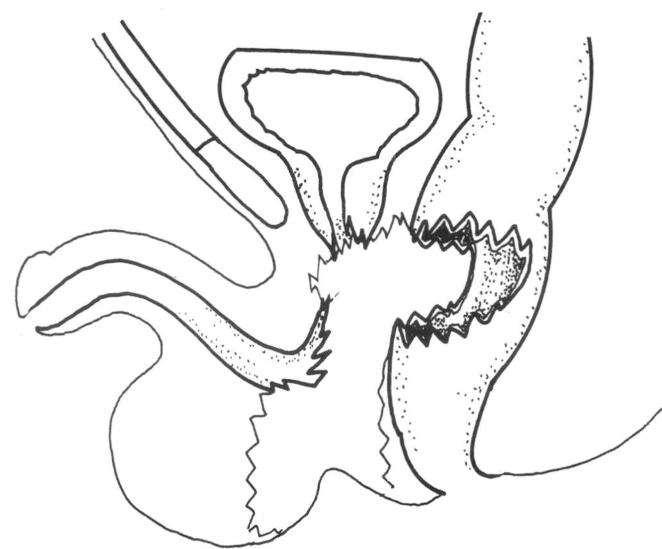

Fig. 20.26. Massive crush injury involving the rectum.

Management. In this kind of injury every artifice to save life is deployed. Massive transfusions, emergency amputations, and the most skilled intensive care sometimes results in a live patient. The next stage is to get the faeces away from the crushed perineum. A colostomy is essential, and must be done as an emergency. The soft tissue injuries are then treated by debridement and delayed primary suture, i.e. at first all the crushed and devitalized tissues are removed, but no attempt is made to suture them. Then several days later, the wound is closed with the minimum of tension. The wound will not heal if urine continues to leak from it, and it may be necessary to perform bilateral nephrostomies or an ileal conduit (see p. 197) to allow the perineal wound to heal.

When the wound has finally healed, then the lost part of the urethra can be reconstructed by some form of urethroplasty (see below).

Impotence after urethral injuries

About one half of the patients with severe pelvic fractures and urethral injuries are impotent afterwards. The cause is either that the nerves of the penis, which lie just on either side of the prostate, have been injured, or that the blood supply to the penis from the terminal branches of the internal iliac artery has been divided. In most of the cases it seems that it is nerve injury which is responsible, and for this reason when undertaking any repair or reconstruction great care must be taken to preserve the neurovascular bundle.

TRAUMA TO THE BLADDER

Intraperitoneal rupture of the bladder

External injury

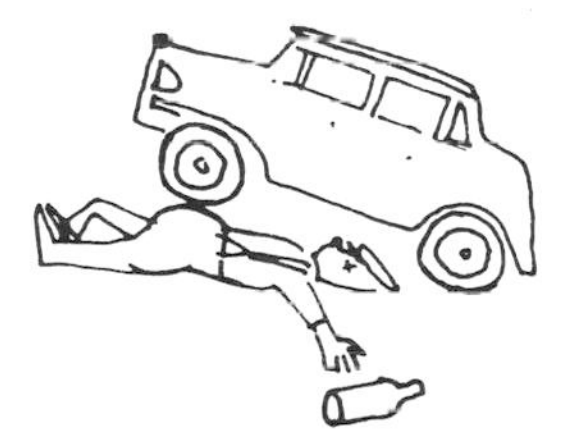

Fig. 20.27.

The typical patient is drunk with a distended bladder when he is run over (Fig. 20.27). The bladder bursts into the peritoneal cavity. Enormous volumes of dilute (and therefore unirritating) urine escape into the peritoneum. There may be good reasons for performing laparotomy, e.g. the suspicion of internal bleeding or a bloody aspirate on 4-quadrant paracentesis, and a tear in the bladder is found when the abdomen is opened. It is easily recognized. The bladder is sutured and drained with a catheter and the outlook is good.

Silent perforation

This odd condition should be borne in mind in any elderly person without a story of injury, but who has recently undergone treatment for carcinoma of the bladder by biopsy or diathermy and returns with abdominal pain, or who is self-catheterizing him- or herself regularly. The clinical signs of urine in the peritoneum are notoriously misleading for unless the urine is infected or very concentrated it is at first not irritating, and the chemical peritonitis may take several days to make itself apparent. At first there may only be vague discomfort and maybe an absence of bowel sounds. The diagnosis can sometimes only be made by a cystogram and even this may require a very large volume of contrast medium before the leakage is detected. These patients seldom need treatment other than an indwelling catheter: so long as the urine is uninfected the peritoneum will absorb it and the hole in the bladder will heal on its own.

Surgical perforation of the bladder

It is very easy to perforate the bladder despite taking the greatest care when performing transurethral resection of a bladder tumour. It is recognized by failing to recover the irrigating fluid from the bladder, by a black hole at the site of resection and, in the very rare case, by recognizing loops of intestine through the resectoscope. In hysterectomy when the uterus is difficult to separate from the bladder a hole may be made. Whatever the case, if the bladder is sewn up and provided with catheter drainage, it heals perfectly: the important thing is to recognize the damage and repair it at once.

Extraperitoneal rupture of the bladder

The bladder wall may be damaged outside the peritoneum along with damage to the urethra and other viscera in fractures of the pelvis where the bladder is lacerated by a spike of bone (Fig. 20.28). There are usually good reasons to perform laparotomy at which the nature and extent of the damage is readily discovered. The pieces of bone are replaced or removed and the wall of the bladder closed with adequate free drainage.

Small extraperitoneal perforations of the bladder are often made when resecting tumours on the trigone and base of the bladder: unless very large they can be disregarded. They heal with catheter drainage and there is very seldom any need to drain a local collection of fluid.

INFLAMMATION OF THE URETHRA AND URETHRAL STRICTURE

Aetiology

A very few strictures of the urethra are congenital (see above); many are due to healing of injury, but in the long history of surgery, stricture was almost synonymous with gonococcal urethritis. Socrates joked about it;

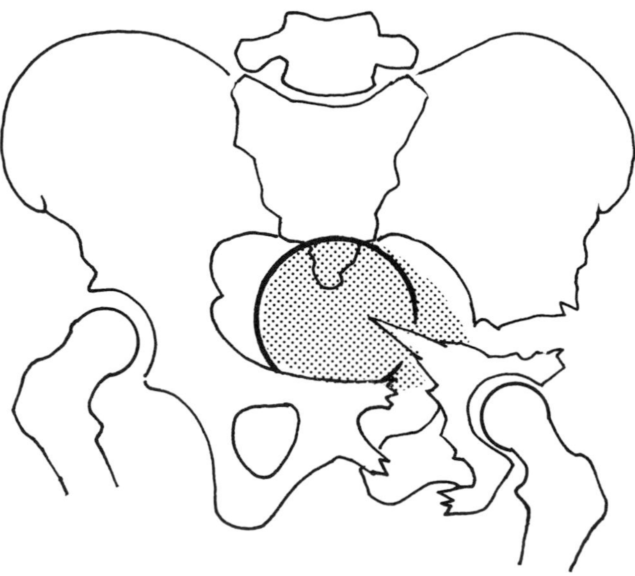

Fig. 20.28. Extraperitoneal rupture of the bladder.

Celsus described operations for it; the Pharoahs took catheters with them to the after life because of it. In children, urethritis of unknown aetiology may cause urethral bleeding and small granulomatous polypi may be found which heal with a stricture. In adults, *Neisseria gonorrhoeae* and *Chlamydia trachomatis* may also give rise to strictures.

Causes of stricture

1 Congenital.
2 Traumatic.
3 Inflammatory.
4 Malignant.
5 Other (e.g. Balanitis xerotica obliterans).

Congenital strictures. These have been described above: they include the anterior urethral valve or double-barrelled urethra and the congenital mid-bulbar stricture.

Traumatic. These follow the injuries described above, and in addition, a much larger group are caused by a catheter. Pressure of a catheter on the wall of the urethra produces a zone of ischaemia just like a bedsore, which is followed by healing with a scar (Fig. 20.29). These tend to occur where the urethra is most narrow (e.g. at the external meatus) amd where the urethra is apt to be angulated (e.g. at the penoscrotal junction) (Fig. 20.30).

Inflammatory. These include strictures resulting from gonorrhoea, chlamydia, and chemical urethritis (Fig. 20.31).

Neoplastic. Carcinoma may arise in the urethra, usually upstream of a long-standing stricture, where urinary stasis has given rise to squamous cell metaplasia. Rare in Britain, it should be considered as a possibility in anyone with a long-standing stricture.

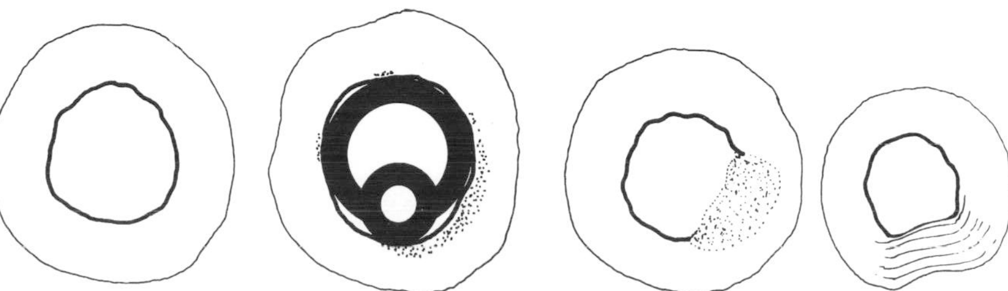

Fig. 20.29. Too large a catheter causes a patch of ischaemia which heals with a scar.

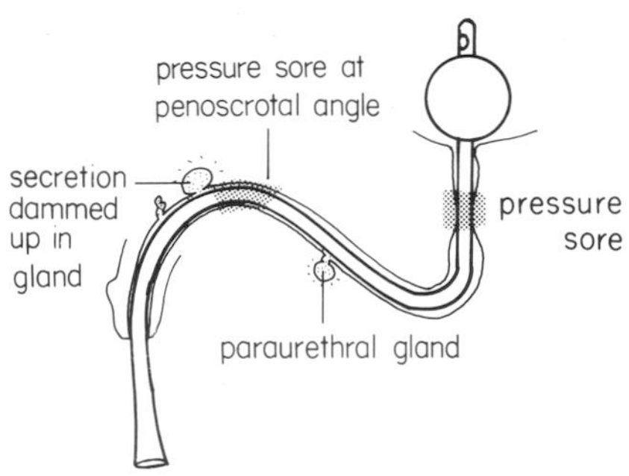

Fig. 20.30. Dangers of a snugly-fitting catheter: it gives rise to pressure sores inside the urethra; or it blocks off the openings of the para-urethral glands, inviting infection and abscess formation. Always use the smallest catheter that will do the job.

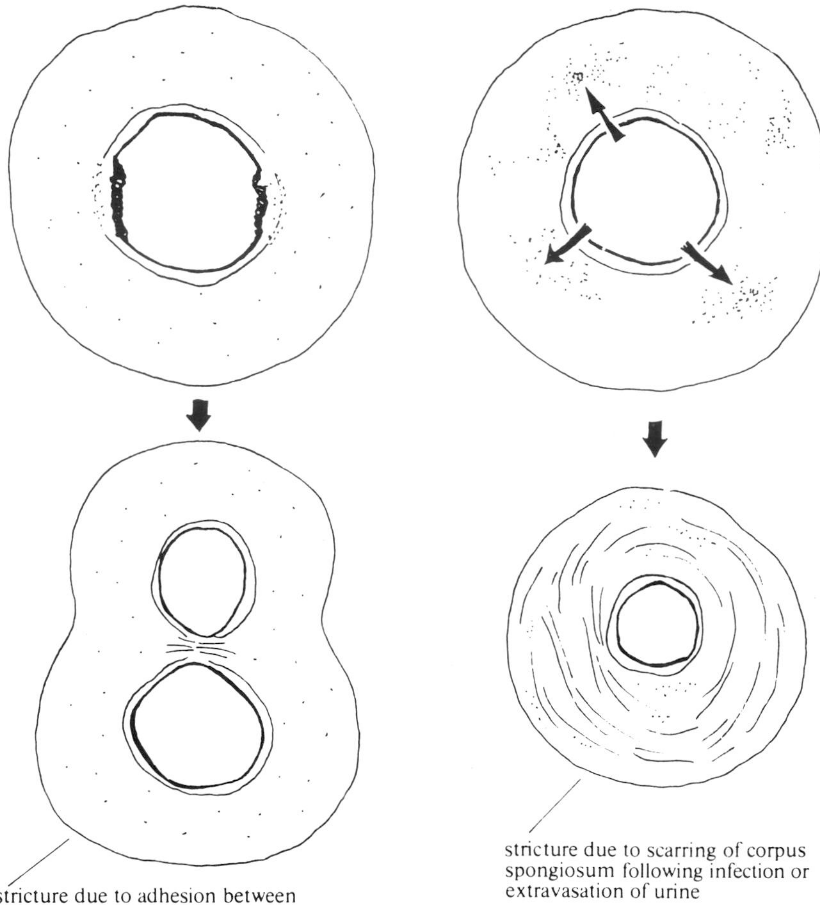

Fig. 20.31. Diagram of urethral strictures.

Balanitis xerotica obliterans. This obscure skin disorder, known elsewhere in the body as *lichen sclerosus et atrophicus* causes a stiff white change in the skin of the prepuce and glans penis, which result in a narrowing of the external urinary meatus. It may also occur in skin grafted into the urethra in order to enlarge it at *urethroplasty*. Fortunately, this is a rare complication, because we do not know how to prevent it. Squamous cell carcinoma occurs in a small proportion of cases of Balanitis xerotica, so they should all be followed up.

Clinical features of urethral stricture

In the absence of a clear history of injury or urethritis the symptoms are similar to those of outflow obstruction caused by enlargement of the prostate. There is a poor flow-rate, and dribbling after the patient thinks he has finished passing water. Sometimes there is a spraying or forked stream.

Complications of urethral stricture (Fig. 20.32)

Residual urine may give rise to *infection* and *epididymitis. Obstructed ejaculation* may result in such a restricted ejaculate that the patient may be infertile. Each time the patient passes urine pressure builds up upstream of the stricture, forcing urine (which is often infected) into the corpus spongiosum where it sets up inflammation. The inflammation may be followed by scarring which contracts longitudinally and produces *chordée* — named after the cord of a bow. It may cause abscesses in distended paraurethral glands (*paraurethral abscess*) which may burst through the skin to form *fistulae. Stones* not uncommonly form inside these abscesses and fistulae. Continuing increase in pressure forces infected urine into the ducts of the prostate to give rise to episodes of *prostatitis.* Finally (and most rare of all) continuing infection causes the lining mucosa to become changed into squamous epithelium, in which *squamous carcinoma* has been estimated to arise in about 1% of patients with long-standing urethral strictures.

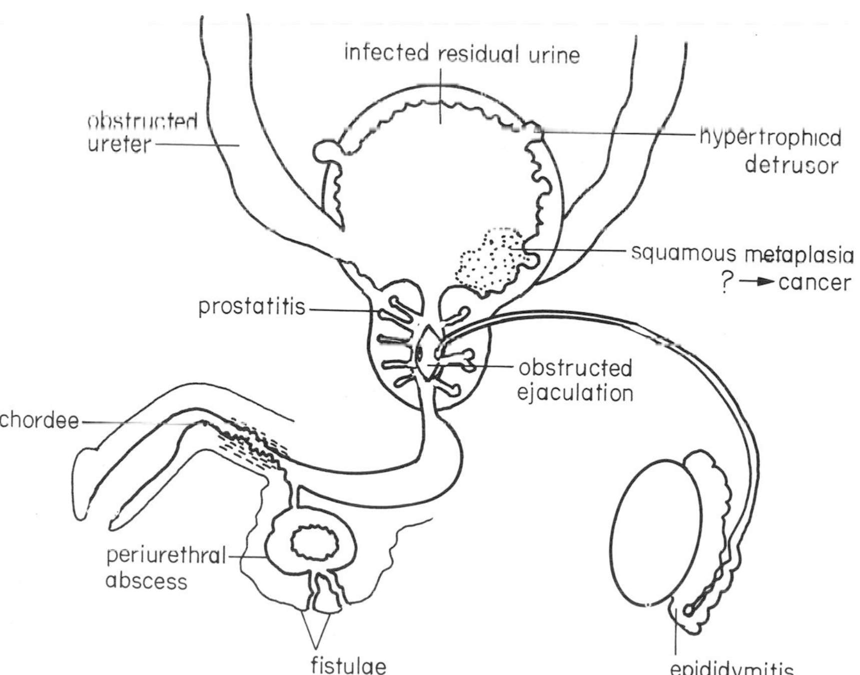

Fig. 20.32. The complications of urethral stricture.

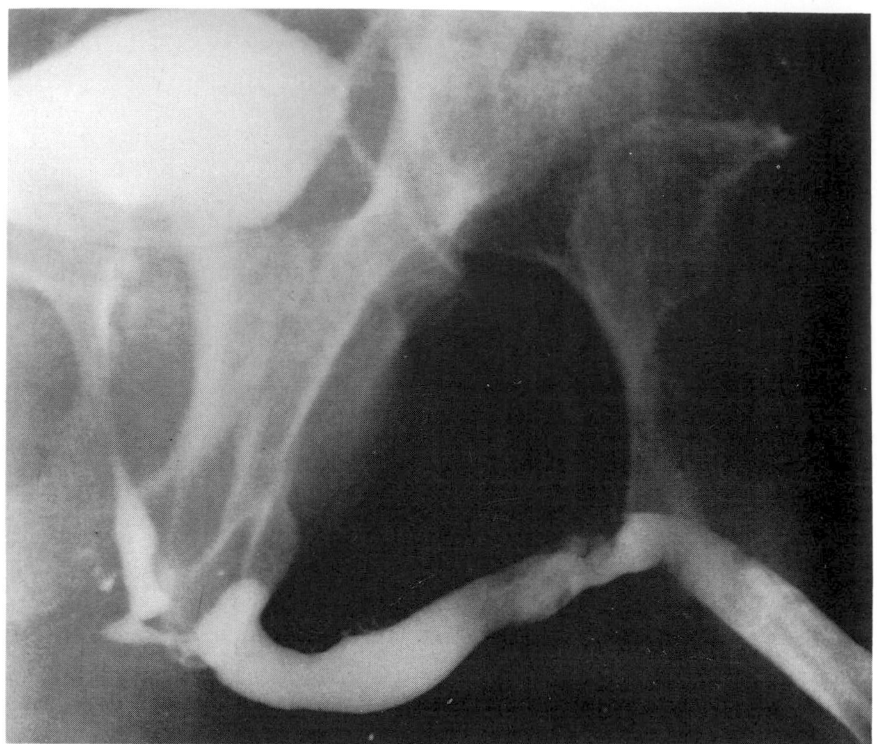

Fig. 20.33. Urethrogram showing post-traumatic stricture of the membranous urethra with typical backwards displacement of the upper (prostatic) urethra.

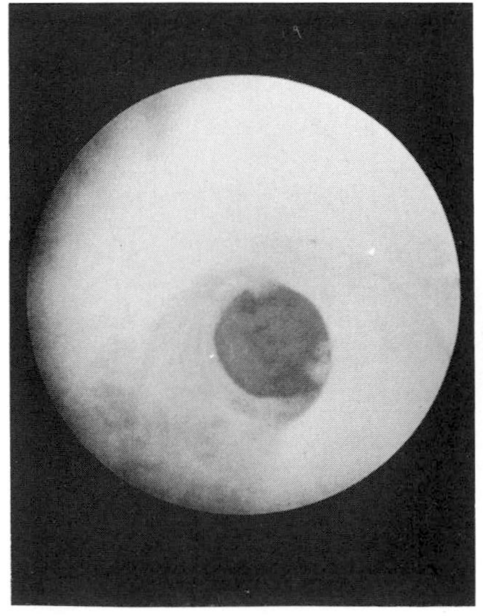

Fig. 20.34. Urethroscopic view of a stricture.

Investigation of urethral stricture

1 Flow rates provide documentation of the stricture, but unfortunately, since flow is proportional to the square of the diameter of the urethra, it needs a very small reduction in the lumen to change a good into a very bad flow-rate.

2 Urethrography (Fig. 20.33).

3 Urethroscopy and endoscopy of the urethra give the best assessment of its extent and severity (Fig. 20.34).

Management of urethral stricture

Once a stricture always a stricture. Even today, for all our modern methods, this ancient dictum is still true. Whenever you read of a new method for treating urethral stricture always ask how long was the follow-up.

Bouginage

Bujiyah is the name of the Algerian town and its adjacent bay renowned from mediaeval times for its honey and its beeswax. For generations its beeswax was prized for making candles and tapers. For as many generations flexible wax tapers were used to dilate strictures, and the French named their tapers after Bujiyah — *Bougie*: and the English copied them. Today bougies are no longer made of wax, but of plastic of very similar consistency and shape.

In ancient days the only way of diagnosing a stone in the bladder was to pass a curved metal instrument which knocked against the stone and *sounded* it. Graduated series of such instruments were very useful to dilate strictures, and so instruments used for dilating strictures were interchangeably called bougies or sounds (Fig. 20.35).

Using instruments of gradually increasing diameter the surgeon gently dilates the stricture hoping to stretch the fibrous tissue of the corpus spongiosum without tearing its mucosa. Urethral bouginage may give rise to bacteraemia: it may tear the urethra and cause bleeding, and if the urethra is forcibly overstretched the resulting extravasation of blood will certainly give rise to worse scarring than ever before.

Classical bouginage was performed at gradually lengthening intervals until eventually the patient only had to undergo dilatation once a year. Nowadays the method has fallen out of fashion — being largely replaced by internal optical urethrotomy: it remains to be seen whether time will ratify this change.

Internal urethrotomy

The scar tissue may be cut rather than stretched. This also is an operation dating from ancient times, but it has been updated by the invention of an

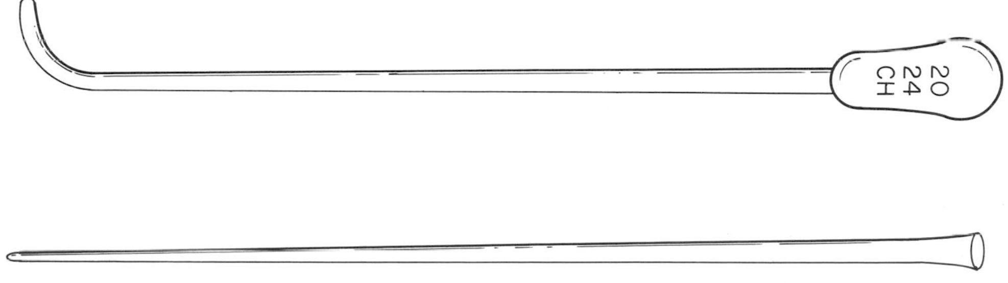

Fig. 20.35. Urethral sound (above) and bougie (below).

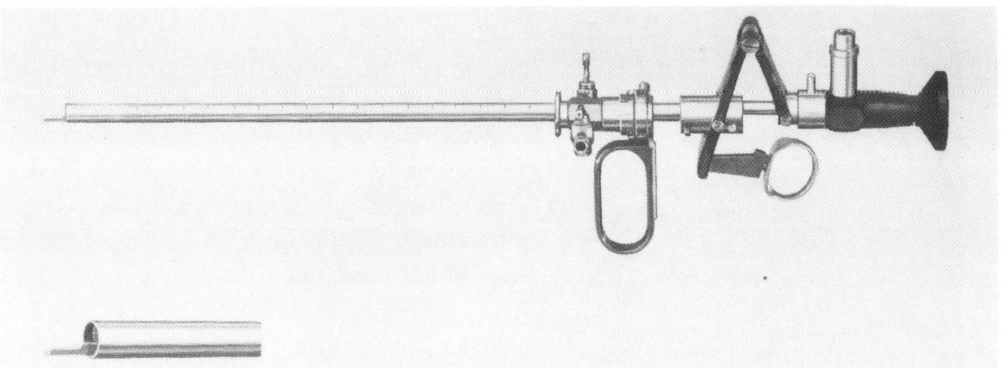

Fig. 20.36. Storz-Sachse internal optical urethrotome. (Courtesy Karl Storz.)

optical urethrotome by Sachse: this elegant instrument allows the surgeon to see where and how deep he is cutting (Fig. 20.36). After urethrotomy a catheter is left in the urethra for a few days to prevent extravasation of urine that might make the inflammatory reaction worse.

Urethroplasty

Sometimes strictures return so quickly, and cause so much pain and misery when they are dilated, that some alternative measure is sought. Sometimes neither bouginage nor internal optical urethrotomy is possible. In these cases a number of operations have been developed to attempt to offer a more permanent cure. One may slit open the urethra and insert a patch of skin — free grafts — either split or full thickness: or pedicled grafts from the prepuce or scrotum.

Anterior urethroplasty. The anterior urethra is exposed through an incision which avoids cutting into the skin of the shaft of the penis. The narrow zone in the urethra is slit open (Fig. 20.37) and a template is made from tinfoil of the right size to patch the defect. To match this template a patch of skin is outlined in the scrotum, provided with a pedicle of the dartos muscle, and sewn into the defect. A catheter is left in position for about 2 weeks.

Posterior urethroplasty. The posterior part of the urethra, including the bulb, is best exposed through an n-shaped incision which gives access like a trapdoor. The narrow part of the urethra is slit up, and a suitably sized patch (made with a tinfoil template) is made from the tip of the n-shaped flap. It is sewn into position over a suitable catheter (Fig. 20.38).

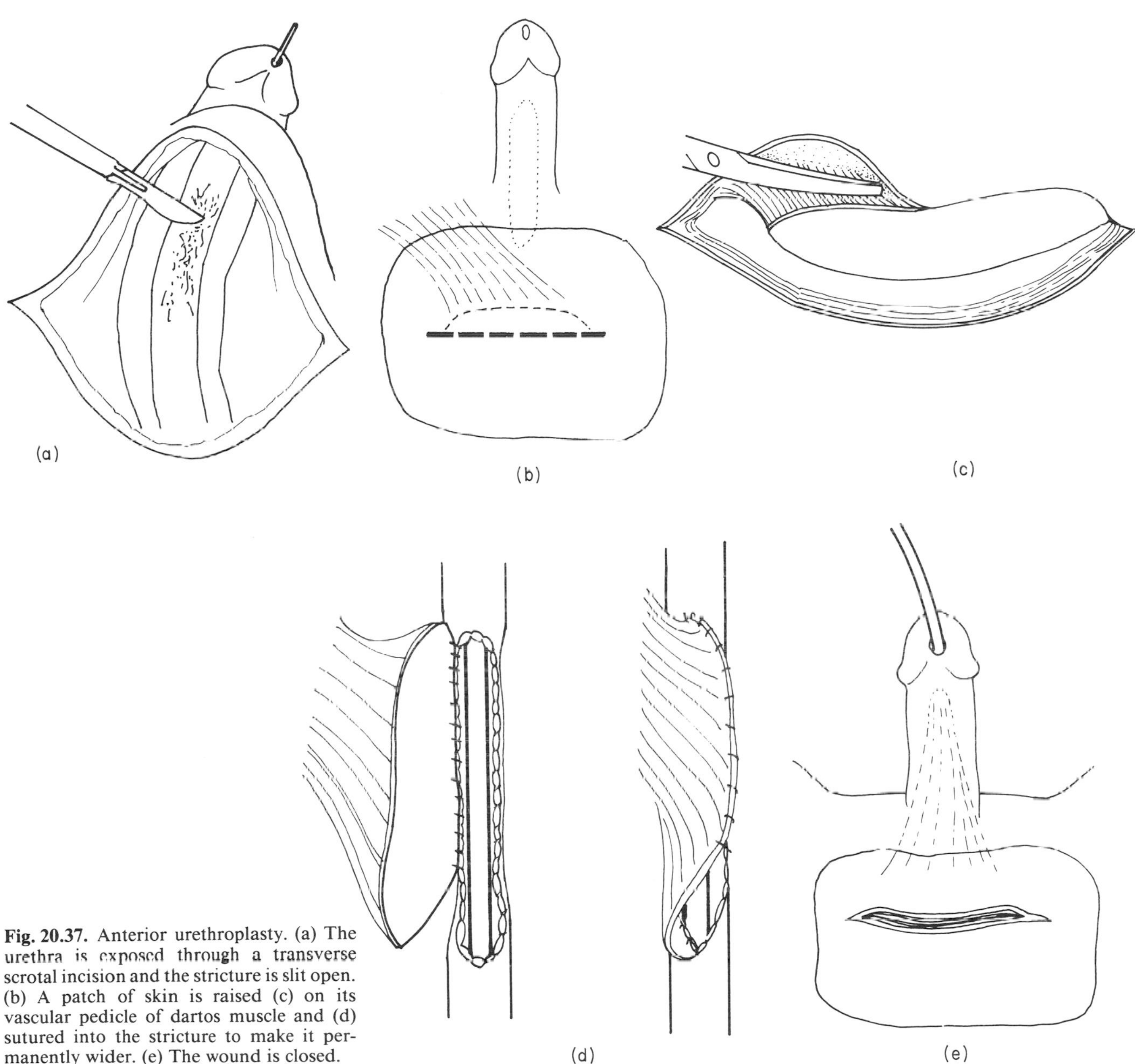

Fig. 20.37. Anterior urethroplasty. (a) The urethra is exposed through a transverse scrotal incision and the stricture is slit open. (b) A patch of skin is raised (c) on its vascular pedicle of dartos muscle and (d) sutured into the stricture to make it permanently wider. (e) The wound is closed.

Full length urethroplasty. When the entire length of the urethra has been replaced by a tight stricture, it is possible to enlarge it with a pair of patches, one for the anterior and one for the posterior urethra.

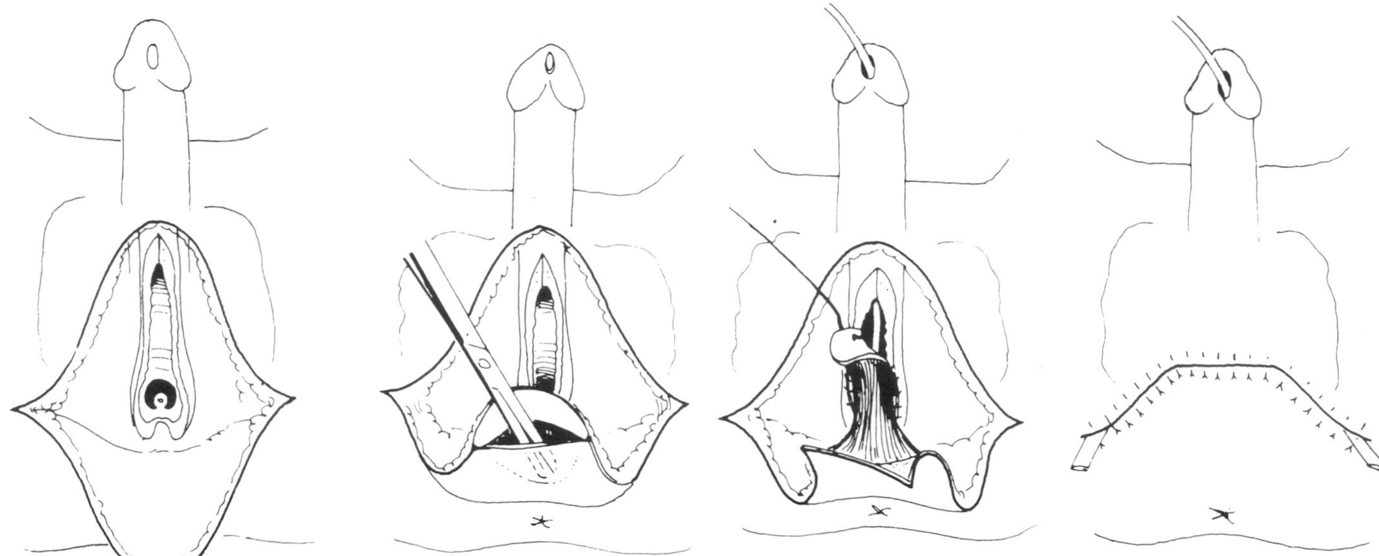

Fig. 20.38. One-stage, island-patch urethroplasty for posterior strictures, based on the tip of a scrotal flap.

Strictures of the membranous urethra. Although the dartos-pedicled patch can be used to bridge the gap caused by a stricture in the posterior urethra, this is not so successful as end-to-end anastomosis.

FURTHER READING

Ahlering TE & Lieskovsky G (1988) Surgical treatment of urethral cancer in the male patient. In: Skinner DG & Lieskovsky G (Eds) *Diagnosis and Management of Genitourinary Cancer*. WB Saunders, Philadelphia. pp. 622–33.

Blandy JP (1986) *Operative Urology*. 2nd Ed. Blackwell Scientific Publications, Oxford. pp. 206–37.

Chilton CP, Shah PJR, Fowler CG, Tiptaft RC & Blandy JP (1983) The impact of optical urethrotomy on the management of urethral strictures. *British Journal of Urology* **55**, 705–10.

Cobb BG, Wolf JA & Ansell JS (1968) Congenital strictures of the proximal urethral bulb. *Journal of Urology* **99**, 629–31.

Corriere JN jr & Sandler CM (1988) Mechanisms of injury, patterns of extravasation and management of extraperitoneal bladder rupture due to blunt trauma. *Journal of Urology* **139**, 43–4.

Fowler JW, Watson G, Smith MF & MacFarlane JR (1986) Diagnosis and treatment of posterior urethral injury. *British Journal of Urology* **58**, 167–73.

Glass RE, Flynn JT, King JB & Blandy JP (1978) Urethral injury and fractured pelvis. *British Journal of Urology* **50**, 578–82.

Hehir M, Duff FA & Kelly DG (1984) Gunshot injuries of the urinary tract. *British Journal of Urology* **56**, 574–6.

Levine RL (1980) Urethral cancer. *Cancer* **45**, 1965–72.

Lowe D & McKee PH (1983) Verrucous carcinoma of the penis (Buschke-Loewenstein tumour): a clinical pathological study. *British Journal of Urology* **55**, 427–9.

Morehouse DD (1988) Management of posterior urethral rupture — a personal view. *British Journal of Urology* **61**, 375–81.

Oeirich TM (1980) The urethral sphincter muscle in the male. *American Journal of Anatomy* **158**, 229–46.

Somerville JJF, Adeyemi OA & Clark PB (1985) Long-term results of two stage urethroplasty. *British Journal of Urology* **57**, 742–5.

21 The Penis

SURGICAL ANATOMY

The penis is made up of three distensible spongy sacs, two corpora cavernosa and a corpus spongiosum ending in the glans penis. Distension of these three sacs within the rigid Buck's fascia results in a firm erection. The spongy spaces of the two corpora cavernosa intercommunicate but those of the corpus spongiosum are virtually distinct (Fig. 21.1).

Blood supply to the penis

The penis receives its blood supply from the terminal branches of the internal pudendal artery, but in addition, in 70% of patients there are accessory pudendal arteries from the obturator and inferior vesical arteries. Each pudendal artery divides into three — a large artery in the middle of the corpus cavernosum, which is the most important artery for the purposes of erection, a smaller dorsal artery and a pair of 'bulbourethral' arteries which run along the length of the corpus spongiosum (Fig. 21.2).

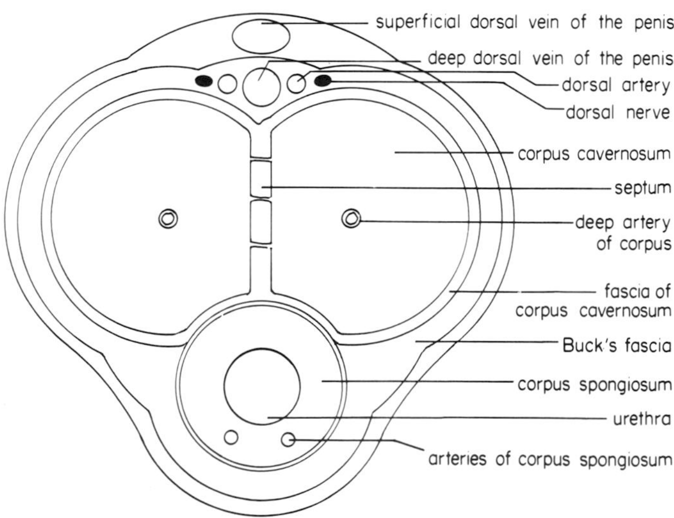

Fig. 21.1. Diagrammatic transverse section through the penis.

Veins

There are three groups of veins (Fig. 21.3):

1 The *cavernous* veins which are the chief drainage of the corpora cavernosa, and empty into a large plexus of veins under the arch of the symphysis which is continuous with those in front of the prostate and bladder.

2 The *superficial* veins just under the skin, which include the superficial dorsal vein of the penis, mostly drain into the saphenous vein (curiously — mostly on the left side).

3 Finally there is an *intermediate* system of veins deep to Buck's fascia which collect the blood behind the glans penis, and communicate both with the superficial and the deep system.

Nerve supply to the penis

The somatic sensory nerve supply of the penis is carried in the dorsal nerve of the penis, just lateral to the dorsal arteries and deep to Buck's fascia. It supplies the skin of the glans penis and is a branch of the pudendal nerve.

The highly important *cavernous nerves* consist of a fine network of autonomic nerves which surround the deep artery of the corpus cavernosum. They are branches of the pelvic parasympathetic nervous system, and they enter the penis in two discrete bundles that run in the neurovascular tissue on either side of the prostate and urethra. It is possible to remove the prostate without injuring these nerves (see p. 237).

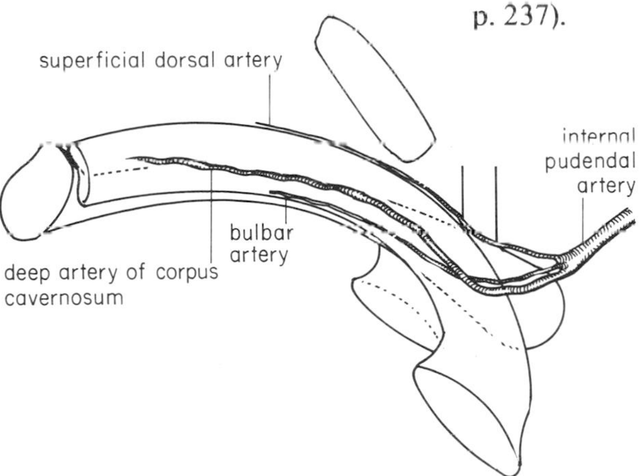

Fig. 21.2. The only important arteries of the penis are those of the corpus cavernosum: the other two branches—the dorsal and the bulbar arteries—are insufficient to maintain erection.

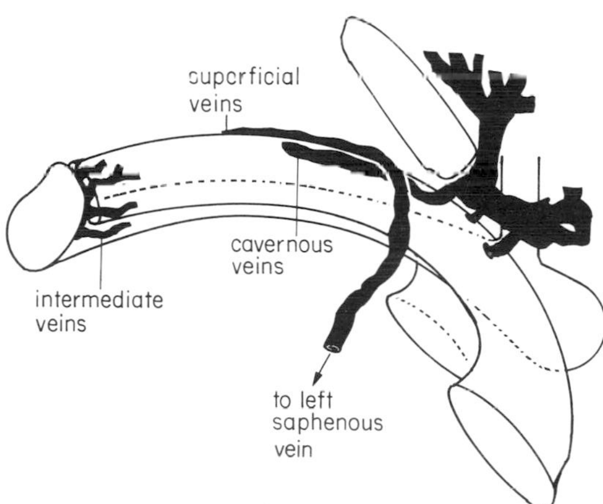

Fig. 21.3. Venous drainage of the penis.

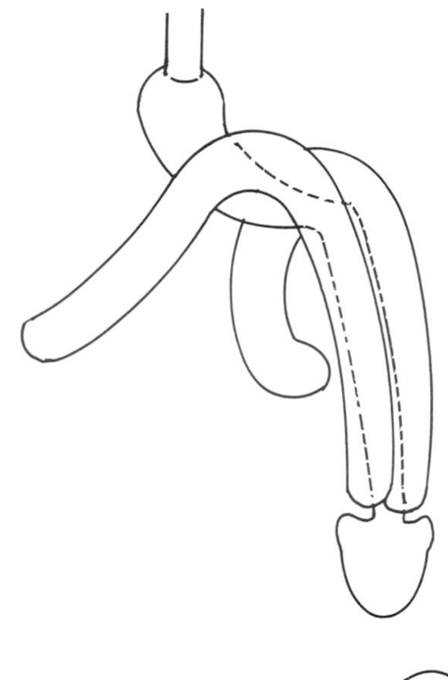

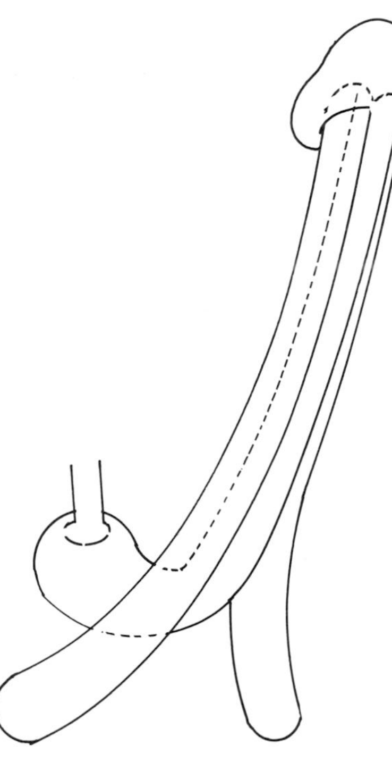

Fig. 21.4. Penis flaccid and erect.

The physiology of erection

There are two phases in erection (Fig. 21.4). In the first phase, the spongy spaces of the corpora cavernosa fill up. This is due to a dilatation of the small branches of the arteries of the corpora cavernosa, mediated by the parasympathetic, involving neurotransmitter substances whose action can be imitated by papaverine or phentolamine. This period of filling of the cavernous tissue produces an increase in the size and length of the penis — *tumescence*. During this phase the pressure inside the penis rises to about 40 mmHg.

In the second phase — *rigidity* — the penis becomes hard and the pressure inside the corpus cavernosum rises to > 150 mmHg. This second phase is the result of closure of the venous drainage from the corpora.

Ejaculation

The process of ejaculation has been studied in volunteers whose seminal vesicles and vasa have been filled with contrast medium. At climax, the seminal vesicles are seen to become dilated, and to pump up with several strokes (Fig. 21.5). Then the vasa deferentia empty into the common ejaculatory duct, pushing out the sperms in a volume of fluid estimated to be about 0.5 ml. Finally the seminal vesicles empty themselves, driving the sperm rich fraction of the semen before them. Contraction of the bulbospongiosus muscles helps to empty the urethra. Ejaculation requires an intact bladder neck muscle to stop semen refluxing back into the bladder.

The contraction of the seminal vesicles, and the shutting-off of the bladder neck, is mediated by alpha-adrenergic sympathetic nerve fibres which reach the base of the bladder from the presacral nerve, accompanying the inferior vesical vessels.

Investigation of the mechanism of erection

Nocturnal penile tumescence

During deep sleep when the eyes show rapid eye movements, the EEG detects alpha-rhythms, and people dream — it is normal for erections to occur. In most men these erections occur three or four times during the night. A simple way to detect whether these erections occur is to stick a strip of postage-stamp paper or a special strip of tape around the penis: if the paper has torn in the morning, erection has occurred (Fig. 21.6).

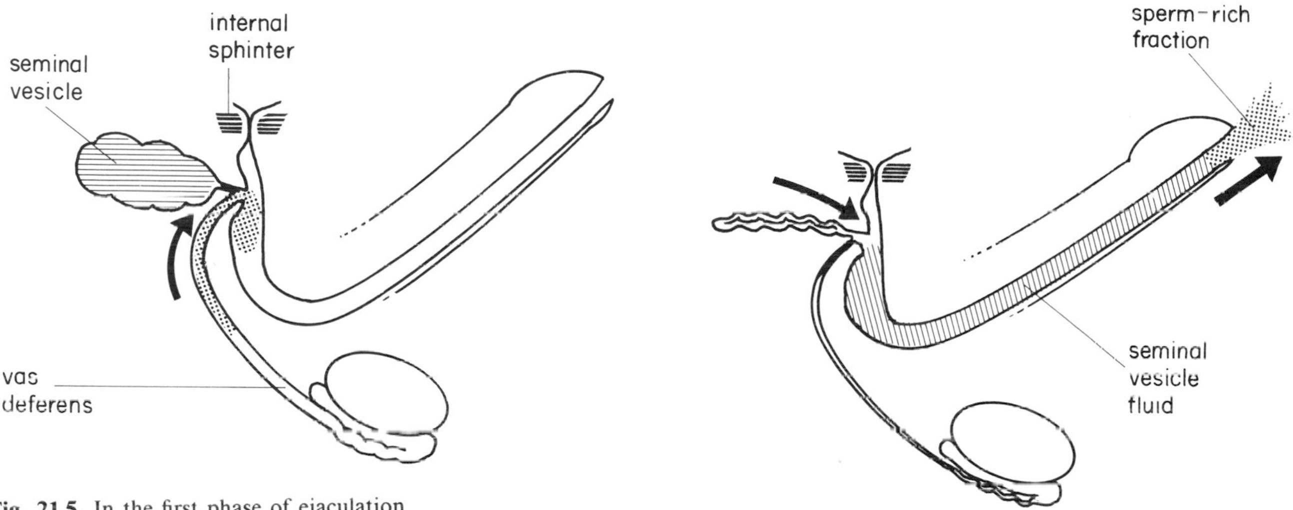

Fig. 21.5. In the first phase of ejaculation the epididymes and vasa deferentia empty the sperms into the prostatic urethra. In the second phase the seminal vesicles squirt their contents down the urethra, pushing the sperms before it.

Using a pair of strain gauges fitted snugly around the penis, connected to a tape recorder (Fig. 21.7), it is possible to record not only the increase in the circumference of the penis but also its length.

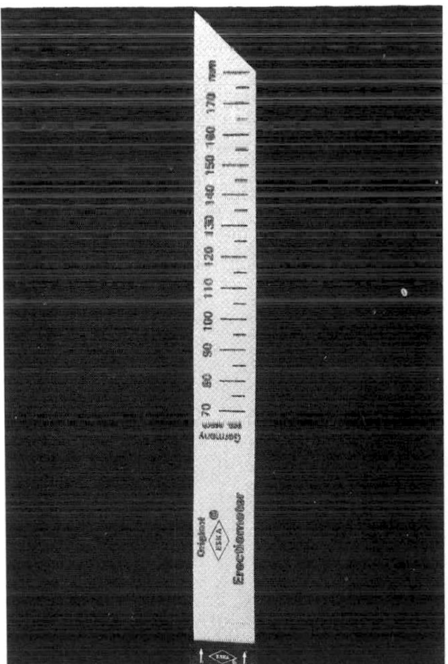

Fig. 21.6. A snap band designed to yield at known tension supplies evidence that an erection has occurred during sleep.

Doppler studies

Using a Doppler ultrasound sensor, the pulsations in the deep artery of the corpus cavernosum can be detected, and the blood pressure can be measured and compared with that in the arm (*Peno-Brachial Index or PBI*). These measurements are simple to perform and can be done in the office.

Injections of papaverine

Papaverine is injected directly into the corpus cavernosum. If the blood supply is intact, this will produce an erection.

Cavernosography and pressure measurements

A fine needle is placed in each corpus cavernosum: one is connected to a manometer, the other to a bottle of contrast medium, while the penis is observed on the image intensifier (Fig. 21.8). In normal erection the contrast medium distends the corpora in the first tumescent phase of erection and the pressure rises to about 40 mmHg: this is followed by the second rigid phase when the pressure should exceed 150 mmHg.

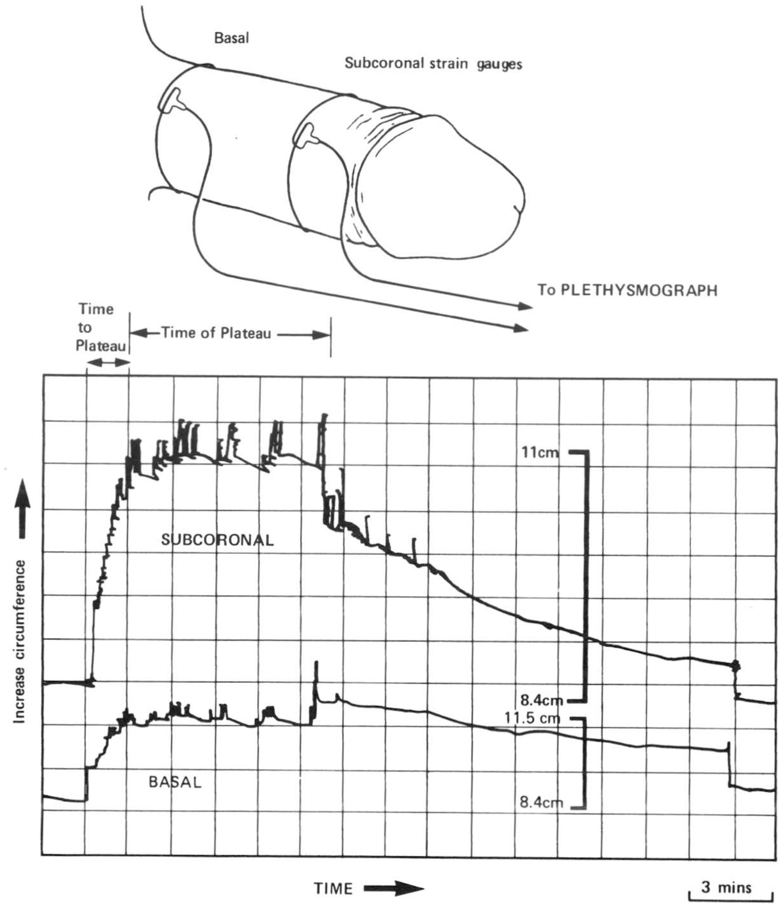

Fig. 21.7. Nocturnal tumescence study using a pair of strain gauges on the penis. (Courtesy of Mr Peter Blacklay.)

Angiography of the internal iliac artery

Through an angiogram catheter passed up one femoral artery contrast is injected into the internal iliac artery, and with the help of *digital vascular imaging* the pudendal artery and its branches are depicted. Since they are very small and concealed behind the bony pelvis this is a difficult investigation.

CONGENITAL LESIONS OF THE PENIS

Phimosis

The two layers of skin which form the foreskin do not separate until about the age of three years. After that age it is necessary to be able to

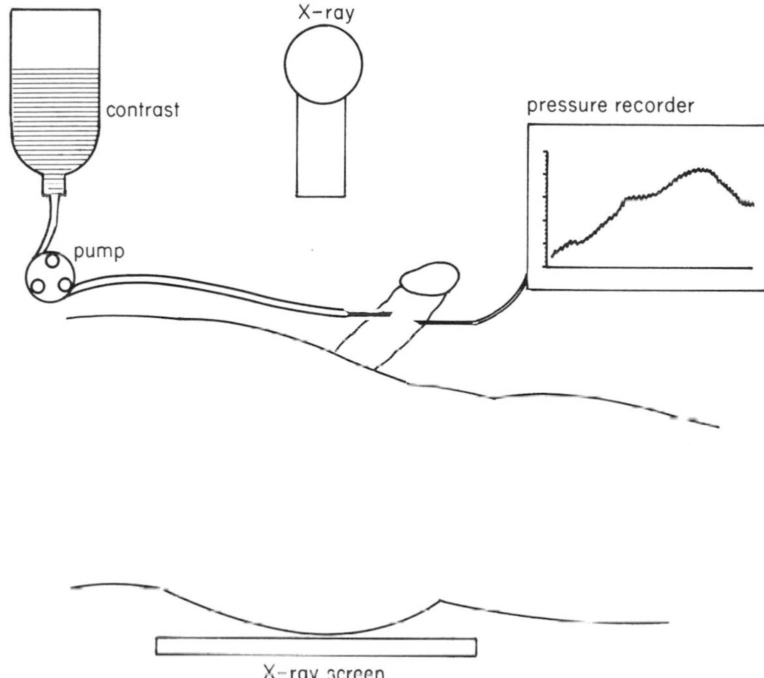

Fig. 21.8. Dynamic cavernosography. Contrast is pumped at a constant rate into the corpus cavernosum while the pressure is measured and venous drainage monitored radiographically.

draw back the prepuce in order to keep it clean, and if the prepuce cannot be drawn back, circumcision is indicated (Fig. 21.9).

Hypospadias

Failure of the embryonic genital folds to fuse in the midline leads to incomplete formation of the distal part of the urethra which may take several forms. Adults may have *chordée* — a shortening and narrowing of the distal urethra, though it may end in the normal position at the tip of the meatus. During erection the penis is bent. More often the distal part of the urethra is a mere fibrous streak, and the urethra opens nearer the perineum. There are different degrees of severity (Fig. 21.10): often the external meatus opens just behind the glans, and the foreskin is cleft. This is *glandular hypospadias* and it seldom causes any disability.

Glandular hypospadias can be remedied by Duckett's MAGPI ('meatus advancement glanduloplasty') operation (Fig. 21.11).

In *coronal hypospadias* there is a considerable chordée and the opening of the meatus is further down towards the scrotum. Repair of these more advanced forms of hypospadias calls for considerable skill

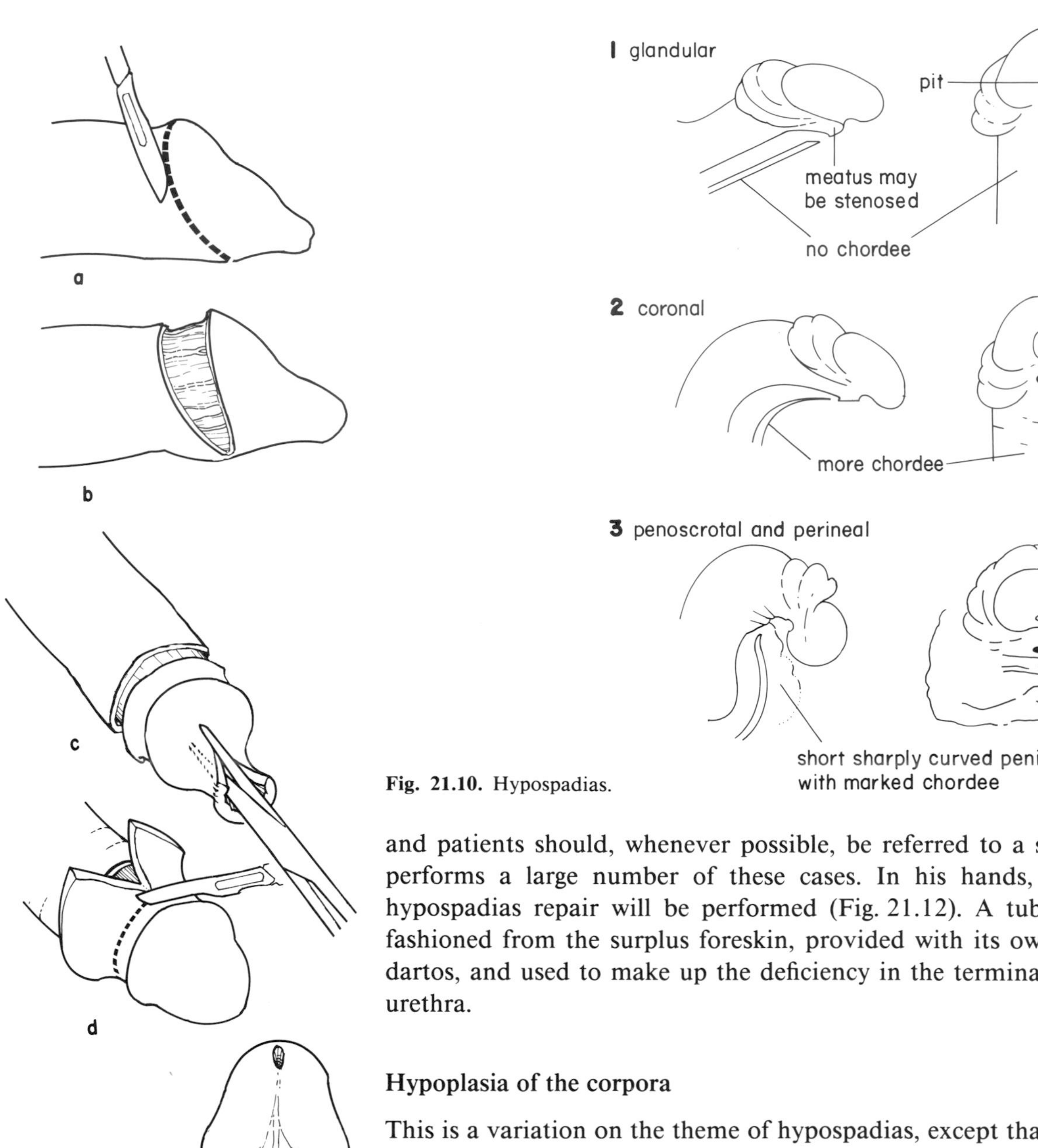

Fig. 21.10. Hypospadias.

Fig. 21.9. Stages of circumcision.

and patients should, whenever possible, be referred to a surgeon who performs a large number of these cases. In his hands, a one-stage hypospadias repair will be performed (Fig. 21.12). A tube of skin is fashioned from the surplus foreskin, provided with its own pedicle of dartos, and used to make up the deficiency in the terminal part of the urethra.

Hypoplasia of the corpora

This is a variation on the theme of hypospadias, except that it is one of the corpora cavernosa which fail to grow rather than the corpus spongiosum. The result is that, during erection, the penis is twisted sideways. It is treated as for Peyronie's disease (see below).

Epispadias and exstrophy

Here there is a defect in the formation of the lower part of the abdominal wall arising from an anomaly in the cloacal membrane (see p. 166).

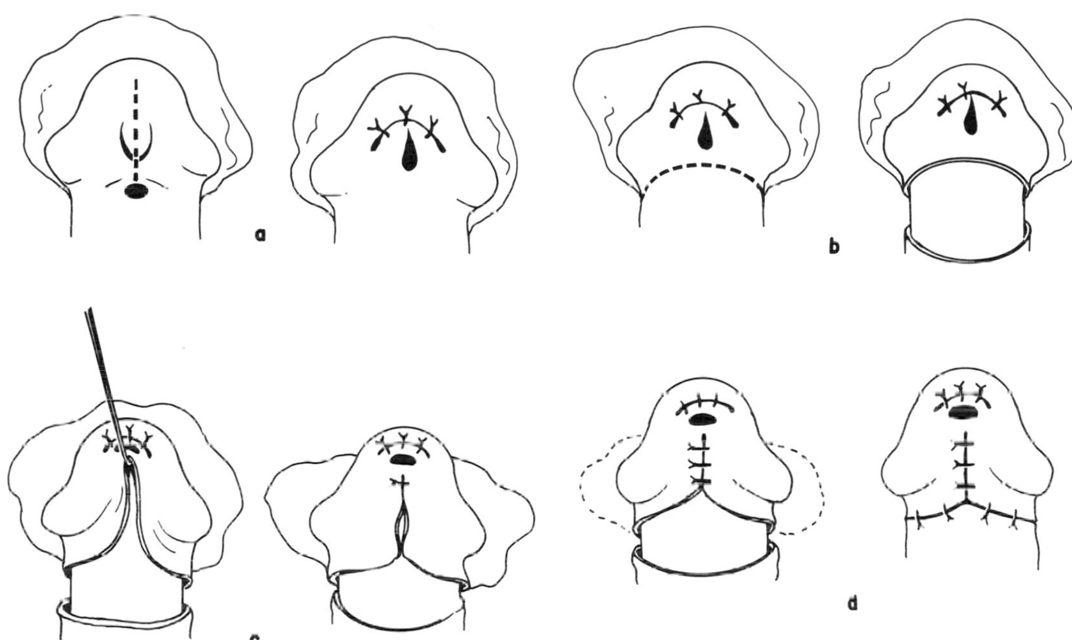

Fig. 21.11. MAGPI operation for glandular hypospadias.

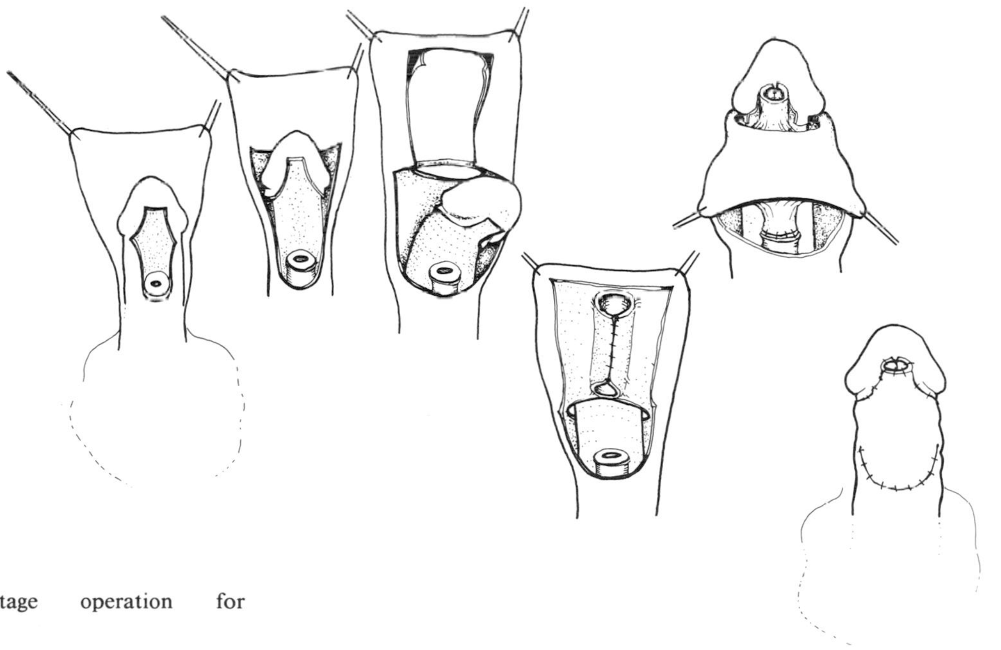

Fig. 21.12. One-stage operation for hypospadias.

TRAUMA

The foreskin is often caught accidentally in zip-fasteners and less often in industrial and other accidents: bizarre degloving injuries have been reported by men who have put their penis into the pipe of a vacuum cleaner. Self-injected paraffin and silicone have caused granulomas in the penis and scrotum.

Accidental amputation of the penis has been reported as a result of criminal or lunatic assault, or in the course of a ritual circumcision. If the detached part is saved, promptly placed in ice, and if there is not too long a delay, the deep artery can be repaired using microsurgical techniques and the penis can be saved.

The corpus cavernosum is sometimes ruptured in intercourse: it is usually recommended that the haematoma should be repaired promptly though cases have been reported where spontaneous healing has taken place.

INFLAMMATION

Inflammation of the glans penis (*balanitis*) usually involves the prepuce as well (*posthitis*). It is common in little boys who cannot retract their prepuce, and may occur from allergy to a condom, from herpes genitalis, or in men with diabetes mellitus where the infecting agent is often *Candida albicans*.

Specific lesions on the glans include the classical Hunterian chancre of primary *syphilis*, the soft painful exuberant chancre of *Haemophilus ducreyi* infection, infected scabies, lymphogranuloma venereum and granuloma inguinale — all lesions that must be distinguished from syphilis by a specialized venereologist. Diagnosis by dark field examination may not be too difficult but tracing contacts and making sure of the efficacy of a course of treatment, let alone investigating (or not investigating) for AIDS requires special training and skill. The penalty for ineffective amateur treatment may be disaster.

Recurrent non-specific balanitis is often cured by circumcision — allowing the glans to become dry and cornified seems to increase its resistance to infection.

In adults *balanitis xerotica obliterans* — a skin condition of unknown aetiology — causes the prepuce to become stiff, white and shrunken. Sometimes the foreskin is trapped behind the glans penis during erection — paraphimosis — which can be very painful (Fig. 21.13). Sometimes the opening of the foreskin becomes so narrow that it gives rise to obstructed urination, or, more often, to recurrent attacks of infection in the urine that is trapped in the space between foreskin and glans penis (*balanoposthitis*). In either event, circumcision is indicated.

When the stenosis affects the external urinary meatus a *meatoplasty* may be needed (Fig. 21.14).

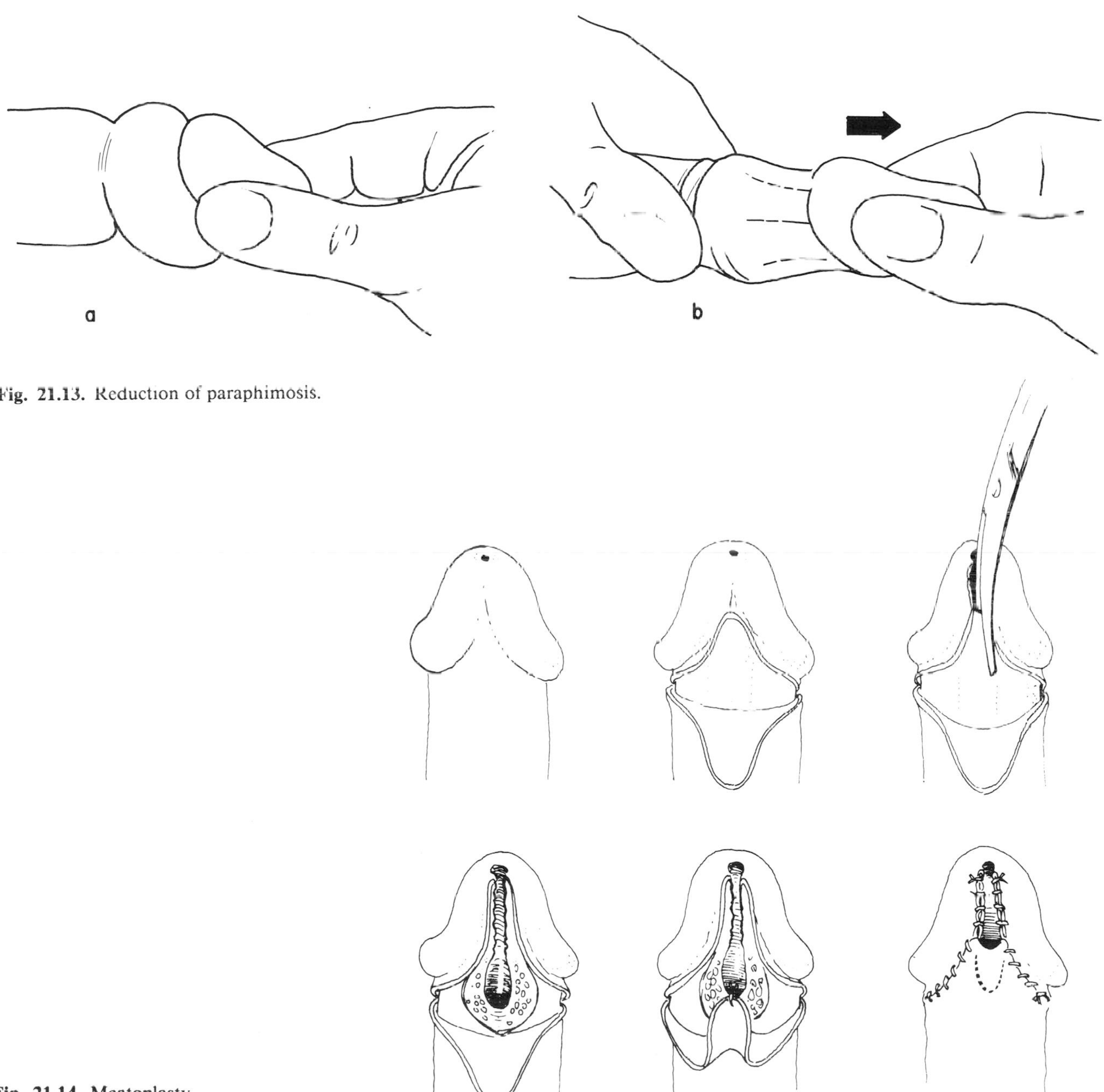

Fig. 21.13. Reduction of paraphimosis.

Fig. 21.14. Meatoplasty.

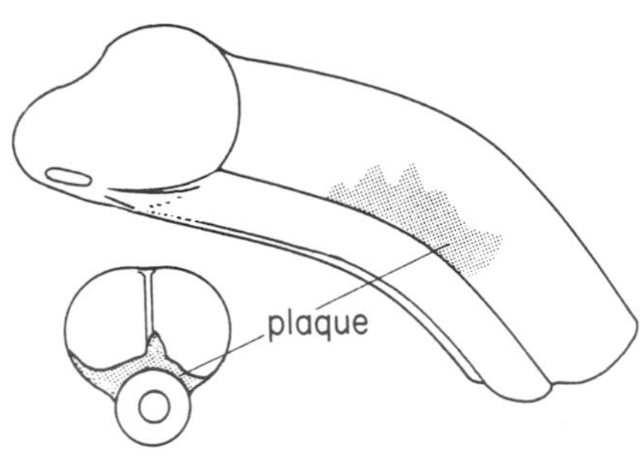

Fig. 21.15. Peyronie's disease.

Peyronie's disease

Described by the founder of the French equivalent of the Royal Society in 1743, we still do not know its cause or cure. A hard plaque of otherwise normal fibrous tissue forms in Buck's fascia or the septum between the corpora. There may be similar lumps in the ear lobes, the palmar fascia (*Dupuytren's contracture*) and the retroperitoneal tissue (*idiopathic retroperitoneal fibrosis*).

Innumerable medications have been used but whenever they are compared with controls they show no difference. The plaques may resolve spontaneously, but this does not always occur and takes several years. The plaque prevents the corpus cavernosum on the affected side from filling, and may prevent blood reaching the spongy tissue distal to it (Fig. 21.15). The result is that the penis is bent during erection. This is sometimes painful. Dissecting away a particularly dense plaque of fibrous tissue and replacing it with a patch of dermis or some other synthetic material would seem logical: it has often been tried but the results are indifferent. More reliable is Nesbit's operation where tucks are taken out of Buck's fascia on the opposite side (Fig. 21.16) until the penis is seen to be straight on artificial erection.

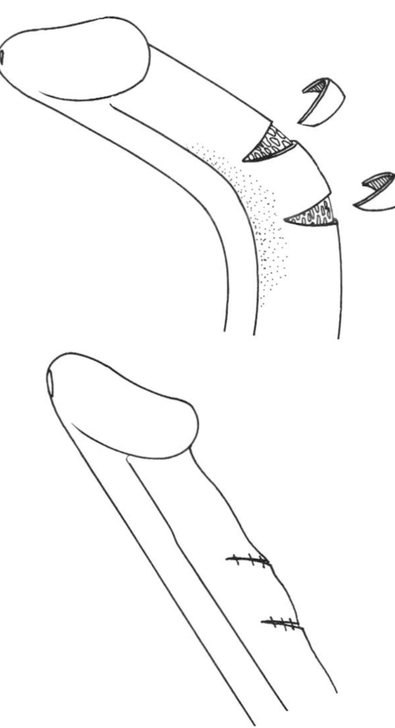

Fig. 21.16. A series of tucks are made in Buck's fascia on the side opposite to the plaque of Peyronie's fibrosis to straighten out the penis.

CARCINOMA OF THE PENIS

Cancer of the penis is only seen in uncircumcized men and usually in those who are old and unwashed, and cannot pull back the foreskin to clean it. In Africa it is particularly common and may occur in young men. It may well be related to previous infection with the human papilloma virus.

Erythroplasia of Queyrat is a precancerous condition — carcinoma *in situ* — of the skin of the glans penis which resembles non-specific balanitis. Biopsy shows *in situ* cancer. Unless treated vigorously with local irradiation or 5-fluorouracil cream it leads on to invasive cancer.

Benign warts occur on the penis — *condyloma acuminata* (Fig. 21.17). They are caused by a virus which is immunologically very similar to that which causes warts on the hands and feet. Like warts elsewhere, they respond to treatment with podophyllin, diathermy, freezing, the neodymium-YAG laser, etc.

Gigantic warts are seen from time to time which undoubtedly have an origin in a condyloma, but end up as a malignant and invasive cancer. They were first described by Buschke and Loewenstein and are often (erroneously) thought to be benign.

Pathology of carcinomas of the penis

These are all squamous cell cancers. They can be graded, like squamous cell cancers elsewhere, into three grades of malignancy, but a more useful guide to their prognosis is given by their pattern of growth — the *cord* pattern does badly, the *solid* ones do well (Fig. 21.18).

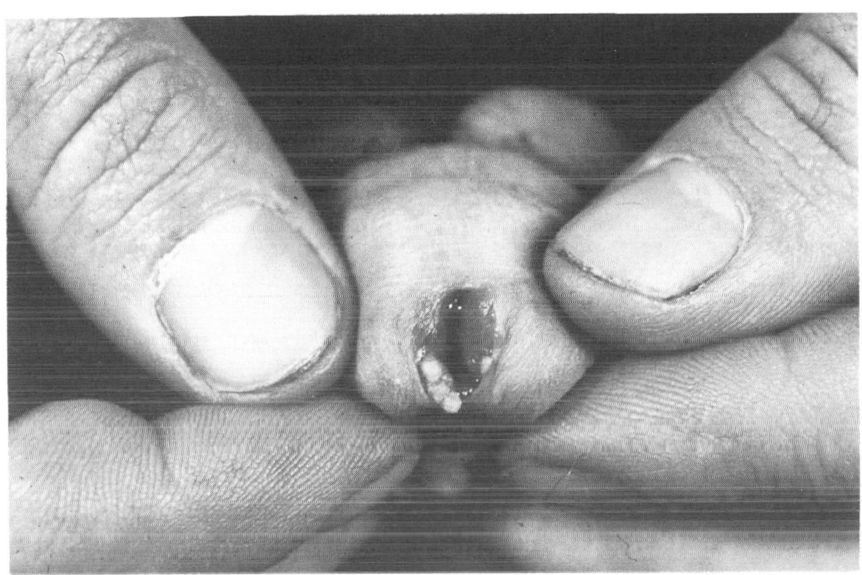

Fig. 21.17. Condyloma acuminatum in the meatus.

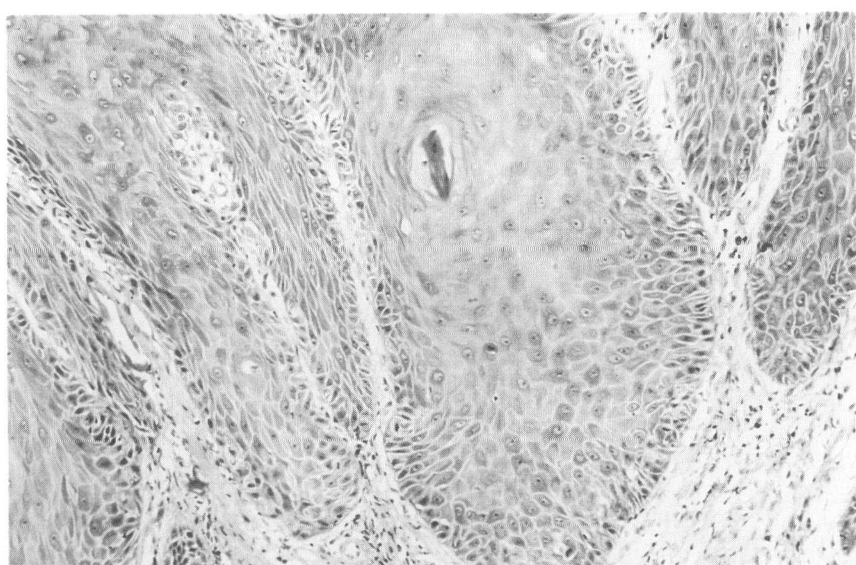

Fig. 21.18. Well-differentiated squamous cell cancer of penis with invasion of stroma. (Courtesy of Dr Jo Martin, London Hospital Institute of Pathology.)

Staging of cancer of the penis

Cancer of the penis usually arises on the glans or the foreskin and spreads locally. When it invades the vascular spaces of the spongy tissue it may disseminate in the veins, but at first tends to spread only in lymphatics, invading first those in the inguinal region, later those in the pelvis (Fig. 21.19).

Stage I. The cancer is confined to the foreskin or glans penis.

Stage II. The cancer has begun to invade the shaft of the penis.

Stage III. The tumour has invaded right back to the scrotum.

Stage IV. The inguinal nodes are involved.

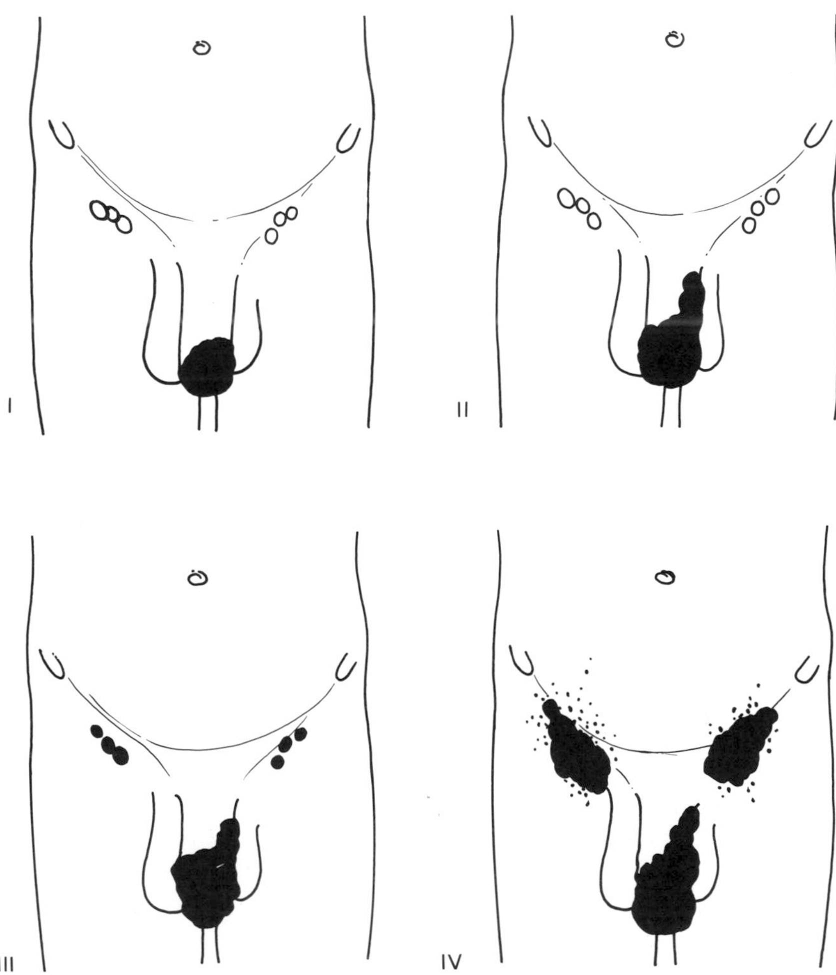

Fig. 21.19. Staging of carcinoma of penis.

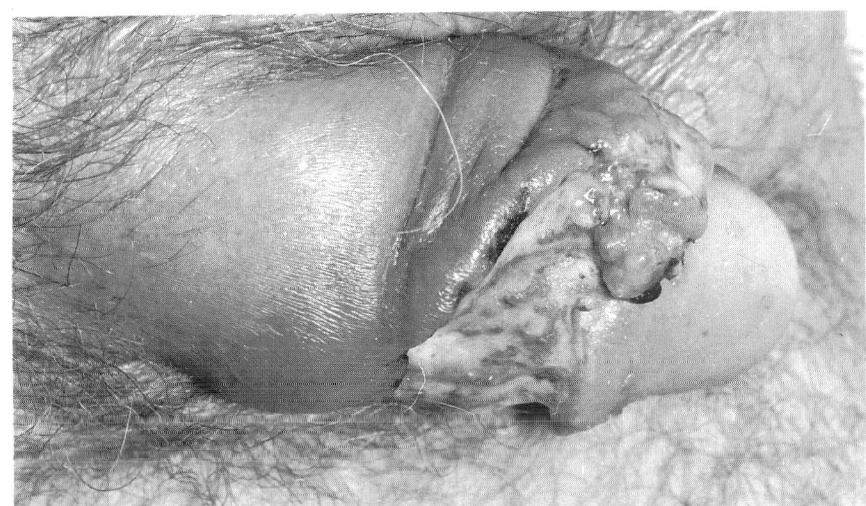

Fig. 21.20. Ulcerated carcinoma of penis revealed when the prepuce was retracted after a dorsal slit.

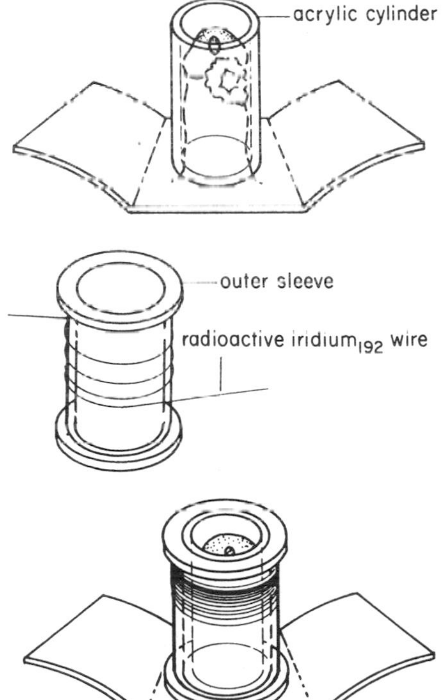

Fig. 21.21. Radioactive Iridium[90] wire is wound on a removable applicator to irradiate the glans penis for Stage I carcinoma.

Clinical features

The elderly unwashed uncircumcized man comes up with a discharge from beneath a swollen inflamed foreskin (Fig. 21.20). Secondary infection is always present, and the inguinal glands are always enlarged and often tender. At this stage it is impossible to tell whether they are enlarged from inflammation or cancer.

Management of carcinoma of the penis

The first task is to make the diagnosis. Any suspicious lesion on the penis must be biopsied: all foreskins removed in adults must be examined histologically. In most cases it is necessary to perform a circumcision in order to reveal the lesion, and a biopsy is taken at this time.

In Stage I cases where the lesion is confined to the prepuce, it may have been possible to remove it all with a safe margin by the operation of circumcision. More often it is not. Residual tumour confined to the glans penis can be treated with local radiotherapy using radioactive Iridium[192] on a special applicator (Fig. 21.21). This gives a good chance of cure without any deformity or loss of function, but local recurrence must be expected in about 20% of patients and will require partial amputation (Fig. 21.22).

In Stage II, where the corpus spongiosum is invaded, it is worth trying the Iridium[192] applicator, but local recurrence calls for partial amputation in as many as half of these patients: the long-term survival is however excellent, and probably improved by the preliminary radiation.

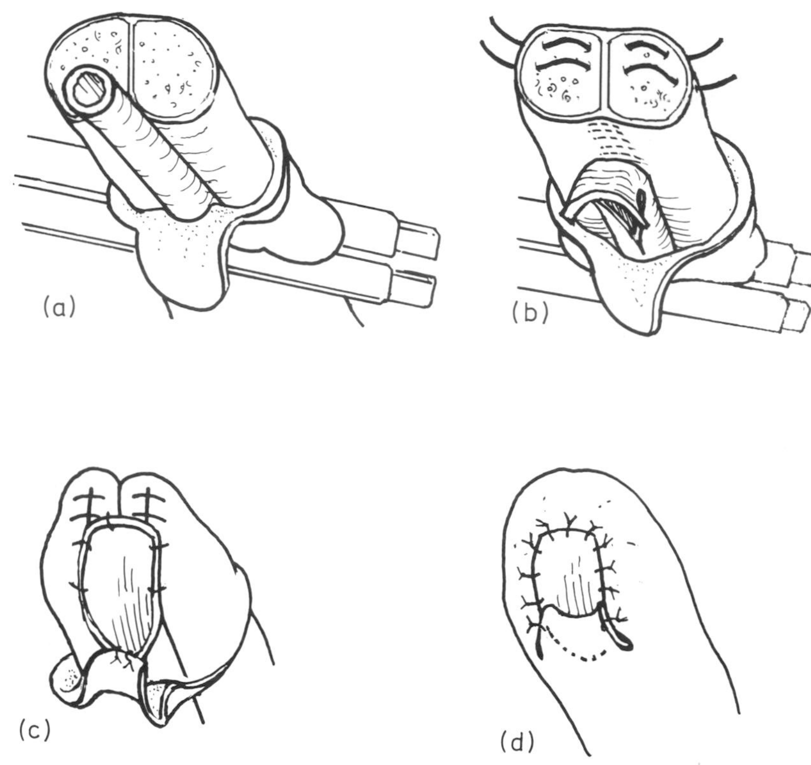

Fig. 21.22. Partial amputation of the penis.

In Stage III where the scrotum is involved, local treatment with radiation is not feasible. A radical amputation is performed and the urethra reconstructed with a scrotal flap (Fig. 21.23).

In Stage IV where the inguinal nodes are involved, preliminary radiation may be attempted, but it usually fails, and a block dissection of the inguinal lymph nodes is then worth while, so long as CT scanning shows that the pelvic lymph nodes are not involved. Once the inguinal lymph nodes are invaded the outlook is poor, but not hopeless.

Chemotherapy for tumours of the penis has been very disappointing. Claims that *bleomycin* was a specific cure for penile cancer have not stood the test of time.

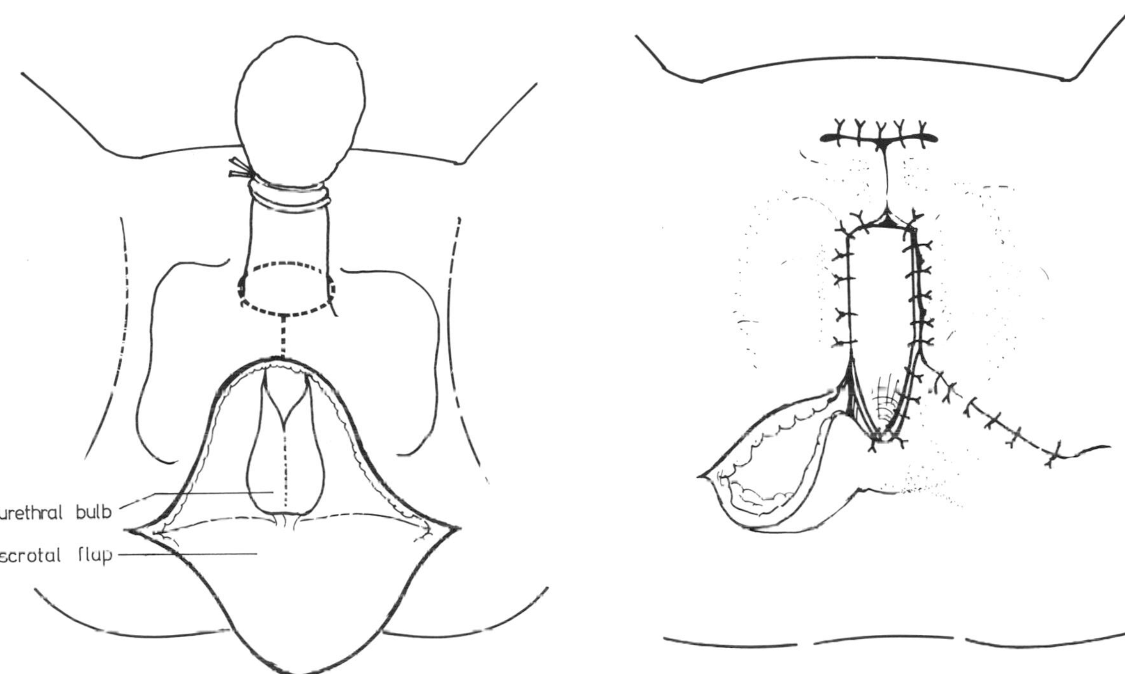

Fig. 21.23. Radical amputation of the penis

IMPOTENCE

When a patient is referred with the complaint of impotence, listen patiently to his story to discover exactly what has gone wrong. You may be able to distinguish five patterns.

1 Too high hopes

Some men have exaggerated notions of what a 'normal' performance should be: they forget that in this as in all physical attributes, performance diminishes with age. Many elderly men seek some wonder-working pill or injection from their doctor, who has none to offer. Do not be bullied into prescribing useless androgens, stimulants or aphrodisiacs: none of them work.

2 Wrong partner

Other men have normal ejaculation, but coitus is unsatisfactory. They can masturbate and may have wet dreams, but cannot make love to one particular partner. Such a patient should be referred to a doctor with special skill and training in psychosexual counselling.

3 Erection normal: ejaculation unsatisfactory

(a) *Premature ejaculation*

Here the trigger is set too delicately. It is a normal phenomenon as can be confirmed by a visit to the monkey cage in the zoo. The patient needs sympathetic reassurance. Let the couple have a rest and try again. Often all that is needed is some information about the techniques of civilized lovemaking. There is no pill that replaces informed understanding.

(b) *Ejaculation inhibited*

Feelings of guilt, anxiety, a squeaky bedstead or fear of discovery (as every novelist knows) may inhibit the progress of lovemaking. When this occurs repeatedly it may blight an otherwise loving and happy relationship. Patient explanation by a skilled counsellor will often bring the problem into the open: all ghosts dissolve in daylight.

(c) *No ejaculation*

(i) *Sympathetic paralysis.* If the last two lumbar sympathetic ganglia, or the presacral nerve have been removed surgically (e.g. for hypertension, removal of malignant lymph nodes in testis tumour, or in surgery of the aorta), then the seminal vesicles are paralysed and the bladder neck fails to shut off. The same effect can result from alpha-blockers given to control hypertension, and in some unhappy young men with diabetic neuropathy.

(ii) *Retrograde ejaculation.* If the bladder neck has been removed surgically, or is congenitally unable to close, then the semen may be pumped out of the vesicles, but wells up back into the bladder. In these cases the semen can be recovered from the urine, and utilized to achieve pregnancy. (In these cases it helps to make the urine alkaline with a dose of sodium bicarbonate before collecting it.)

(iii) *Blocked ejaculatory ducts.* This is difficult to diagnose, but if ejaculation is painful one should suspect that the semen is dammed up behind stenosed ejaculatory ducts. The diagnosis is confirmed by injecting contrast medium down the vasa and showing that it does not enter the urethra. Occasionally it is possible to unblock the ejaculatory ducts transurethrally.

4 No desire

Such a patient can obtain an erection and wakes with one in the morning but has no desire. This may be a feature of *overwork* — the so-called *Barristers' impotence* (barristers are by no means the only young ambitious workaholics who bring their work home, have no time for anything else and find their wife less exciting than their work). Frustration, alcohol and divorce are common clinical features of the syndrome. A careful history usually reveals this condition, and the remedy is a good holiday away from the telephone, but by the time they complain to the doctor more expert psychosexual counselling may be needed.

This condition may need to be distinguished from *depression* with which it shares many features, and will respond to expert psychiatric treatment.

5 No erection

A careful history is the most important part of the investigation, and will reveal some of the conditions referred to above. But it may still be difficult to distinguish the kind of impotence that is caused by psychogenic causes from that due to a disorder of the veins or blood supply of the penis.

In making this distinction the measurement of nocturnal penile tumescence (see above) will settle the matter.

Diabetes must be looked for as well as other evidence of small artery disease, e.g. hypertension or a history of coronary artery disease.

Doppler studies, the measurement of the penile blood pressure, and a test injection of papaverine will show whether there is arterial filling of the penis. If there is none, then it suggests that there is a neurological cause for the impotence. Such patients may be offered a *penile prosthesis.* There are several varieties of these: some are permanently semi-stiff (Fig. 21.24); others contain a silver wire that can be bent down or up according to need (Fig. 21.25), still others can be pumped up or let down (Fig. 21.26). These require a good deal of care and are only appropriate for the well-motivated patient with some manual dexterity.

If there is some filling of the penis, but it is incomplete — and especially if there is a failure to achieve the second phase of erection where the penis finally becomes rigid — then there may be a vascular

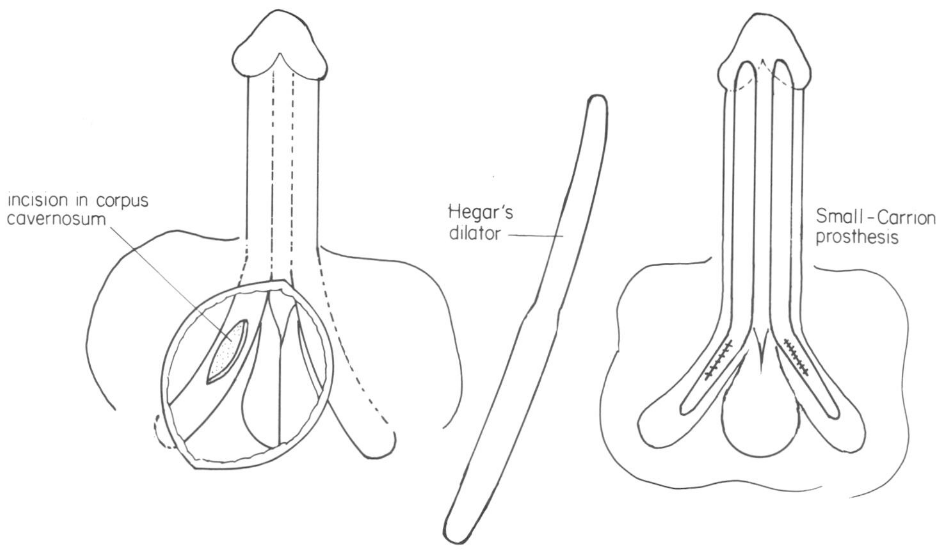

Fig. 21.24. Small-carrion prosthesis.

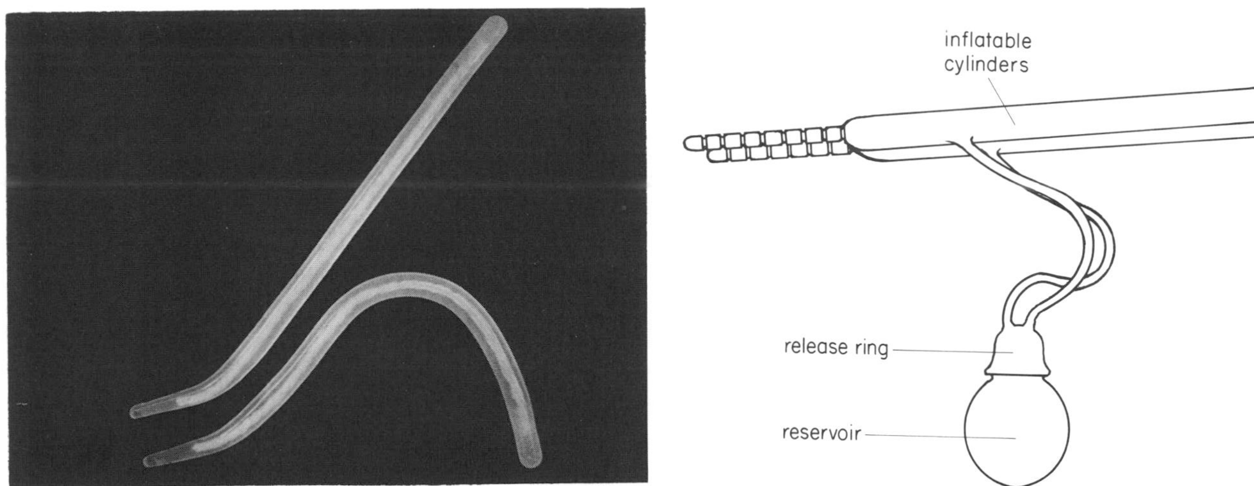

Fig. 21.25. Jonas flexible prosthesis.

Fig. 21.26. Inflatable prosthesis. (Mentor.)

cause. Angiography may be indicated, and if there is a blockage of the pudendal artery, success has sometimes followed microvascular reconstruction whereby the inferior epigastric artery is anastomosed to the proximal end of the dorsal artery of the penis, allowing blood to run up to the junction and down to the artery of the corpus cavernosum (Fig. 21.27).

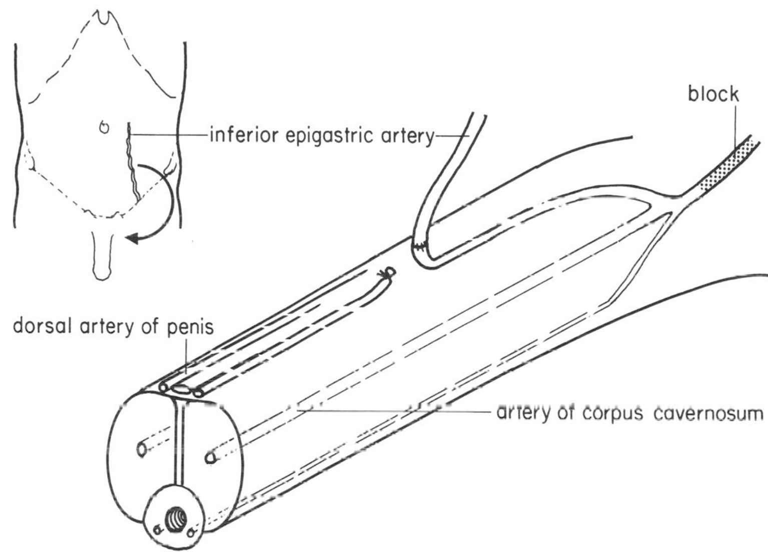

Fig. 21.27. Revascularization of the penis by anastomosis between the inferior epigastric artery and the dorsal artery of the penis.

In other cases, pressure cavernosography may show a venous leak. In some men there is a congenitally anomalous vein which allows the blood to enter the saphenous vein and if this is tied, normal erections may return. In others, the venous leakage is probably caused by failure of the closing mechanism inside Buck's fascia, and surgical efforts to close off the superficial or deep veins are disappointing.

Patients for whom the injection of papaverine results in a useful erection can be provided with a supply of papaverine and taught how to make the injection themselves. It requires care, and there is a risk of causing a haematoma afterwards with resulting fibrosis in the cavernous tissue rather like Peyronie's disease. There is also a risk that the injection may bring on an erection that will not lie down — priapism — so that it is necessary to provide an emergency service for this complication.

PRIAPISM

Priapism may occur after normal intercourse, in sickle cell disease, leukaemia, and in some patients on haemodialysis. Nowadays it is also seen in patients giving themselves papaverine injections.

The first remedy is to aspirate the penis with a wide-bore needle introduced under local anaesthesia: the blood in a priapism is thick and dark, but never clots. The aspiration and irrigation of the penis is continued until the blood becomes bright red. This is then followed by an

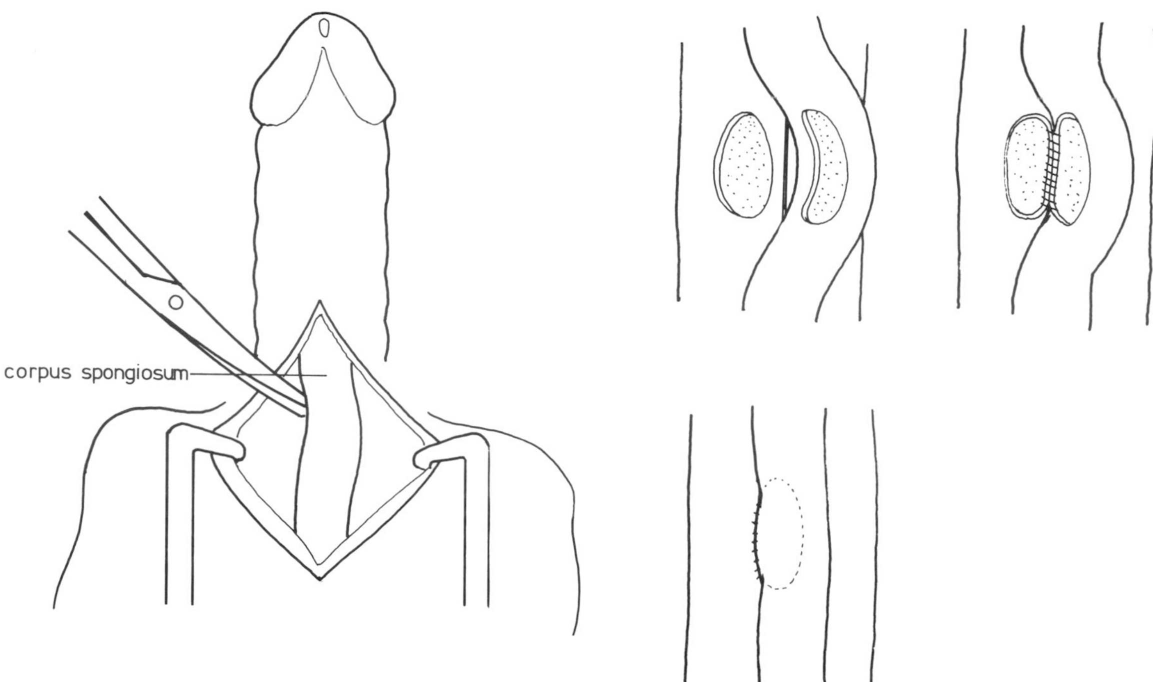

Fig. 21.28. Corpus–corpus anastomosis for priapism.

injection of 2 mg metaraminol in 4 ml saline. A careful watch must be kept on the patient's blood pressure.

If this fails to cure the priapism, it may be necessary to perform a *corpus-corpus shunt* (Fig. 21.28), allowing blood to pass from the distended corpora cavernosa into the flaccid corpus spongiosum.

FURTHER READING

Ahlering TE & Lieskovksy G (1988) Surgical treatment of urethral cancer in the male patient. In: Skinner DG & Lieskovsky G (Eds) *Diagnosis and Management of Genitourinary Cancer*. WB Saunders Co., Philadelphia. pp. 622–33.

Bailey MJ, Yande S, Walmsley B & Pryor JP (1985) Surgery for Peyronie's disease: a review of 200 patients. *British Journal of Urology* **57**, 746–9.

Bennett AH (1982) *Management of Male Impotence*. Williams and Wilkins, Baltimore.

Blandy JP (1986) *Operative Urology*. 2nd Ed. Blackwell Scientific Publications, Oxford. pp. 198–9.

Brindley GS (1986) Sexual and reproductive problems of paraplegic men. In: Clarke JR (Ed) *Oxford Reviews of Reproductive Biology 8*. Clarendon Press, Oxford. pp. 214–22.

Brindley GS (1986) Sacral root and hypogastric plexus stimulators and what these models tell us about autonomic actions on the bladder and urethra. *Clinical Science* **70**, 41s–4s.

Brindley GS (1986) Maintenance treatment of erectile impotence by cavernosal unstriated muscle relaxant injection. *British Journal of Psychiatry* **149**, 210–5.

Bunney MH (1986) Viral warts: a new look at an old problem. *British Medical Journal* **293**, 1045–6.

Crawford ED & Dawkins CA (1988) Cancer of the penis. In: Skinner DG & Lieskovsky G (Eds) *Diagnosis and Management of Genitourinary Cancer.* WB Saunders, Philadelphia. pp. 549–63.

El-Demiry MIM, Oliver RTD, Hope-Stone HF & Blandy JP (1984) Reappraisal of the role of radiotherapy and surgery in the management of carcinoma of the penis. *British Journal of Urology* **56**, 24–8.

Gairdner D (1949) The fate of the foreskin. *British Medical Journal* **2**, 1433–7.

Lemberger RJ, Bishop MC & Bates CP (1984) Nesbit's operation for Peyronie's disease. *British Journal of Urology* **56**, 721–3.

Pryor JP & Lipshultz LI (Eds) (1987) *Andrology.* Butterworth, London.

Wiles PG (1988) Successful non-invasive management of erectile impotence in diabetic men. *British Medical Journal* **296**, 161–2.

22 The Testicle and Seminal Tract

SURGICAL ANATOMY

By tradition testis and epididymis are together included in the term 'testicle'. They lie in the scrotum, the testis in front of the epididymis, slung from the external inguinal ring by the spermatic cord. In front of the testis, and nearly surrounding it, is a thin-walled sac, which is the remnant of the peritoneum: this is the tunica vaginalis, and it contains a trace of fluid (Fig. 22.1).

The testicular artery is a branch of the aorta arising below the level of the renal arteries; it passes lateral to the inferior epigastric vessels along the inguinal canal (Fig. 22.2). Many large veins drain the testicle, forming the pampiniform plexus: these merge into the spermatic veins which on the left enter the left renal vein and on the right, the vena cava.

The testis is composed of sets of tubules which drain into the rete

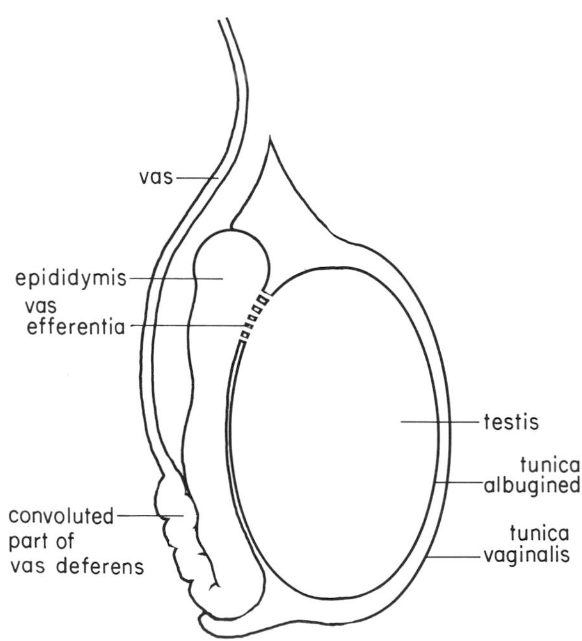

Fig. 22.1. Surgical anatomy of the testicle.

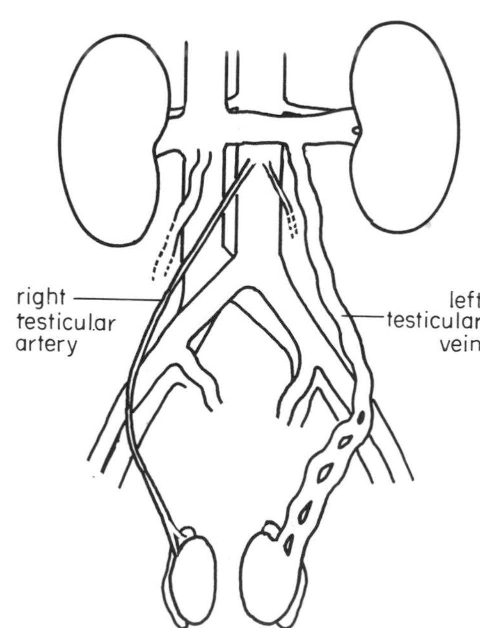

Fig. 22.2. Arteries and veins of the testicle.

testis, and thence along the vasa efferentia into the epididymis, which is a long coiled tube lined with ciliated epithelium that issues into the vas deferens (Fig. 22.3).

The vas deferens runs behind the spermatic cord, curls around the inferior epigastric vessels, crossing the ureter, and dives down through the prostate to emerge beside the utriculus masculinus at the side of the verumontanum in the prostatic urethra (Fig. 22.4).

HISTOLOGICAL STRUCTURE OF THE TESTICLE

Each testicular tubule has a thin basement membrane within which one finds two types of cell: the germinal cells and the Sertoli cells (Fig. 22.5). Packed between the tubules are Leydig cells. The germinal cells subdivide into primary and secondary spermatocytes, spermatids, and finally spermatozoa. The Sertoli cells appear to play an important role in the final preparation of spermatids, grooming and streamlining them into spermatozoa. They probably make oestrogens, androgen binding protein, and *inhibin* which regulates the output of follicle-stimulating hormone by

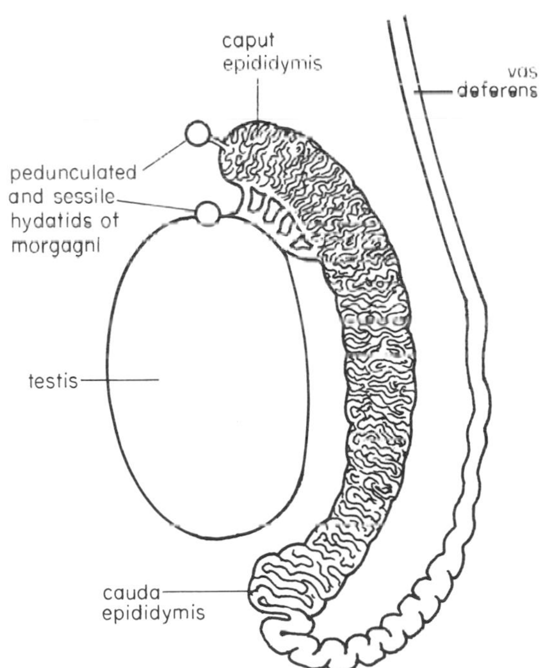

Fig. 22.3. Structure of testis and epididymis.

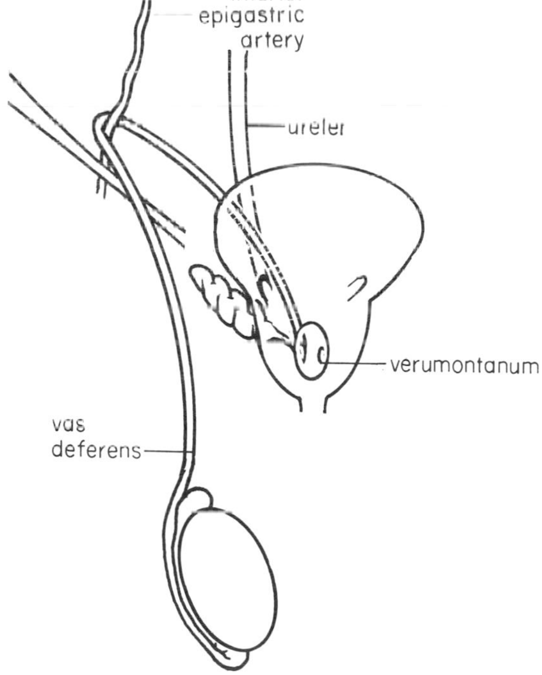

Fig. 22.4. Surgical anatomy of the vas deferens.

the pituitary. In turn, it is thought that follicle-stimulating hormone works through the Sertoli cells to increase spermatogenesis (Fig. 22.6).

The Leydig cells (interstitial cells) manufacture testosterone which is necessary for the development of male secondary sexual characteristics as well as for spermatogenesis.

EMBRYOLOGY

The most imaginative author of scientific fiction would balk at presenting the story of the development of the human testicle on the grounds that it was far too improbable. The germ cells can be found in the yolk sac of the embryo (Fig. 22.7) and then make an extraordinary journey by means of their amoeboid movements, along the umbilical cord, across the primitive coelom, to the genital ridge where they creep through the endothelium and burrow into the gonadal mesenchyme to form what are destined to become the seminiferous tubules. There they proliferate and bulge into the peritoneum, becoming surrounded by a peritoneal covering which will be the tunica albuginea testis (Fig. 22.8).

The tubules join up with adjacent mesonephric tubules to form the

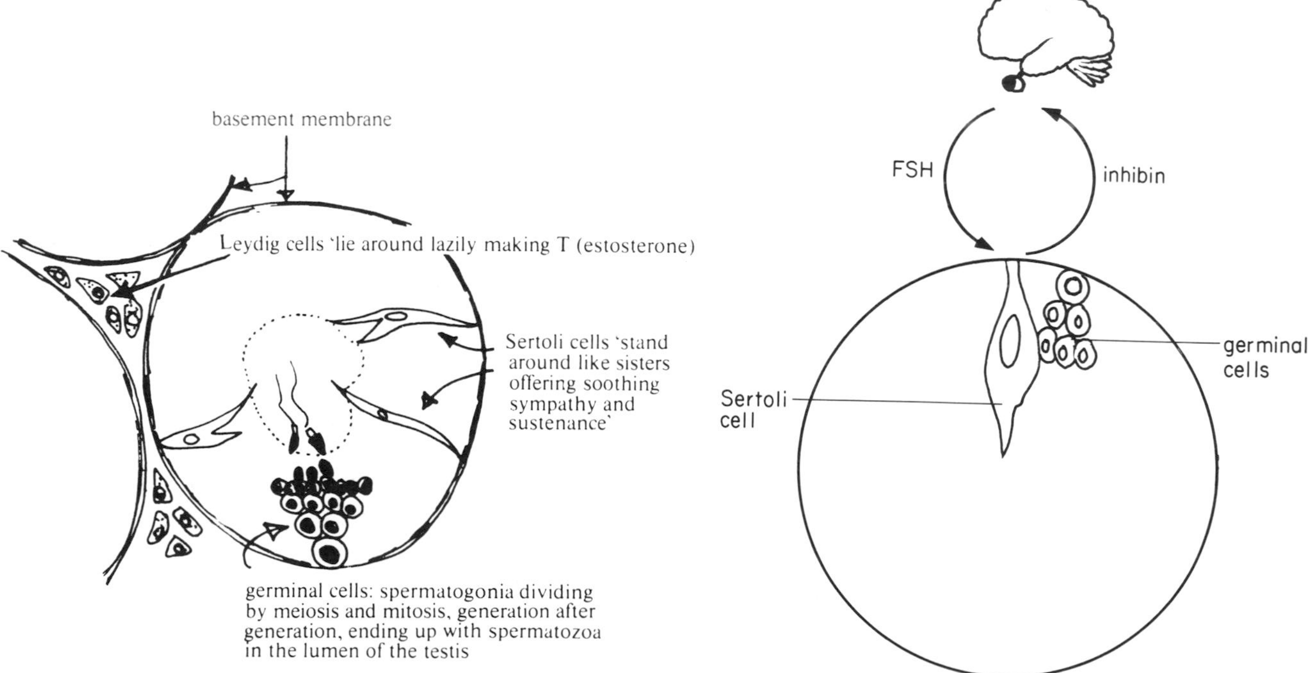

Fig. 22.5. Histology of the testis.

Fig. 22.6. The relationship between the pituitary and the Sertoli cells.

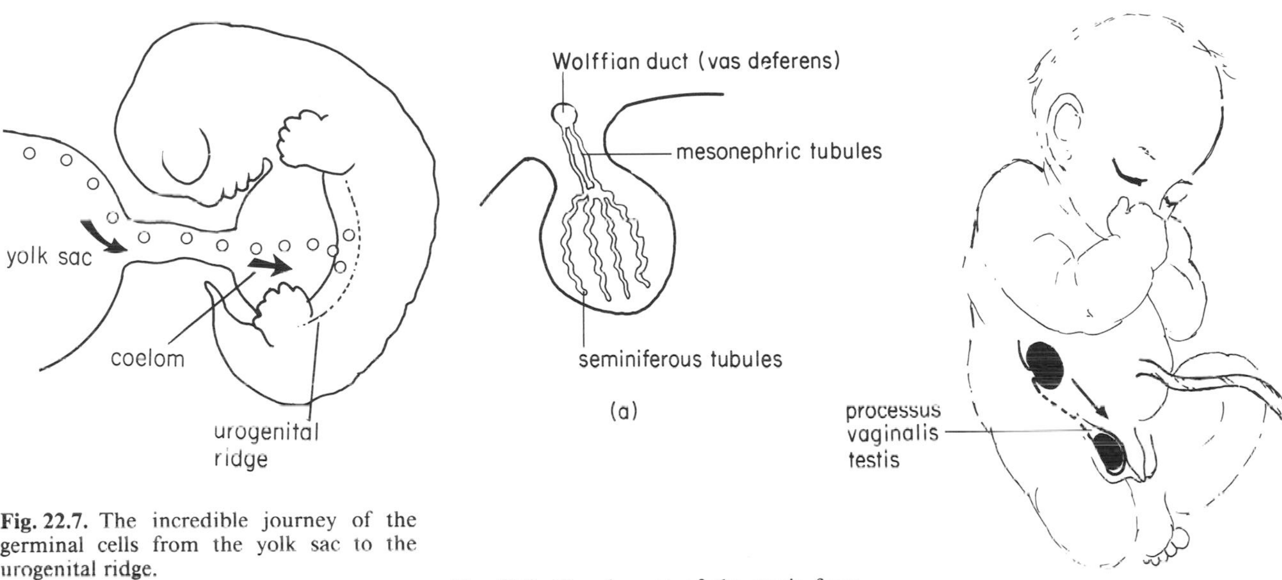

Fig. 22.7. The incredible journey of the germinal cells from the yolk sac to the urogenital ridge.

Fig. 22.8. The descent of the testis from the gonadal ridge to the scrotum.

vasa efferentia testis and these in turn enter the Wolffian duct to become the epididymis.

Shortly before birth, the testis makes another journey from the back of the peritoneal cavity to the bottom of the scrotum. This journey is not complete in all mammals: in elephants the testicles stop just near the kidneys; in whales they fetch up near the bladder; in hedgehogs just inside the abdominal wall; in pigs they lodge in a shallow sac without a definite neck and in sheep and man they hang at the bottom of a pendulous scrotum.

Undescended testicle

In making this migration into the scrotum the testicle is preceded by a gelatinous body which seems to dilate the tissues to make way for the testicles to follow: this is called the *gubernaculum* (Fig. 22.9). The gubernaculum does not always reach the right place, and one classifies undescended testicles according to whether the gubernaculum has taken a wrong course, or has not completed it (Fig. 22.10).

1 The gubernaculum takes a wrong direction. The gelatinous lump of gubernaculum may wander off into the root of the penis, the thigh, the fat of the abdominal wall, or the perineum, and when the testicle follows it into one of these abnormal positions, it is called *ectopic*.

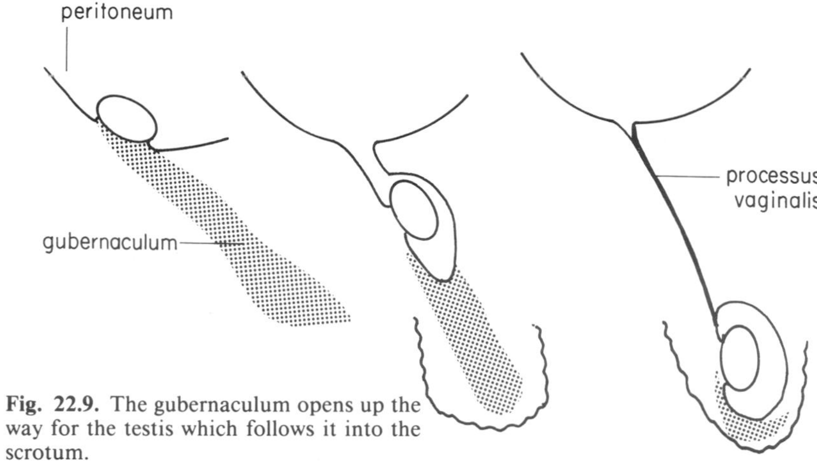

Fig. 22.9. The gubernaculum opens up the way for the testis which follows it into the scrotum.

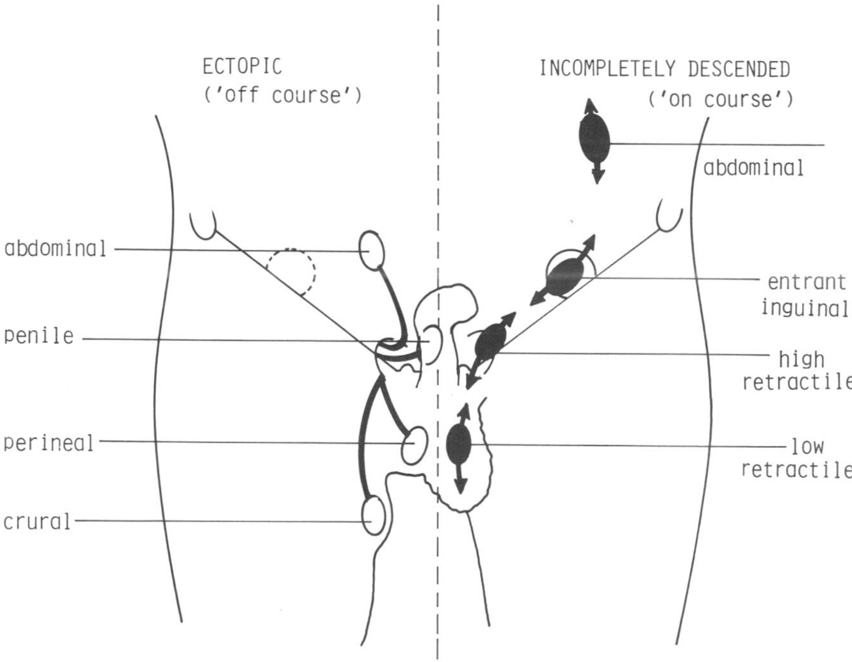

Fig. 22.10. The maldescended testis may either be off course or on course, i.e. ectopic (left) or incompletely descended (right). All types other than the 'low retractile' need orchidopexy.

2 The gubernaculum does not reach its destination. These are 'incompletely' descended rather than 'ectopic' testicles. Like the normal testicle they all have a certain normal range of movement. They are classified as *abdominal, inguinal,* or *retractile.*

Abdominal testes are usually found just inside the internal ring. Inguinal testes lie in the inguinal canal, where they cannot usually be felt under the tight covering of the external oblique muscle. It is the retractile testicles which cause most of the difficulty: they are very common. High retractile testicles ride up and down from the external ring to the upper part of the scrotum: low retractile testicles can be persuaded to reach the bottom of the scrotum.

In little boys the testicles are normally very apt to be drawn up to the external ring, probably as a protective reflex, and it can be quite difficult to make the distinction between the high retractile testicle which will not settle at puberty in the scrotum and the low retractile which will, and does not need an operation. Gentleness and warm hands are essential, but the diagnosis can only be made in some boys with general anaesthesia.

Complications of undescended testicles

There is nearly always a rather large sac of peritoneum — *tunica vaginalis* — associated with an undescended testicle, and an *inguinal hernia* is often present. In this baggy sac, the testicle may lie on a kind of stalk upon which it may twist (Fig. 22.11), hence *torsion* of the testicle is associated with imperfect descent of the testicle. The high lying testis is less likely to produce sperms than the testis in the scrotum, perhaps because the latter is a cooler environment, and *infertility* is common when both testes are affected, though it is not any more common in unilateral undescent.

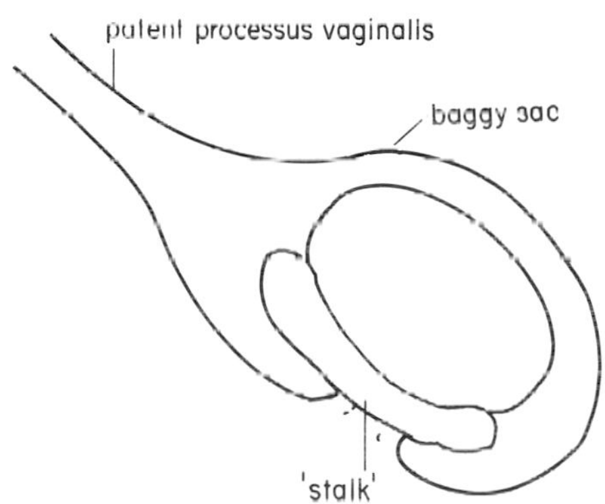

Fig. 22.11. The big baggy peritoneal sac associated with the undescended testis encourages torsion.

Malignancy is more common in undescended testicles: about one in ten of all testicular tumours arise in association with cryptorchidism.

Orchidopexy

Indications

All ectopic, and all incompletely descended testicles other than the low retractile ones, should be brought down surgically. The timing of the operation is governed by two considerations: (i) the hope of fertility and (ii) the risk of cancer.

1 *Fertility.* In the normal testicle, at the time of birth there are spermatogonia inside the tubules which are surrounded by primitive Sertoli cells, and between the tubules there are Leydig cells. By six months after birth the Leydig cells are disappearing, and until the age of 3 years the testis is more or less dormant. After the age of 3 the tubules seem to enlarge, more spermatogonia appear and by the age of 8 one can find primary spermatocytes. By 11, secondary spermatocytes and spermatids can be seen and the Leydig cells begin to reappear after their long absence. With the onset of puberty the testicular tubules begin to show complete and active spermatogenesis.

In the undescended testicle at the age of 3, when the dormant testis ought to awaken, everything seems to lag behind. The spermatogonia fail to increase or divide, and as the years pass by the basement membrane begins to thicken and become fibrotic. The Leydig cells hypertrophy as if to stimulate the sleeping tubules with an excess of androgens. By the age of 6 irreversible damage can be identified even under light microscopy, while the electron microscope is said to be able to show significant changes even before the age of 3.

2 *The risk of malignancy.* Cancer of the testicle is very rare before puberty, but from then on it is a significant risk in the undescended testicle, and either the testicle should be brought down into the scrotum where it can be examined from time to time, or it should be removed.

In consequence there has been a change in the age at which orchidopexy is now offered to little boys. Most surgeons with experience of the problems prefer to see orchidopexy completed before the age of 3. What evidence there is suggests that this may improve the subsequent chances of fertility, and minimize the risk of development of cancer later on.

If there is an associated hernia, then the operation is performed as soon after birth as possible, since there is a significant risk of strangulation in a neonate.

Hormone therapy

By giving gonadotrophins one may bring on a premature puberty at the cost of early fusion of the epiphyses and a stunted growth. The logic of the treatment is that it will cause low retractile testes to stay down in the scrotum where they would have lodged anyway at puberty. When in doubt examination of the scrotum under anaesthesia distinguishes the low retractile testes, and anyway, to put off making the decision until near puberty is to lose the chance of preserving the function of the testis. The use of gonadotrophins appears quite illogical today.

Technique of orchidopexy

Through an incision in the skin crease sited over the internal inguinal ring the external oblique is slit open, the peritoneal sac separated from the cord, and the plane between peritoneum and cord opened up by dividing several crescentic bands of fibrous tissue (Fig. 22.12). This usually allows the testicle to be brought right down to the scrotum without any tension. Occasionally it helps to divide the inferior epigastric vessels, or bring the testicle out medial to them.

Very rarely the vessels of the spermatic cord are still too short even after this mobilization. As a rule the testicle is then left just outside the external ring. One or two years later a second operation is performed at which it is usually found that the vessels of the cord have elongated and now allow the testis to be brought without tension into the scrotum.

To fix the testicle in position a sac is made between the dartos muscle and the skin of the scrotum. There is no need to fix the testicle to the thigh for there should never be any tension.

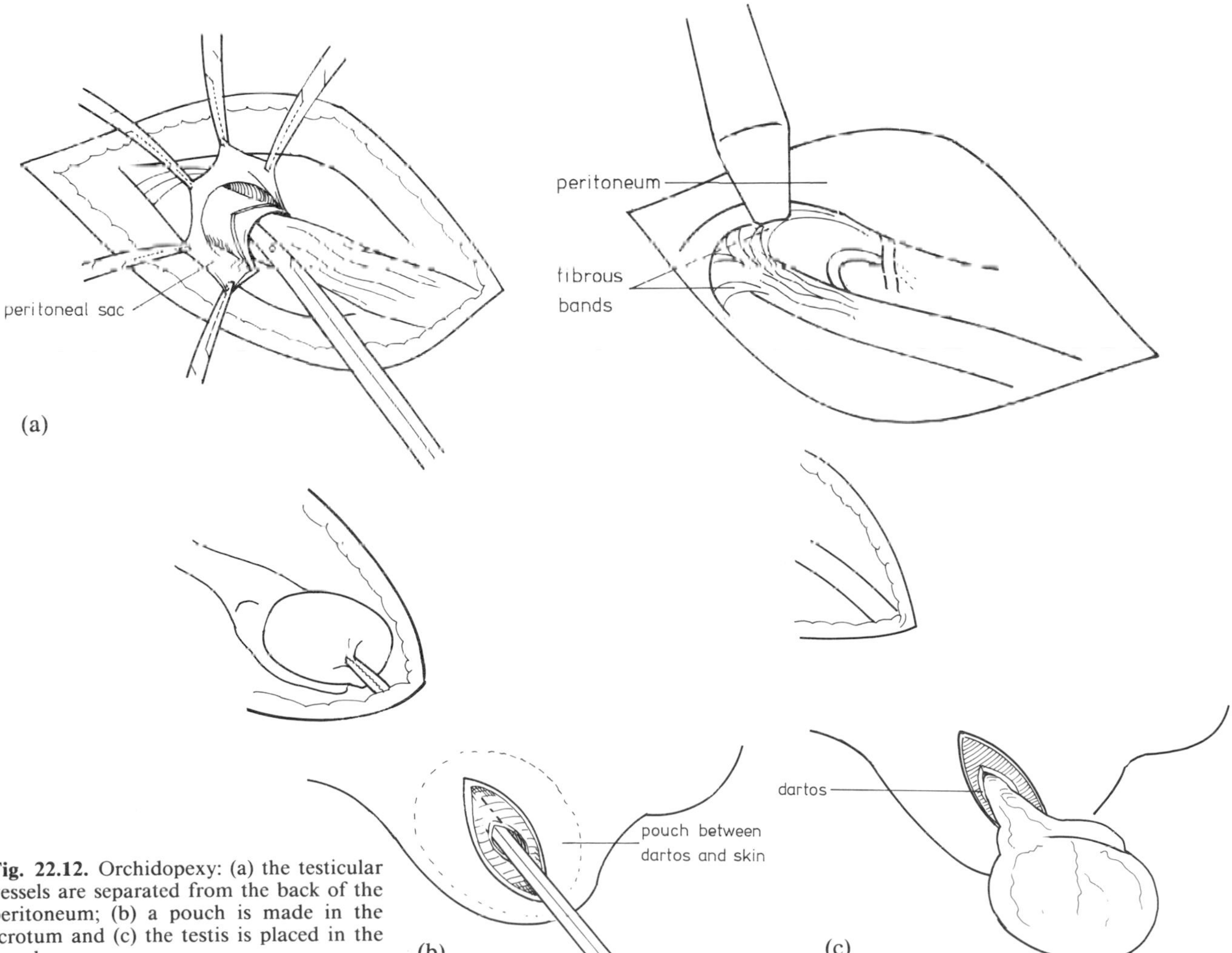

Fig. 22.12. Orchidopexy: (a) the testicular vessels are separated from the back of the peritoneum; (b) a pouch is made in the scrotum and (c) the testis is placed in the pouch.

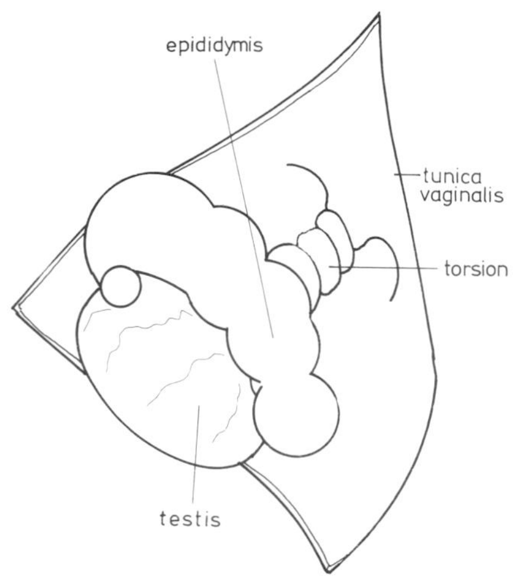

Fig. 22.13. Torsion of the testicle.

TORSION OF THE TESTICLE

A baggy tunica vaginalis may occur even in a completely descended testicle and allows the testis to rotate on a kind of stalk, causing obstruction first to the veins, then to the arteries, and finally death by infarction (Fig. 22.13). These patients often have warning attacks of pain that come on suddenly and equally suddenly are relieved. Torsion may occur at any age but is most common around puberty. It helps to remember that epididymitis is very rare in children and mumps orchitis never seen before puberty. So in a boy with a swollen painful testicle, torsion should be the first consideration, and requires urgent treatment. Today the diagnosis may be confirmed by Doppler studies which will show absence of blood flow into the testicle, but when in doubt, it should be explored. While waiting for the opportunity to get the boy to the operation room, it is worth attempting to untwist the testis manually: rotate it first one way, then the other. If successful there is a distinct 'click; and the pain is relieved.

The signs of torsion are indistinguishable from other causes of infarction, acute epididymo-orchitis and the 10% of cancers which present with features of inflammation.

Operation for torsion of the testicle

The testis is exposed through the scrotum, the tunica opened, and the twist undone. If the testis is thought to be alive, it is returned to the scrotum.

Since the other side may also have the same baggy hydrocele and the same tendency to undergo torsion, it is always necessary to explore the other side, if not there and then, at least within a few days, to fix it and prevent bilateral torsion.

Torsion of the appendix testis

There are tiny pedunculated remnants of the Müllerian duct sitting on the top of the testis which can twist on a stalk (Fig. 22.14) producing pain almost identical to that of torsion of the testis. Sometimes one can see a distinct bluish, pea-sized tender swelling through the skin of the scrotum: more often there is so much inflammatory oedemia that the diagnosis can only be made when the testis is explored and the tunica vaginalis opened.

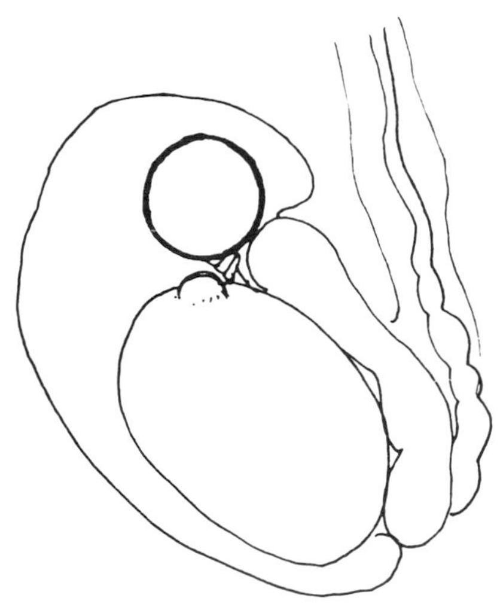

Fig. 22.14. Torsion of the appendix testis.

VARICOCELE

The veins issuing from the testis and epididymis are so remarkably tortuous and complicated (Fig. 22.15) that they are believed to serve as a heat-exchanger mechanism to keep the testicle cool, and by inference, a varicocele is thought to depress spermatogenesis. It is widely believed that division of these veins may improve spermatogenesis, and even though controlled studies fail to show any difference in the patterns of spermatogenesis whether varicoceles are operated on or not, the operation is still widely performed.

HYDROCELE

Fluid may accumulate in the cavity of the tunica vaginalis testis as a result of obstruction to the lymphatic drainage of the tunica and cord, or

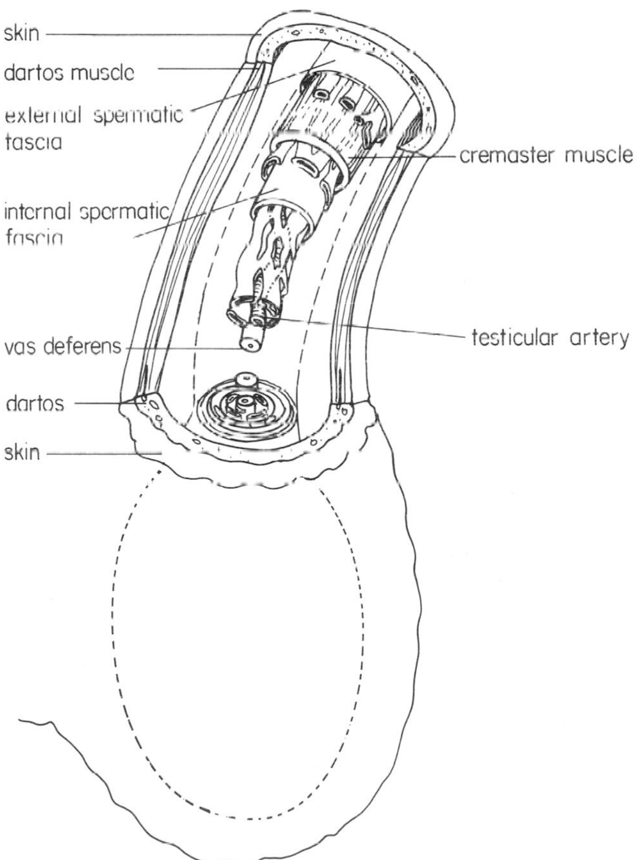

Fig. 22.15. The spermatic cord is made of several sleeves between each of which run numerous veins — the pampiniform plexus.

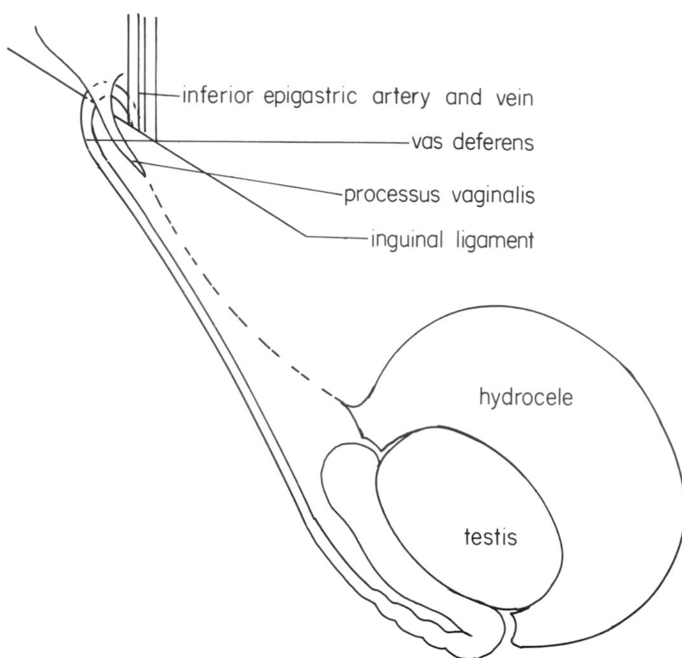

Fig. 22.16. Structure and anatomical relations of a hydrocele.

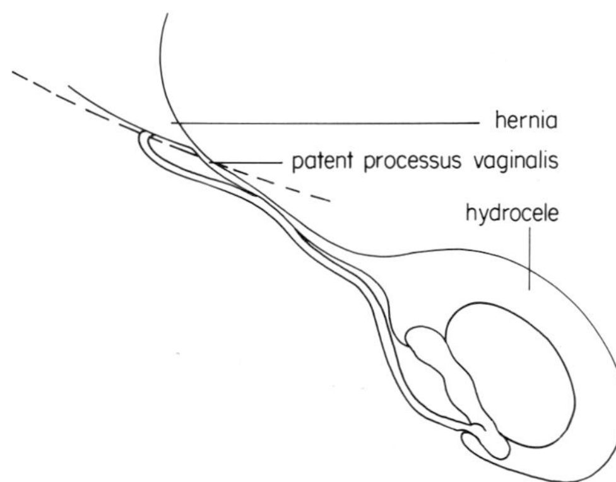

Fig. 22.17. Hydrocele in an infant—the processus vaginalis is patent so that it alters in size. A hernia is often associated.

as a response to some pathological process in the testis and epididymis — in this the accumulation of fluid follows exactly the same rules as for ascites (Figs. 22.16, 22.17).

The lymphatic drainage of the testicle begins as spaces between the tubules which drain into the lymphatics of the cord. It is common to find hydroceles in patients with cardiac failure or in those who have undergone surgical removal of the retroperitoneal lymph nodes in nephrectomy for cancer of the kidney or have developed post-radiation fibrosis or idiopathic retroperitoneal fibrosis. In the tropics, lymphatic obstruction may occur from infestation with *Wuchereria bancroftii* — a microfilarial worm which resides in the veins of the pampiniform plexus and obstructs free drainage.

The majority of hydroceles have no identifiable cause: they are labelled ‘idiopathic’ and they are innocuous unless meddled with. Secondary hydroceles occur in tumours, epididymitis, mumps, and acute orchitis. It may be necessary to aspirate them in order to make sure that the underlying testis does not contain a tumour.

Hydroceles are treated when they are so big that they cause discomfort or embarrassment.

Aspiration (tapping) a hydrocele

Under local anaesthetic a plastic trochar and cannula is inserted into the sac, the trochar is removed and the fluid drawn off with a syringe (Fig. 22.18). It is said that injection of various sclerosant solutions (e.g. tetracycline) will cause obliteration of the sac and prevent recurrence. In practice this is painful and by no means always successful.

Operation for hydrocele

Through the scrotum the testicle is delivered: the sac is opened, everted and secured behind the testicle with one or two sutures — Jaboulay's operation — (Fig. 22.19). An alternative is to bunch up the surplus tunica with a series of sutures — Lord's procedure — (Fig. 22.20). When the sac is thick, it is excised: careful haemostasis is secured by a running catgut suture along the thick edge of the hydrocele (Fig. 22.21). After all these operations there is nearly always a considerable swelling caused partly by oedema and partly by effusion of blood, and the patients need to be warned of this.

CYSTS OF THE EPIDIDYMIS AND SPERMATOCELE

Most men over the age of 40 have tiny cysts in the sulcus between epididymis and testis. These are diverticula of the collecting tubules of

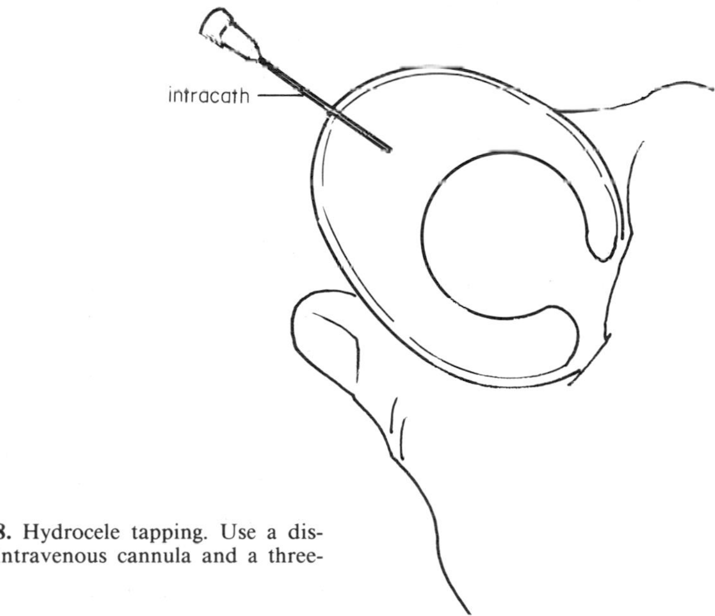

Fig. 22.18. Hydrocele tapping. Use a disposable intravenous cannula and a three-way tap.

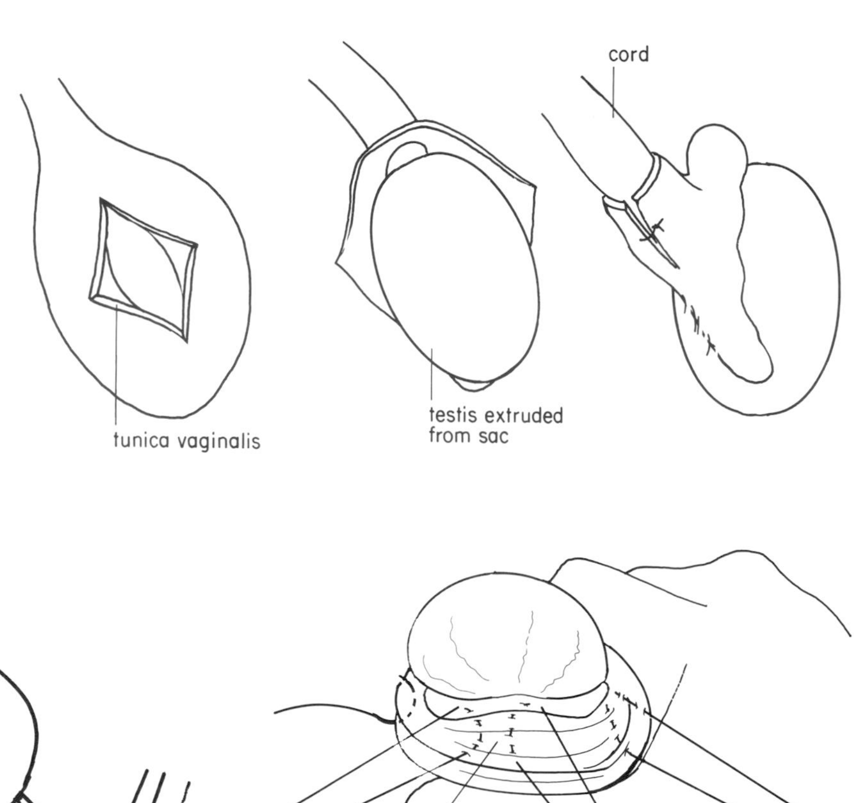

Fig. 22.19. Jaboulay or bottleneck operation. The hydrocele is opened, turned inside out, and sewn up behind the cord.

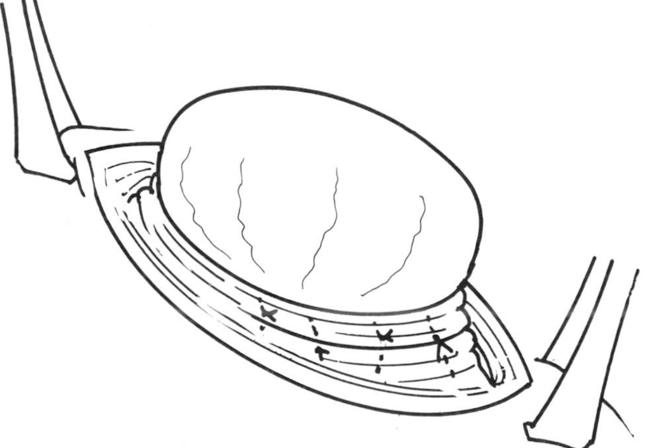

Fig. 22.20. Lord's operation for plication of a hydrocele.

the vasa efferentia testis. When they enlarge they form translucent cysts, often multiple, like a bunch of grapes, lying behind the testis (Fig. 22.22). They contain varying numbers of sperms, sometimes so many as to cause their fluid to look like cream — *spermatocele*. Clinically, they present as a fluctuant translucent lump behind the testis. Nothing should be done about them unless they are causing difficulty in wearing trousers. If they are operated on, the vasa efferentia testis are likely to be obstructed and the patient to be made infertile on that side just as if with a vasectomy. Claims are made that aspiration and injection of sclerosants will cure them, but they are usually multilocular and sclerosants cause considerable discomfort. If very large, these cysts are easily removed at operation.

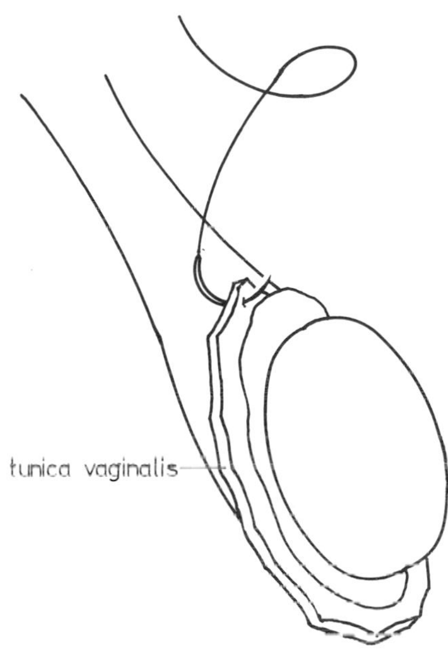

Fig. 22.21. Radical cure of hydrocele: the sac is excised and its edge oversewn to stop bleeding.

TRAUMA TO THE TESTICLE

The testicle is easily injured in sport or at work. There is usually a split in the visceral layer of the tunica vaginalis through which blood and testicular tubules protrude like cotton wool. The cavity of the tunica vaginalis fills with blood (*haematocele*). If left alone the blood clot gradually reabsorbs but not before it has compressed the testis and caused irreparable damage. To avoid this the testicle should be explored as soon as possible, the clot evacuated and the tear in the tunica sewn up (Fig. 22.23).

INFLAMMATORY DISEASES OF THE TESTICLE

Acute orchitis

Most acute infections in the testis are caused by viruses, usually mumps, sometimes Coxsackie and other viruses. Mumps orchitis is usually

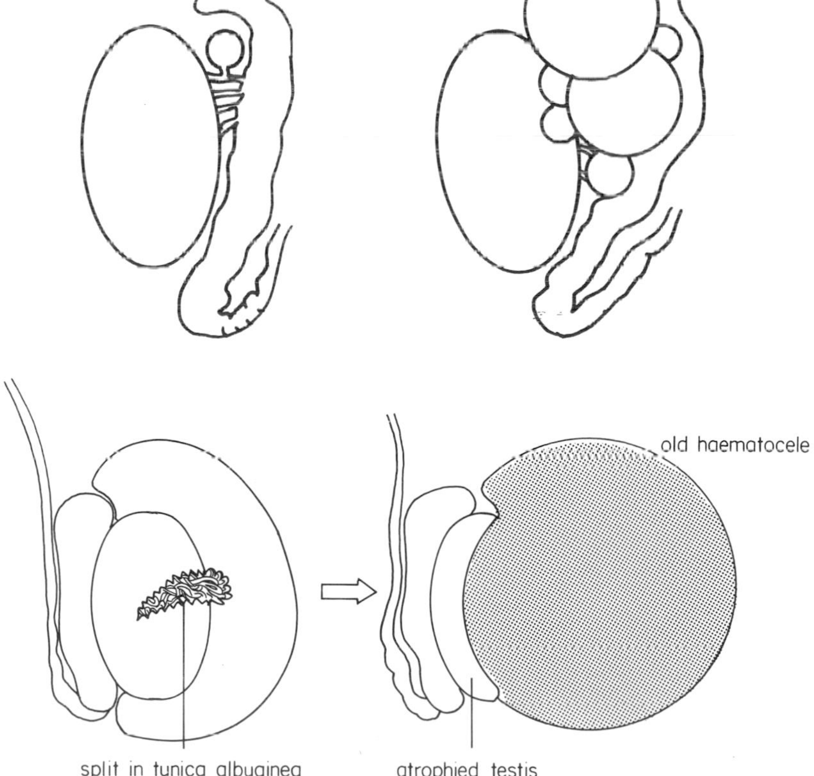

Fig. 22.22. Cysts of the epididymis.

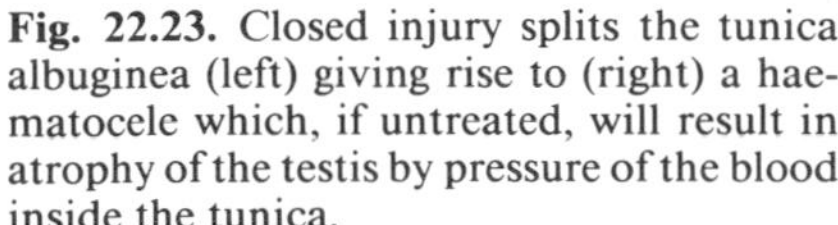

Fig. 22.23. Closed injury splits the tunica albuginea (left) giving rise to (right) a haematocele which, if untreated, will result in atrophy of the testis by pressure of the blood inside the tunica.

unilateral and never occurs before puberty. Rarely it is bilateral and can cause atrophy of both testes. It is a common complication of mumps in adults, occurring in 15–20% of cases. Unless there is an epidemic it is difficult to distinguish orchitis from torsion. Doppler studies may help, but as a rule it is wise to explore the testicle. It has been claimed that in mumps, incision of the swollen tunica albuginea may decompress the testicle and prevent atrophy.

Acute epididymitis

A generation ago acute bacterial infection of the epididymis occurred so often after operations on the urinary tract that vasectomy was a routine preliminary to prostatectomy. It is still a rare but important complication of operations where a catheter is placed in the urethra, and it also occurs without warning in men without any obvious urinary infection.

In some of these patients there is a previous episode of strenuous activity, and it is possible that reflux of urine occurs from urethra to epididymis along the vas to give rise to an extravasation of urine in the epididymis and a chemical epididymitis. In others, aspiration of the epididymis reveals infection with *Chlamydia trachomatis.*

Although it is very rare, every patient with acute epididymitis should have tuberculosis excluded by examination of three early morning specimens of urine — a precaution which is even more important in chronic epididymitis.

Syphilis

Formerly common, gumma is today very rare. It presents as a woody hard lump in the testicle indistinguishable from a cancer, and calls for orchidectomy.

Granulomatous orchitis

In men with repeated attacks of previous urinary infection there can be a hard mass in the testis. This rare type of granulomatous orchitis does not respond to antibiotics: since it is impossible to distinguish it from a cancer, the treatment is orchidectomy.

Chronic epididymitis

Tuberculosis characteristically starts in the head of the epididymis by haematogenous spread rather than along the lumen of the vas. The vas is

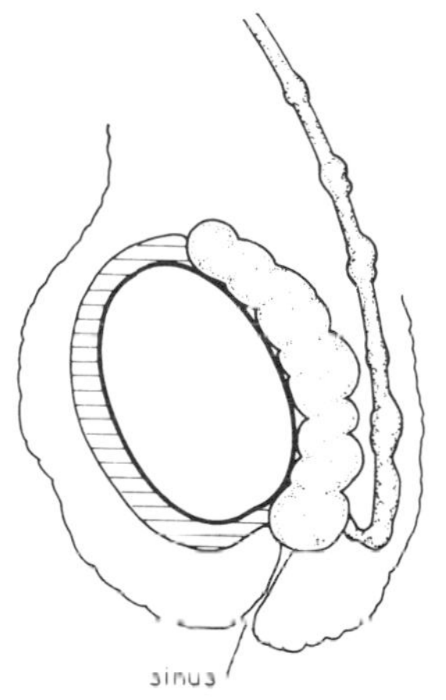

Fig. 22.24. Genital tuberculosis.

found to be beaded and shortened. The epididymis is nodular and hard, thanks to a series of caseating abscesses (Fig. 22.24). Rectal examination reveals similar changes in the prostate and seminal vesicles, and in late cases, the changes extend into the testis as well.

In some patients there is tuberculosis of the urinary tract, but not in all and it may be quite difficult to establish the diagnosis without biopsy.

Extravasation of sperm — sperm granuloma

Today this is a very common cause of painful indurated thickening in the epididymis, and is caused by extravasation of sperm after vasectomy. The sperms are intensely irritating and give rise to a chronic granuloma very similar to that found in tuberculosis.

CANCER OF THE TESTIS

Aetiology

There are about 500 new cases in Britain per annum and tumours of the testis are one of the most common cancers in men under the age of 35. It is rare in men of African ancestry both in Africa and in the United States. Cancer of the testicle is very rare before puberty, and reaches a peak incidence in the early 20s.

Pathology

Testicular tumours arise from the germ cells, the Sertoli cells, or the Leydig cells. The latter are all very rare, and usually benign. The main group of testicular cancers arise from the germinal cells.

Since the germinal cells may, ultimately, give rise to any tissue in the body it is hardly surprising that there is a very broad spectrum of cellular appearances. In addition, testicular tumours display the malignant counterparts of two very interesting primitive types of cells — *trophoblast* and *yolk-sac* cells. When trophoblast is present, it manufactures *beta chorionic gonadotrophin*, and this can be detected in the patient's plasma as well as in the tissues of the tumour by means of immunoperoxidase stains. When yolk sac tissue is present, it makes *alpha-fetoprotein* which can also be measured in the plasma and identified in the tissue. These two proteins are useful *markers* of the tumour, disappearing when the tumour is cured, reappearing if it relapses.

In former times much was made of the distinction between *seminoma* and *teratoma*. The seminoma was thought to arise from spermatocytes,

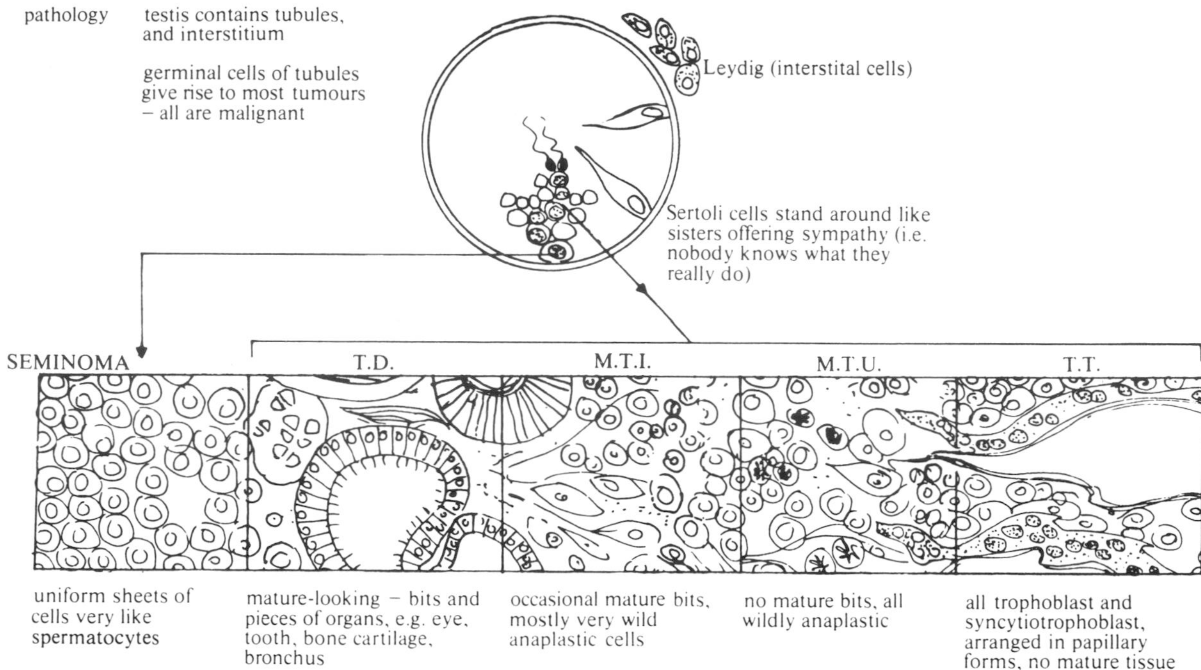

Fig. 22.25. Tumours of the testis.

occurred in older men and was known to be exceedingly sensitive to radiotherapy. Teratomas on the other hand occurred in younger men with a peak age of about 18, were less sensitive to radiation, and had a much worse prognosis.

Today, with the availability of tumour markers, it is now clear that in each tumour there may be a spectrum of different malignant tissues — parts may show seminoma, other parts teratoma.

Before the discovery of the markers there were several classifications of testicular tumours: now they have largely been superseded by systems which attempt to quantify how much of each type of tissue is present in each tumour. By and large, if differentiated tissue is present, the prognosis is better than if yolk-sac or trophoblastic tissue is to be found, and the more of these elements, the worse the outlook. At one end of the spectrum one finds well-differentiated tissues with mature skin, teeth, bones and joints — this is called *Teratoma Differentiated* or *Teratoma*: at the other end there is *choriocarcinoma* and *embryonal carcinoma*. In the British classification the range goes from Teratoma Differentiated (TD), through Malignant Teratoma Intermediate, Malignant Teratoma Undifferentiated to Choriocarcinoma. All of these may or may not be mixed with Seminoma (Fig. 22.25).

Spread of testicular tumours

Testis tumours spread by local invasion into the epididymis and cord, and then usually by lymphatic invasion along the lymphatics which accompany the testicular arteries to the level of the renal arteries, i.e. retroperitoneal para-aortic lymph nodes. Tumours with trophoblast elements tend to invade the veins early and metastasize systematically.

Staging of testis tumours

The TNM system is useful in testis tumours: locally the tumours are classified (Fig. 22.26) according to their spread through the testicle itself T1–4. The lymph nodes are either N1 (involving the para-aortic nodes) or N2 (secondary nodal involvement in the pelvis or mediastinum) (Fig. 22.27). M signifies bloodborne metastases usually to the lungs, sometimes to the brain and liver. In addition, because the response to treatment of the para-aortic nodes depends very much upon their size: the N stages are subdivided into those that are more or less than 2 cm in diameter (as measured in the CT scan).

Clinical features of testis tumours

Most patients complain of a painless lump in the testis (Fig. 22.28). Sometimes there is discomfort. In about 10% of patients the tumour has

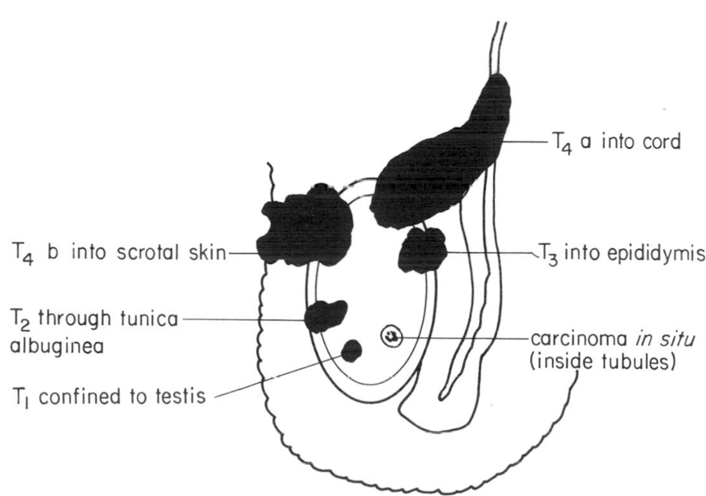

Fig. 22.26. T staging for cancer of testicle.

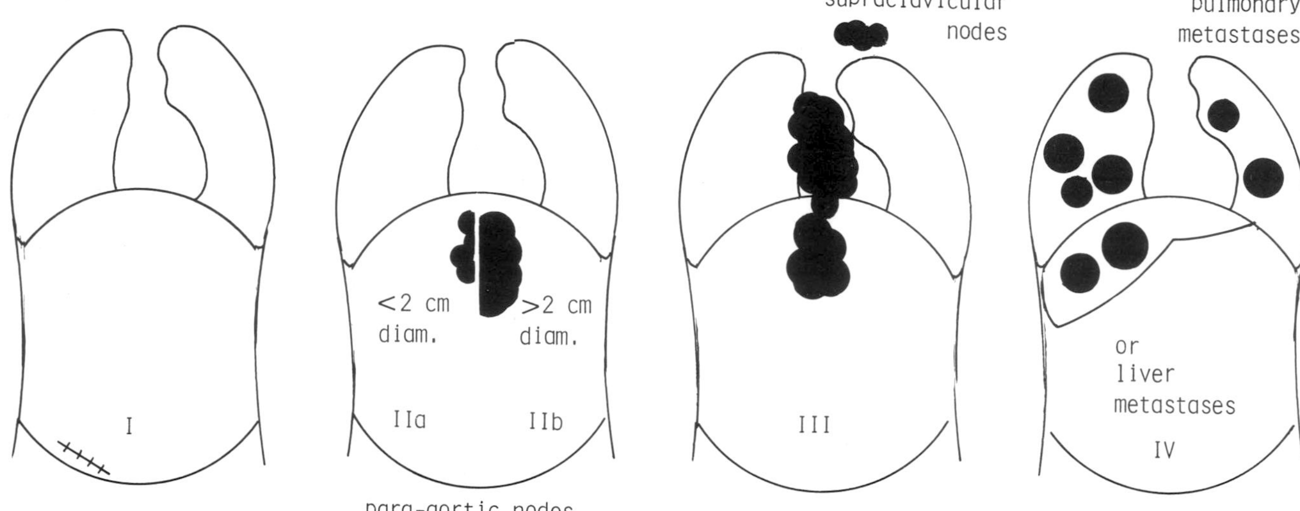

Fig. 22.27. Royal Marsden Hospital Staging of testicular cancer which is in actual clinical use. In the TNM system, I and II = N1, III = N2, and IV = M1.

redness and pain resembling an inflammation and in another 10% the lump is only discovered after an injury. Unfortunately there is a large (about 30%) group of patients who only come up when there are distant metastases.

On examination there is a lump in the body of the testis. Since there are almost no benign conditions which give rise to a lump in the testis, as soon as one has been felt — or as soon as there is a suspicion of one — the testis should be explored. Today the advent of ultrasound examination of the testis may strengthen the surgeon's suspicion, but it is very seldom that it adds anything to what careful palpation has already revealed.

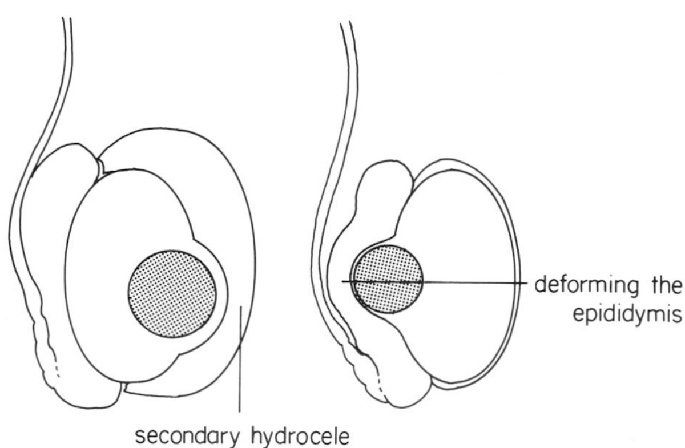

Fig. 22.28. Small lumps in the testis may be misleading if they are smothered by a secondary hydrocele (left) or so near the epididymis that they resemble epididymitis (right).

Investigations

The first investigation is to send blood for tumour markers (alpha-fetoprotein and beta HCG).

The next investigation consists of orchidectomy through an inguinal incision (Fig. 22.29). The inguinal canal is opened and a clamp placed on the spermatic cord to prevent inadvertent dislodgement of tumour tissue up the veins during the handling of the lump. The testis is delivered. If there is still any doubt about the diagnosis a frozen section may be obtained, but as a rule the diagnosis of a cancer is obvious and the cord is transfixed and ligated and the testis removed.

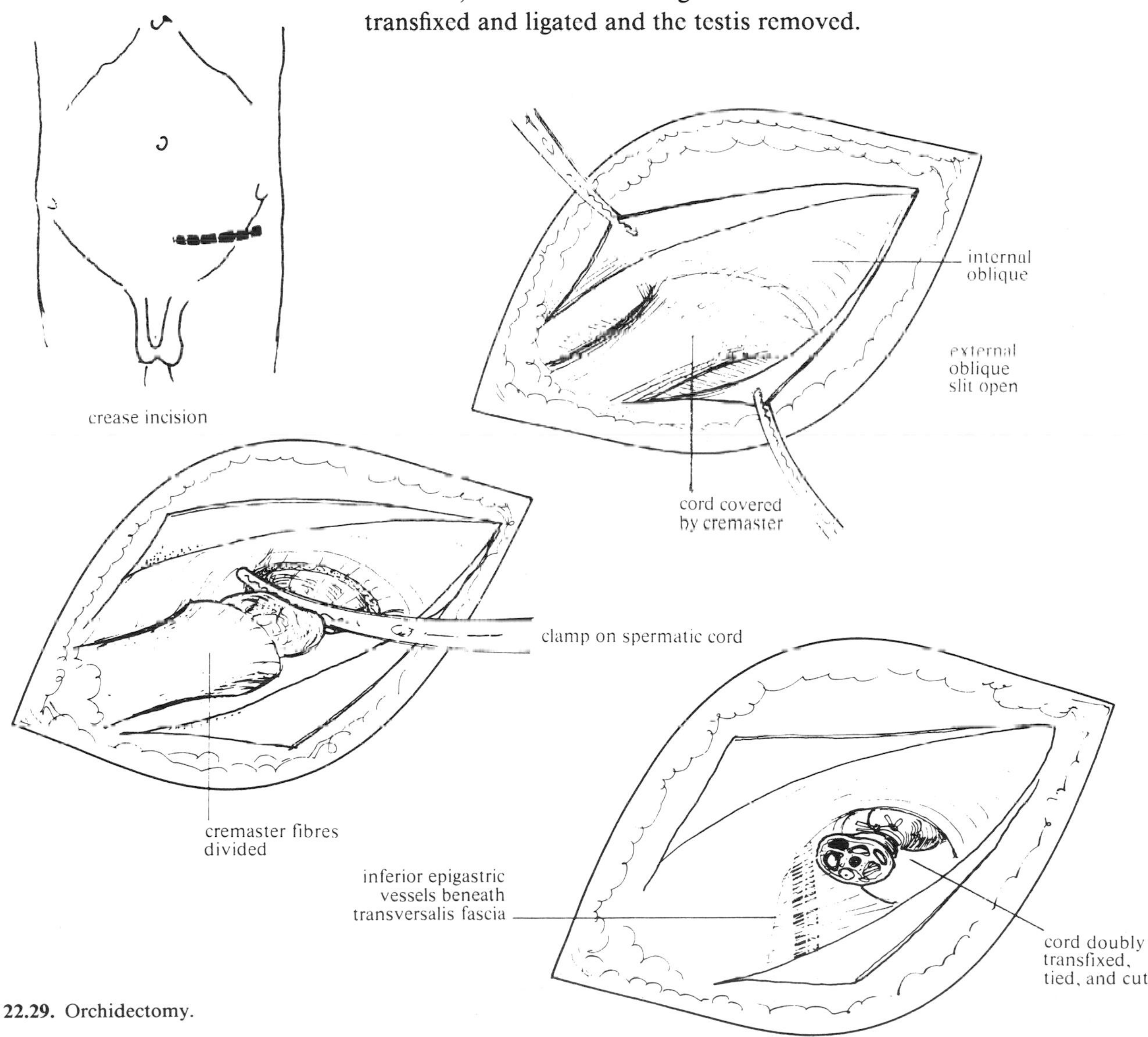

Fig. 22.29. Orchidectomy.

Clinical staging

A CT scan is performed of the lungs, mediastinum and retroperitoneal tissue (Fig. 22.30). This is able to detect small para-aortic deposits of tumour more than 1 cm in diameter. If there is any doubt this may be supplemented by a lymphangiogram but in practice in recent years this investigation has been virtually given up.

Treatment of testis tumours

In patients whose tumour shows only pure seminoma, with negative markers after orchidectomy and no markers to be found in the specimen, and who have no detectable metastases, the standard treatment consists of giving the patient 3000 cGray radiotherapy to the retroperitoneal lymph nodes. With this regime any tiny metastases that might be present will be cured and large series show a 100% survival rate. There are drawbacks to radiotherapy, and in recent years it has been proposed that equally good prophylaxis may be obtained with a short course of single-agent *carboplatin*.

In other non-seminomatous germ cell tumours, where no evidence can be found of retroperitoneal invasion at all, i.e. the post-orchidectomy markers have fallen to zero, and the CT scans are negative, there are two alternative courses of action. The first is to keep the patient under *surveillance*, i.e. they report for 3 monthly markers and CT scans. In this group about 80% escape the need for any further therapy, and in the 20% who show a relapse, treatment (by chemotherapy) can be given without undue waste of time.

The alternative is to perform a radical retroperitoneal node dissection (Fig. 22.31) in order to provide clear-cut biopsy evidence of nodal involvement. This operation can be performed with preservation of the sympathetic nerves so that ejaculation is not affected. If the nodes are negative, then the patient is followed in the usual way: if the nodes are found to contain microscopical metastases the surgery itself may have got rid of them, and in most centres chemotherapy is only given when the specimen is found to contain bulky deposits of tumour.

Whatever the original histology, where there is evidence of retroperitoneal node disease, a series of courses of combination chemotherapy are given, and the patient followed by regular measurements of tumour markers and CT scans. When the bulk of tumour is small, one expects the masses to disappear entirely, and there is almost 100% cure. When the bulk of tumour is large and where there are obvious metastases in the liver or lungs, a mass may remain behind after chemotherapy, which

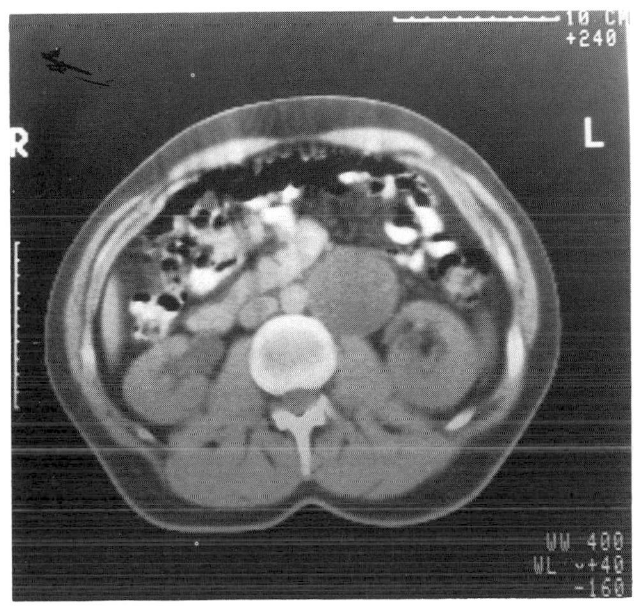

Fig. 22.30. CT scan showing a mass between the left kidney and the aorta.

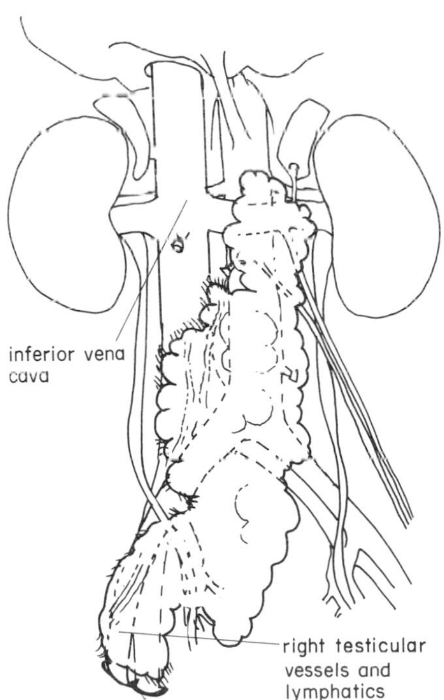

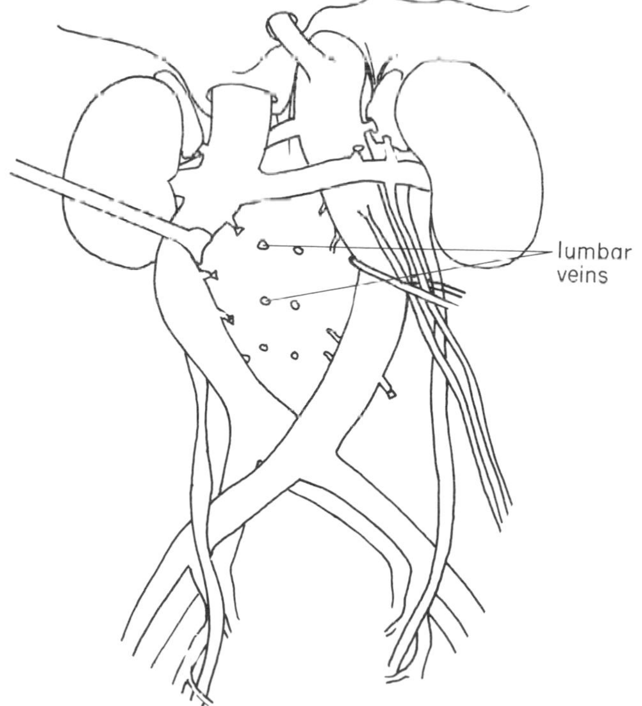

Fig. 22.31. Removal of residual tumour mass from the retroperitoneum.

might contain actively growing cancer, differentiated teratoma, or mere fibrofatty tissue.

In these cases it is necessary to perform a *salvage node dissection*. The procedure is similar to that performed in the early cases, but the technical difficulties of removing the mass of tissue from the aorta and vena cava are much increased. The objective is to remove all the suspect tissue, with a good margin.

If only fibrofatty tissue is found, no further chemotherapy need to be given, and the chance of a long-term cure is very high.

If well-differentiated teratoma is found in the specimen, unless it has all been removed, it will certainly recur within the next 3 years.

If active cancer is present in the tissue that is removed, further chemotherapy is given, and has been shown to result in a cure in about 30% of patients.

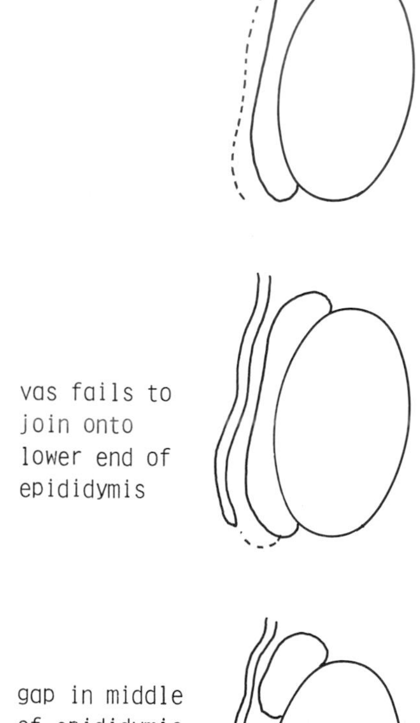

Fig. 22.32. There are many different types of failure of development of the vas and epididymis: absence of the vas, failure of its union with the epididymis and a hiatus in the body of the epididymis are some of the more common varieties.

MALE INFERTILITY

When a couple seek advice because they have been unable to have a child it should be possible to start by investigating both partners from the beginning. In investigating the husband, a gross endocrine deficiency is usually obvious from the beginning: the young man who has normal physique and body hair, and needs to shave daily, has no deficiency of androgens. Rare pituitary tumours which secret an excess of prolactin may be revealed by measurement of the plasma prolactin.

Genetic disturbances may be more difficult to detect: the *XXY Klinefelter syndrome* may occur in an otherwise normal mesomorphic male, but his small testes and a buccal smear showing the Barr body which betrays the extra chromosome will establish the diagnosis.

The testicles must be carefully examined: their size and firmness may be relevant to their function. Previous inguinal scars may mark the site where the vas has inadvertently been injured at herniorrhaphy. The vas deferens may be deficient on both sides, either absent entirely, or failing to join to the lower pole of the epididymis (Fig. 22.32).

Semen analysis

Semen is provided by masturbation into a sterile plastic container. The semen should be kept at 20°C, not in the refrigerator, before it is examined. Normal semen coagulates within a few minutes of ejaculation and liquifies after about another 20 minutes when it may be examined. Its *volume* is measured in a calibrated cylinder and varies from 1–8 ml. Most of the volume of the semen is contributed from the seminal vesicles

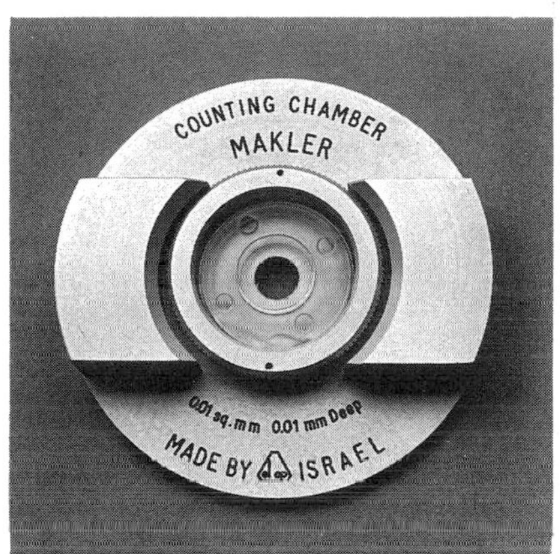

Fig. 22.33. Makler chamber (courtesy of Mr. D. F. Badenoch).

and when they are inflamed, absent or diseased the semen has a very small volume.

Sperm density is measured by the Makler chamber (Fig. 22.33) — a modified haemocytometer: but this measurement is so subject to observer error that more objective measures such as the estimation of DNA content of semen are now being used, and these show that any number of sperms $>1 \times 10^6$ per ml is compatible with normal fertility.

Sperm motility is difficult to measure — only the newer computerized methods of measuring sperm velocity (Fig. 22.34) are repeatible and objective. A good sperm velocity is a useful predictor of fertility so long as there are $>1 \times 10^6$ sperms per ml.

Sperm morphology to give useful information requires expensive scanning electron microscopy. Reports on sperm morphology based on light microscopic features are invalid and should be disregarded.

Readers will note that these observations on the normal semen analysis are at variance with much that has been published previously: they are based on Badenoch's researches which have invalidated the majority of previous work and have set new standards of normality (Table 22.1). In particular this work exposes the fallacy of the concept of 'oligozoospermia'.

Azoospermia

When no sperms can be discovered in the patient's semen at all on repeated testing there is either a blockage at some point in the delivery system between testis and external meatus, or the testis is not making any sperms.

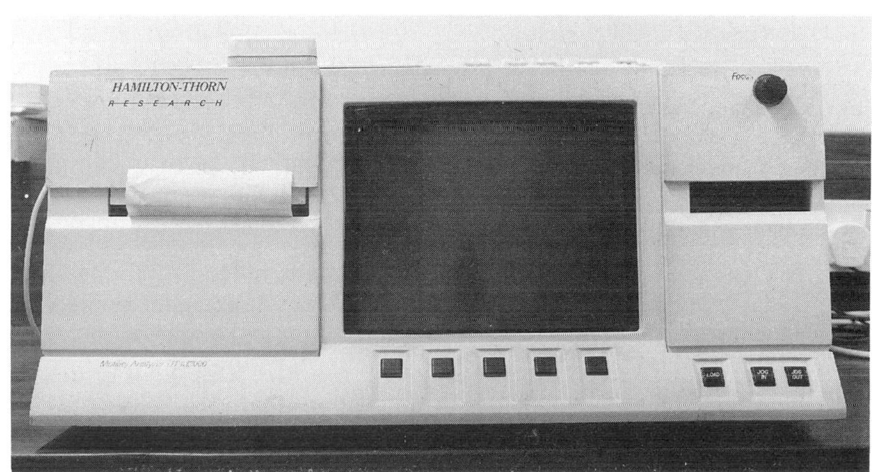

Fig. 22.34. Computerized system of measuring sperm velocity.

Table 22.1. Normal values for semen analysis, found in a series of men whose paternity had been established by HLA analysis of father and child. (Badenoch D.F., DM Thesis, Oxford 1988.)

	Fertile			Infertile		
	Range	Standard deviation	Mean	Range	Standard deviation	Mean
Sperm density	6–281	60.1	91.3	1–275	34.8	26.9
% Motility	10–90	29.9	61.9	0–74	22.8	29.6
Mean sperm velocity	13–834	11.3	44.4	0–33.7	10.4	15.1
% of hamster ova penetrated	0–100	32.9	57	0–100	25.7	10.7

Values from semen analyses on 104 proven fertile males and 52 infertile males.

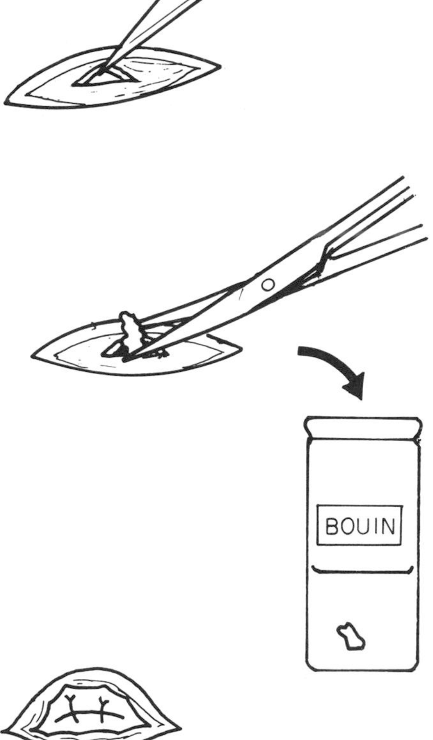

Fig. 22.35. Testis biopsy.

If the testis is not making any sperms, then the Sertoli cells will not be secreting *inhibin*, and in response, the pituitary will be secreting an excess of *follicle stimulating hormone* (FSH) in the effort to stimulate the testis to make sperms. If the plasma FSH is measured and found to be elevated (above 15 mIU/ml) then there is little point in confirming the diagnosis with a testis biopsy. When the values are borderline, or the patient insists on making the diagnosis for certain, a testis biopsy is performed.

Testis biopsy

Under general anaesthesia the testis is exposed through a small incision in the scrotum. A sharp knife punctures the tunica albuginea allowing a few testicular tubules to protrude (Fig. 22.35): these are snipped off with scissors and plunged at once into Bouin's fixative, which contains picric and acetic acids as well as formalin, and prevents distortion of the tubules and allows more accurate identification of the various cells within them. The small hole in the tunica albuginea is closed with a catgut suture. The testis biopsy is examined carefully, and a Johnsen count made according to a scale where in 2 there are no spermatogenic cells and in 7 there are spermatids but no mature sperms. By assigning such a score to all the tubules in the biopsy, and averaging the result, one is provided with an index of the state of spermatogenesis in the testis. In a normal fertile male one expects a mean Johnsen score of about 9: in Klinefelter's syndrome the score is only 1 or 2.

If the biopsy shows that normal spermatogenesis is present inside the tubules, but none are getting into the semen, one must consider the possibility that there is a block. The testicles may then be explored with a view to attempting to bypass the blockage.

Vasography and epididymovasostomy

Under anaesthesia the testis is exposed through a scrotal incision, and a fine cannula is placed in the vas through which contrast medium is injected to fill the seminal vesicles and show that there is no obstruction at that end of the system (Fig. 22.36). This may, very rarely, show an obstruction at the outlet of the ejaculatory duct, or an interruption in the course of the vas deferens, perhaps from some previous hernia repair.

The epididymis is now examined. Its tubules are often seen to be crammed with yellow material consisting of innumerable sperms, and if the epididymis is punctured and a drop of the fluid placed on a slide under a cover-slip, microscopy will identify spermatozoa.

Using magnification, a side to side anastomosis is made between the lumen of the vas deferens and the thin fascia covering the epididymis (Fig. 22.37). Sperms may not appear in the ejaculate for several weeks

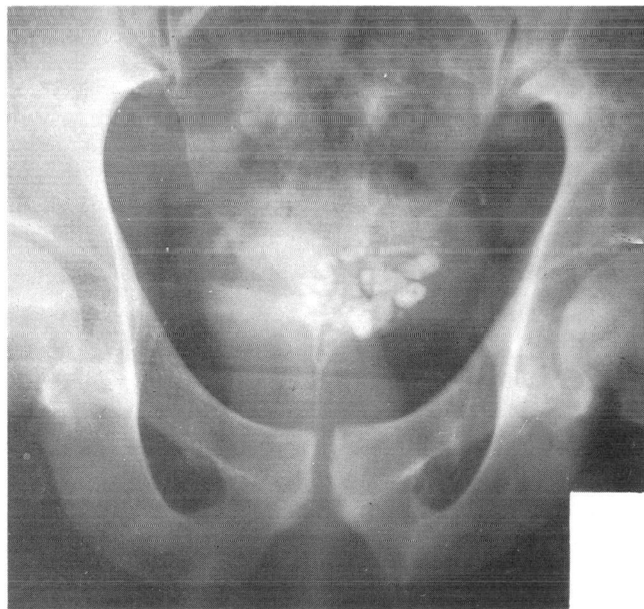

Fig. 22.36. Normal vasogram, showing filling of the vas and seminal vesicle on the left side.

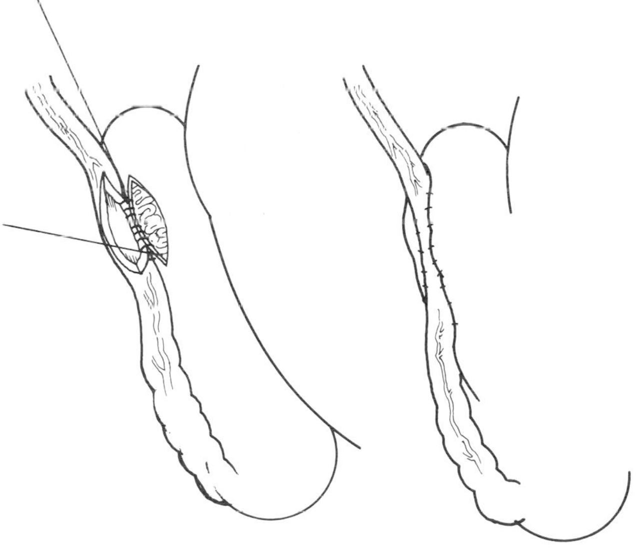

Fig. 22.37. Epididymovasostomy.

What to tell the patient

It is always best to tell the truth, but in this area you must be exceedingly cautious before pronouncing a diagnosis of infertility. Never make this diagnosis on the basis of a few semen analyses purporting to show 'oligozoospermia.' Nevertheless, a couple are entitled to know when the chance of success is poor, so that they can consider alternatives such as adoption or artificial insemination with donor semen. Temper the wind to the shorn lamb: mix frankness with sympathy and whenever possible, offer hope.

VASECTOMY FOR MALE STERILIZATION

Counselling

Both husband and wife must clearly understand that vasectomy may be irreversible, but that there is a small chance (perhaps 1:8000) that the ends will join again spontaneously at some time — perhaps years — after the operation. They must appreciate that after this, as after any other operation in surgery, there may be post-operative complications, e.g. haematoma and wound infection and they must understand that living sperms may remain in the storage system of the vas and seminal vesicle, and that until these sperms have been cleared away the patient may still father a child.

It is the usual rule to require at least two 'clear' specimens of semen from the patient before declaring the operation a success.

Vasectomy should not affect a man's desire or his capacity to make love but occasionally men claim that their libido vanishes after the operation for reasons which must have a deep-seated psychosexual origin.

Anaesthesia

Vasectomy can be performed under local infiltration anaesthesia, but this is unwise if the patient is very anxious, very fat, or has had previous surgery to the testicles or herniae.

The operation of vasectomy

There are many methods in use, and despite the claims made for some of them, there is no evidence that any one technique is superior to any other. The vas is exposed through a short scrotal incision or pair of

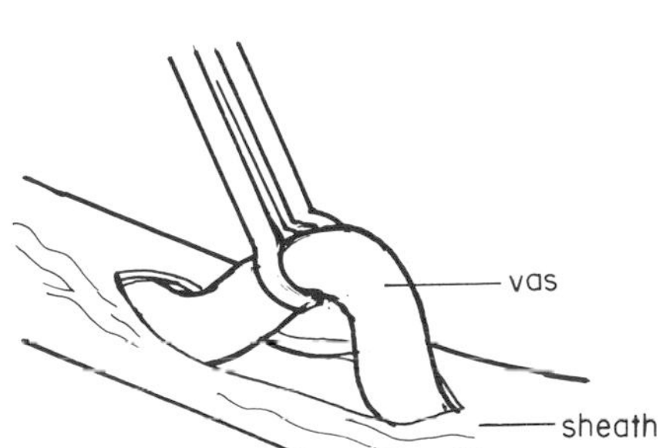

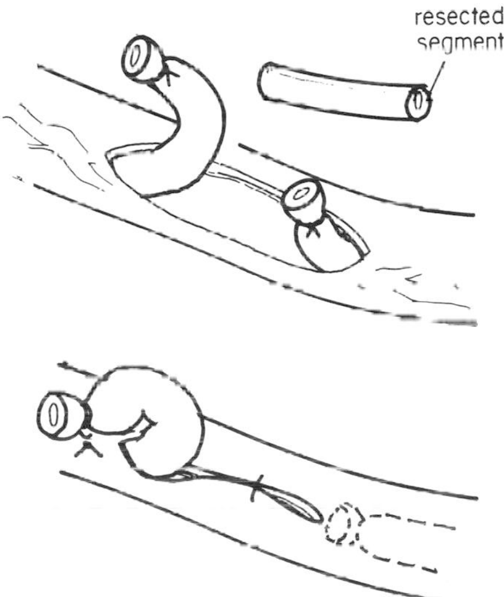

Fig. 22.38. One technique for vasectomy.

incisions. The sheath of the vas is incised, the vas lifted out, its ends ligated with fine catgut and in one popular technique, one end is turned back on itself, and the sheath of the vas closed over the other end to try to prevent spontaneous recanalization — although it does not always do so (Fig. 22.38). In another method the lumen of the vas is coagulated with a diathermy needle to produce obliteration over a length of 1 to 2 cm.

Before the scrotum is closed care is taken to make sure that all the bleeding vessels have been sealed off. The patient rests quietly for 5–10 minutes to make sure there is no reactionary haemorrhage from a vein that may have been sealed by spasm, and will start to bleed again later.

Early complications of vasectomy include: *haematoma* (despite every precaution); *infection* at the site of the skin incision; and unexpected *pain* in the scrotum.

The most important late complication is late *spontaneous recanalization*, which, though exceedingly rare, brings disastrous medicolegal consequences unless the patient has been warned of this possibility. Less important, but increasingly commonly observed, is the development of painful *sperm granuloma* either at the site of the divided vas deferens or in the epididymis. This is caused by the granulomatous reaction to the leakage of sperms into the tissues of the epididymis or around the vas. Fortunately the pain is usually short-lived, because even putting the vasa together again does not always relieve it.

Rejoining the vas after vasectomy

From time to time a couple separate, or a man tragically loses his wife and children in a road accident, and the patient asks to have the vas put together again. This requires time, magnification, and a general anaesthetic. The ends of the vasa are found, opened up, spatulated and anastomosed with very fine nylon. Sperms find their way through the anastomosis in about 80% of patients but only about 50% of their partners are able to become pregnant. The reasons for this are not clear: it is believed that while the vas are obstructed the patient may be autoimmunized against his own sperms.

FURTHER READING

Badenoch DF (1987) *Semen Analysis in Fertile and Infertile Males.* DM Thesis, Oxford University.

Barlow DH (1988) Antisperm antibodies in infertility. *British Medical Journal* **296**, 310–1.

Blandy JP, Oliver RTD (1986) British experience in the management of testicular cancer. In: Javadpour N (Ed) *Principles and Management of Testicular Cancer.* Georg Thieme Verlag, New York. pp. 378–82.

Browne D (1949) Treatment of undescended testes. *Proceedings of the Royal Society of Medicine* **42**, 643–5.

Dennis MJS, Fahim SF & Doyle PT (1987) Testicular torsion in older men. *British Medical Journal* **294**, 1680.

Donohue JP, Rowland RG, Kopecky K, Steidle CP, Geier G, Ney KG, Einhorn L, Williams S & Loehrer P (1987) Correlation of computerized tomographic changes and findings in 80 patients having radical retroperitoneal lymph node dissection after chemotherapy for testis cancer. *Journal of Urology* **137**, 1176–9.

Einhorn LH (1988) Chemotherapy of disseminated testicular cancer. In Skinner DG & Leiskovsky G (Eds) *Diagnosis and Management of Genitourinary Cancer.* WB Saunders, Philadelphia. pp. 526–31.

Giwercman A, Grindsted J, Hansen B, Jensen OM & Skakkebaek NE (1987) Testicular cancer risk in boys with maldescended testis: a cohort study. *Journal of Urology* **138**, 1214–6.

Grant JBF, Costello CB, Sequira PJL & Blacklock NJ (1987) The role of *Chlamydia trachomatis* in epididymitis. *British Journal of Urology* **60**, 355–9.

Hargreave TB (1986) Carcinoma in situ of the testis. *British Medical Journal* **239**, 1389–440.

Hargreave TB, Elton RA, Webb JA, Busuttil A & Chisholm GD (1984) Maldescended testes and fertility: a review of 68 cases. *British Journal of Urology* **56**, 734–9.

Jequier AM & Holmes SC (1984) Aetiological factors in the production of obstructive azoospermia. *British Journal of Urology* **56**, 540–3.

Jequier AM & Ukombe EB (1983) Errors inherent in the performance of a routine semen analysis. *British Journal of Urology* **55**, 434–6.

John Radcliffe Hospital Cryptorchidism Study Group (1986) Cryptorchidism: an apparent substantial increase since 1960. *British Medical Journal* **293**, 1401–4.

London NJM, Joseph HT & Johnstone JMS (1987) Orchidopexy: the effect of changing patterns of referral and treatment on outcome. *British Journal of Surgery* **74**, 636–8.

Oliver RTD, Dhaliwal HS, Hope-Stone HF & Blandy JP (1988) Short-course Etoposide, Bleomycin and Cisplatin in the treatment of mestatic germ cell tumours. Appraisal of its potential as adjuvant chemotherapy for Stage 1 testis tumours. *British Journal of Urology* **61**, 53–8.

Senturia YD (1987) The epidemiology of testicular cancer. *British Journal of Urology* **60**, 285–91.

Smith RB (1988) Testicular seminoma. In: Skinner DG & Lieskovsky G (Eds) *Diagnosis and Management of Genitourinary Cancer.* WB Saunders, Philadelphia. pp. 508–15.

Glossary of Urological Eponyms and Jargon

Albarran, Joaquin (1860–1912). Cuban urologist working in Paris. Described pedunculated 'middle lobe' of prostate and invented the Albarran lever on the catheterizing cystoscope.

albumen. Latin, egg-white.

Alport, Cecil (1880–1959). South African physician.

ampulla. Latin, a flask.

Anderson-Hynes. Method of pyeloplasty devised by James Christie Anderson, urologist, Royal Hospital, Sheffield and Wilfred Hynes, plastic surgeon, United Sheffield Hospitals. (See Anderson J.C. (1963) *Hydronephrosis*. William Heinemann Medical Books, London.)

Avicenna (1037). Abu Ali Hussein Ibn Sina. Iranian physician. Used soft catheters of leather, and of silver. (See Hanafy M. H. *et al.* (1976) *Urology* **8**, 63.)

balanitis. Greek, *βάλανος*, the glans penis, xerotica obliterans (Greek, dry; Latin, obliterating).

Barr, Murray (1908–). Contemporary Canadian anatomist.

Behcet, Hulúsi (1889–1948). Turkish dermatologist. Described a syndrome including ulceration of mouth, genitalia, uveitis, iridocyclitis.

Belfield, W. T. American urologist who probably did the first open prostatectomy intentionally. (See Belfield W. T. (1887) *J. Am. Med. Assoc.* **8**, 303.)

Bellini, Lorenzo (1643–1704). Anatomist of Pisa. Described, among many other things, the straight collecting tubules of the renal papilla.

Bence-Jones, Henry (1814–73). Physician, London.

Benedict, Stanley Rossiter (1884–1936). Biochemist of Cornell University, USA. Described test for sugar in the urine.

Béniqué, Pierre Jules (1806–51). Surgeon of Paris.

Bertin, Exupère Joseph (1712–81). Associate anatomist at the Academy of Sciences in Paris.

Bigelow, Henry Jacob (1818–90). Surgeon of Boston, USA. (See Bigelow H.J. (1879) Lithotrity by a single operation. *Boston Med. Surg. J.* (later *New Eng. J. Med.*) **98**, 259 and 291.)

Bilharz, Theodor Maximilian (1825–62). German physician working in Cairo who first described *Schistosoma haematobium*; hence Bilharziasis

Boari, Achille (1894). Italian urologist who devised bladder flap procedure for bridging gap at lower end of ureter.

Bonney, W.F. Victor (1872–1953). Gynaecologist, The Middlesex and Queen Charlotte's Hospitals, London.

bougie. French, candle (wax 'bougies' were often used to dilate urethral strictures).

Bouin, Paul (1870). Histologist of Strasbourg. Described fixative for testicular biopsies containing picric acid, acetic acid and formalin.

Bowman, Sir William (1816–92). Ophthalmic surgeon of London. Described the capsule of the glomerulus and recognized that it was extruded from the end of the renal tubule.

Braasch, W. F. Urologist of the Mayo Clinic. Described many urological conditions and invented many instruments, of which the bulb-ended ureteric catheter is best known today.

Bricker, Eugene M. Professor of Surgery, Washington University School of Medicine, St. Louis. Described ileal conduit. (See Bricker E. M. (1950) Bladder substitution after pelvic evisceration. *Surg. Clin. N. Am.* **30**, 1511.)

Bright, Richard (1789–1858). Guy's Hospital physician.

Brown-Buerger. One of the best cystoscopes was devised by Tilden Brown and Leo Buerger. (See A new combination observation catheterizing and operating cystoscope. *N.Y. Med. J.* Aug. 25 1917.)

Browne, Sir Denis (1892–1967). Paediatric surgeon at Great Ormond Street Hospital for Children. Invented operation for hypospadias. (See *Postgrad. Med. J.* (1949), **25**, 367.)

von Brunn, A. (1841–95). Professor of Anatomy, Göttingen. Described cell nests in chronic cystitis. (See *Arch. Mikr. Anat.* (1983), **41**, 294.)

Buck, Gordon (1807–77). New York surgeon who described the deep fascia of the corpora cavernosa of the penis.

Calix, Greek, *κάδνλιξ*, cup; 'confused by modern scientific writers with Graeco-Latin *calyx* and written calyx' (OED).

calyx. Greek *κάλυξ*, from root *καλυπτειν*. Often confused with calix, the whorl of leaves forming the outer covering of the flower while in the bud.

Camper, Peter (1722–89). Physician and polymath of Amsterdam.

Cannula. Rigid tube for insertion into a body cavity or vessel. Latin, canna–reed.

Carr, R.J. Contemporary radiologist, Bradford. Described his tiny concretions and worked with Henry Hamilton Stewart in studying the 'stone nest theory' of calculus formation.

carbuncle. Latin, carbolive coal.

catheter. Greek, *καθετηρ*, *καθιεμη*, to send down.

Charrière, Joseph (1803–76). Instrument maker of Paris. Made instruments for Civiale (1792–1867) and many other celebrated French surgeons. Made the first effective lithotrite. Devised the French (logical) metric system of catheter sizes, the number signifying the circumference of the instrument in millimeters.

Chevassu, M. Urologist of Paris. Made many contributions including a useful bulb-ended catheter for the ureter. His thesis (Paris, 1906) first clearly distinguished between seminoma and teratoma and urged early and radical orchidectomy.

chordée. A painful downward concavity of the penis. Originally associated with inflammation of the corpora cavernosa from gonorrhoea (chaudepisse cordée) it is now used more often for the bend associated with hypospadias.

Clutton, Henry (1888). The curved steel bougies named after him were copied from those recommended by Otis (q.v.) and Clutton never pretended otherwise.

Colles, Abraham (1773–1843). Professor of Surgery in Dublin. Described the tough layer of superficial fascia of the perineum. (See *A Treatise on Surgical Anatomy* (1811) Edinburgh.)

Collings, C. W. Early exponent of TUR: knife named after him. (See *J. Urol.* (1926), **16**, 545.)

Conn, Jerome W. (1907–). American physician, described primary hyperaldosteronism.

coudé. French, elbowed, a shape of catheter invented by Mercier of Paris.

Cowper, William (1666–1709). Anatomist and surgeon of London who described the glands sandwiched in the levator ani behind the bulbar urethra.

Culp, Ormond. Chief of Urology, Mayo Clinic.

Cushing. Harvey Williams (1869–1939). Surgeon of Boston, the father of modern neurosurgery.

Denonvilliers, Charles Pierre (1808–72). Surgeon and anatomist of Paris. Remembered for the fascia formed by fusion of the layers of peritoneum between the rectum and prostate. (See L'anatomie due Perinée. *Bull. Soc. Anat. Paris* (1836), **12**, 106.)

detrusor. Latin, detrudere, to push down.

Dietl, Joseph (1804–78). Pathologist of Cracow. Described the episodes of pain of intermittent hydronephrosis — the so-called Dietl's crises.

dilate. Latin, dilatare, whence *dilatation*. The shorter 'dilation' is wrong.

Doppler, Christian Johann (1803–53). Austrian physicist.

Dormia, Enrico. Contemporary assistant Professor of Urology, Milan. Devised his basket for dislodging stones, and now celebrated for methods for dissolving calculi with continuous ureteric irrigation.

Ducrey, Augosto (1860–1940). Dermatologist of Rome. Described the *Haemophilus ducreyi* which causes soft chancre.

Duplay, Simon (1836–1921). Surgeon of Paris. Devised an operation for urethral stricture similar to that of Denis Browne. (See Injuries and disease of the urethra. *Int. Encycl. Surg.* (1886), **6**, 487.)

ectopic. Greek εκτώπος, displaced.

enuresis. Greek, ένουρειν̆, incontinence of urine. Today generally applied to bed-wetting, which should strictly be called nocturnal enuresis.

epididymis. Greek, ε'πι upon, and διδυμοι, twins (testes).

epispadias. Greek, ε'πι and σπάδον, a rent or tear.

Escherich. Theodor (1857–1911). Paediatrician of Munich who described *Bacillus coli*, now named *Escherichia coli* in his memory.

exstrophy, Greek, εξοτρεφειν, to turn inside out.

Fabricius. ab Acquapendente (Girolamo Fabrizio) (1537–1619). Teacher of Harvey at Padua. Bursa of Fabricius — outgrowth of chick embryo cloaca resembling thymus. Hence B-lymphocytes.

Falloppius, Gabriel (1523–62). Polymath of Padua, favourite pupil of Vesalius.

von Fehling, Hermann Christian (1812–85). German chemist.

Fenwick, Hurry (1856–1944). Surgeon at St Peter's and The London Hospital. Introduced the new-fangled electric cystoscope to England, founded the International Society of Urology and pioneered retrograde urography.

Foley, Frederic Eugene Basil (1891–1966). Urologist of Minneapolis-St. Paul. Devised self-retaining balloon catheter and a method of pyeloplasty.

fossa. Latin, ditch.

Fournier, Jean Alfred (1832–1914). Venereologist and dermatologist at Hôpital St. Louis, Paris. Described Fournier's gangrene.

fraenum, fraenulum. From Latin, fraenum, a bridle.

Freyer, Sir Peter J. (1851–1921). Surgeon at St. Peter's Hospital. Brilliant Irish surgeon. Won international fame by litholapaxy in children in India and later perfected the method of transvesical prostatectomy now named after him.

Fuller, Eugene (1858–1930). New York urologist. Made many contributions to urology including the transvesical operation. (See *J. Cutan. Genit. Dis.* (1895), **13**, 229.)

fundus. Latin, bottom. The bottom or the part furthest from the orifice.

Gerota, Dumitru (1867–1939). Anatomist of Budapest. Described the posterior fascia of the kidney. (See *Arch. Anat. Leipsig* (1895), 265.)

Gersuny, Robert (1844–1924). Surgeon of Vienna. Attempted to devise method of urinary bladder substitution using rectum for urine, and bringing faecal stream through anal sphincter (his case died).

Gibbon, Norman. Contemporary urological surgeon. Sefton Hospital, Liverpool. Devised narrow plastic catheter for use in paraplegics.

Gil-Vernet, J. M. Contemporary Spanish surgeon of Barcelona. Devised extended pyelolithotomy through renal sinus.

Gimbernat, Don Manuel Louise (1734–1816). Professor of Anatomy in Barcelona. Surgeon to the King of Spain.

Giraldes, Joachim (1808–75). Professor of Surgery, Paris. (See *C.R. Soc. Biol. Paris* (1859), 123.)

glomerulus. Little ball (Latin, glomus, ball).

Goodpasture, Ernest William (1886–1960). American pathologist. Described glomerulitis associated with haemoptysis.

Grawitz, Paul Albert (1850–1932). Pathologist of Greifswald. (See *Virchow's Archiv.* (1983), **93**, 39.)

gubernaculum. Latin, helm-rudder. Lump of jelly which steers the testicle into the scrotum. Described by John Hunter and sometimes called Hunter's gubernaculum.

gum elastic. Catheters formely made of silk, woven and impregnated with gum. Invented by Bernard (a Parisian jeweller) in 1779.

Guthrie, Sir George James (1785–1856). Hero of Waterloo and Surgeon to the Westminster Hospital, Pioneer of TUR.

Harris, Samuel Henry (1880–1937). Urologist of Sydney, Australia, who published first safe and antiseptic transvesical, one-stage prostatectomy series. (See *Brit. J. Surg.* (1933), **21**, 434).

Helmstein, Karl. Contemporary Swedish urologist, Stockholm.

Henle, Fredrich (1809–85). Anatomist of Berlin.

Henoch, E. (1820–1910). Paediatrician, Berlin.

Hilum. Latin, 'little thing' applied to eye of bean or seed hence to hilum of kidney.

Hopkins, Professor Harold. Contemporary Professor of Optics, University of Reading. Devised modern rod-lens system and flexible fibre-optic cable used throughout modern urology.

Hounsfield, Godfrey Newbold. Wartime radar expert. Designed the first transistorized computer. Invented CT scanner. Nobel Prize 1979.

Hunner, Guy Leroy (1868–1951). Gynaecologist at Johns Hopkins Hospital, Baltimore. Described interstitial cystitis. (See Hunner G.L. *Boston Med. Surg. J.* (1914), 660.)

hyaline. Greek υ″αλοϑ, glass.

hyatid. Greek υ″δωρ, drop of water.

hydrocele. Greek κήλη, swelling, like κόλακοϑ, belly: often misspelt hydrocoele, from confusion with κόλοϑ, hollow, hence coelom means watery swelling.

hypospadias. Greek υπο, below, σπάδον, a rent or tear.

Jaboulay, Mathieu (1860–1913). Surgeon of Lyons.

Jaques, Frère Jacques de Beaulieu (1651–1714). Itinerant lithotomist through lateral approach. (See Barret (1949) *Ann. Roy. Coll. Surg. Eng.* **5**, 275.)

Jaques, James Archibald (1815–78). Works manager, William Warne and Co. Ltd., Barking, Essex. Improved and patented soft rubber catheter.

Johanson, Bengt. Contemporary surgeon, Stockholm. Pioneer of urethroplasty.

Kidd, Frank, S. (1878–1934). London Hospital surgeon. Invented the 'big-ball' diathermy cystoscope.

Klinefelter, E.W. Contemporary radiologist, Massachusetts General Hospital.

Kolff, W.J. Contemporary nephrologist. Pioneer of first effective artifical kidney in Holland during Nazi occupation, 1944. Now at Cleveland.

Leadbetter, Wyland (1911–74). Distinguished urologist of Boston.

Leydig, Franz von (1821–1908). Anatomist and zoologist of Bonn.

litho. Greek λιθος, stone, *-tripsy*, Greek τριβειν, wear away, τομή, cut, λάπαξιν, evacuation.

Littre, Alexis (1658–1726). Anatomist of Paris.

Loewenstein-Jensen. Culture medium for tuberculosis. Ernst Loewenstein (1878), pathologist of Vienna and Carl Oluf Jensen (1864–1934), pathologist of Copenhagen.

Lord, Peter, Contemporary English Surgeon. High Wycombe. Vice-President RCS.

Lewsley, O.S. (1884–1955). New York urologist.

Mackenrodt, Alwin (1859–1925). Professor of Gynaecology, Berlin.

McCarthy, Joseph Francis (1874–1965). New York urologist. Inventor of the foroblique lens, and the 'panendoscope'.

malakoplakia. Greek μαλακός, soft and πλαλε̂α, plaque.

Malécot, Achille Etienne (b. 1852). Described his winged self-retaining catheter in 1892. (See Outwin E.L. (1955) The development of the modern catheter. *J. Am. Surg. Tech.* **1**, 8.)

Malpighi, Marcello (1628–94). Anatomist, physician, polymath of Rome and Bologna. Described just about everything.

Marchetti, A. A., see below.

Marion, Georges (1869–1960). French urologist of Paris. Described many conditions, especially 'prostatisme sans prostate', i.e. bladder neck stenosis, which is sometimes called after him, though it was described by John Hunter, Morgagni, Valsalva and Ambroise Paré beforehand.

Marshall, Victor F. Contemporary urologist at New York Memorial Hosptial. (See Marshall V. F., Marchetti, A.A. and Krantz K.E. (1949) The correction of stress incontinence by simple vesicourethral suspension. *Surg. Gynec. Obstet.* **88**, 509.)

meatus (pl. meatus). Latin, a passage or channel.

micturition. From Latin, micturire, derived from mingere, to mix (originally meant the desire to make water, implying 'a morbid frequency in the making of urine: often erroneously the action of making water'. OED).

Millin, Terence. Irish urological surgeon. Described retropubic prostatectomy. (See Livingstone E. & S. (1947) *Retropubic Urinary Surgery* Edinburgh.)

Morgagni, Giovanni Battista (1682–1771). Anatomist and pathologist of Padua.

Morris, Sir Henry (1844–1926). Surgeon trained at Guy's Hospital, London, worked at the Middlesex Hospital. Did the first deliberate removal of a calculus from the kidney. (See *Invest. Urol.* (1973), **11**, 170.)

Müller, Johannes (1801–58). Physiologist of Berlin. Described the paramesonephric ducts and the organs derived from them.

navicularis, Latin, having the shape of a small boat.

Neisser, Albert Ludwig Siegmund (1855–1916). Dermatologist of Breslau. (See *Centr. Med. Wiss.* (1879), **17**, 497.)

neph. *νεφροῦ*, Greek, kidney;-ectomy,-itis,-stomy, etc.

nexus, Latin, a tying together (like connected, knitted, etc.).

Nitze, Max. Professor of Urology in Berlin, invented the first incandescent lamp cystoscope in 1877.

nocturia. The discharge of an abnormally large quantity of urine at night.

Otis, Fessenden Nott (1825–1900). American urologist who devoted his life to the study of the urethra.

Page, I. Harriet. American physician, Cleveland clinic. Produced hypertension by wrapping kidney in cellophane; showed how the same could occur when kidney surrounded by fibrosis.

Paget, Sir James (1814–99). Surgeon, St. Bartholomew's Hospital, London. (See *St. Barts. Hosp. Rep.* (1874), **10**, 87.)

pampiniform. Shaped like a tendril, Latin pampinus tendril.

Papanicolaou, G. N. (1883–1962). Greek pathologist working in New York. (See Cytology of the urinary sediment in neoplasms of the urinary tract. *J. Urol.* (1974), **57**, 375.)

papilloma, Latin papilla, a nipple and Greek, -oma, tumour.

Parks, Sir Alan Guyatt (1923–84). Surgeon, The London Hospital.

Petit, Jean Louis (1674–1760). Surgeon, Paris. Elected to Royal Society of London.

Peyronie, François de la (1678–1747). Surgeon of Paris.

Pfannenstiel. Hermann Johann (1862–1909). Gynaecologist of Breslau. Described the lower abdominal incision named after him.

piezo-electric. Greek, *πιεζεν* — to press.

Politano, Victor. Contemporary urologist, Miami, Florida.

polyuria. Greek *πὸλυ*, much, and *ὀυρια*. An increase in the amount of urine excreted, usually implies frequency.

posthitis. Greek, *πόσΘε* foreskin.

Queyrat, L. Dermatologist of Paris. (See Queyrat, L. (1911) Erythyroplasie du gland. *Bull. Soc. Franç. Derm. Syph.* **22**, 378.) Described carcinoma *in situ* of penis, already described by Paget (1874).

Randall, Alexander (1883–1951). Urologist of Philadelphia. Made many contributions including the description of the various lobes of the prostate and the 'bar at the neck of the bladder', as well as the Randall's plaques on the renal papillae.

Rehn, Ludwig (1849–1930). Surgeon of Frankfurt. Noticed workers in factory making fuchsin got bladder cancer.

Retzius, Andreas Rolf (1796–1860). Anatomist, Karolinska Hospital, Stockholm. Described the retropubic space.

Riches, Sir Eric. Late Consulting Urologist, Middlesex Hospital.
Riedel, Bernhard Moriz Cark Ludwig (1846–1916). Anatomist, Jena.
Rovsing, N. T. (1862–1927). Professor of Surgery, Cophenhagen.
Sachse, Hans. Contemporary German urologist: invented optical urethrotome.
Santorini, Giovanni Domenico (1681–1737). Anatomist, Venice. Described the plexus of veins in the pelvis.
Scarpa, Antonio (1747–1832). Professor of Anatomy at Pavia, Italy.
schistosoma, Greek, *σχιστω* — split, *σωμα* — body.
Schönlein, Johann L. (1793–1864). German physician.
Sertoli, Enrico (1842–1910). Physiologist of Milan.
spermatozoa. Greek, *σπερμα* — seed, *ζωιον* — animal.
Stewart, Henry Hamilton (1904–70). Urologist of Bradford. One of the pioneers of punch resection in England; inventor of numerous, ingenious, plastic, urological procedures for urethral stricture, hydronephrosis, etc.
strangury. From Greek *στράγξ*, drop squeezed out, and *ουρον*, urine. Slow and painful emission of urine.
teratoma. From Greek *τέρας*, monster.
testis. Latin, witness.
Thompson, Sir Henry (1820–1904). Great stone-crusher. (See *Invest. Urol.* (1973), **11**, 263.)
Tiemann, G., and Co, Instrument makers of New York.
trichomonas. *θριξ*, a hair, *μονοζ*, unit (though it has three to five hairs!).
trochar. French. Trois carrés; three sided sharp perforator used to introduce a cannula.
urachus. From Greek *ουρωε* -urine. Noted by Hippocrates, who thought it was the urinary canal of the fetus.
urethra. Greek, *ουρηθρα*.
utriculus. Latin, small bag.
varicocele. Varix — tortuous vein (Latin, varus — bent); Greek, *κηλε*, — swelling.
vas. A vessel, deferens, carrying.
verumontanum. Latin veru, a spit; montanus, mountainous.
vesicle. Latin, a little bladder.
vulva. Latin, a wrapper.
Wilms, Max (1867–1918). Surgeon of Heidelberg. Nephroblastoma was previously described by Rance (1814).
Wolff, Kaspar Friedrich (1733–94). German anatomist and embryologist, working in St. Petersburg.
xanthogranuloma. *ξανθός*, Greek, yellow.
Young, Hugh Hampton (1870–1945). Urologist of Baltimore. Inventor of the first cold punch, and a method of perineal prostatectomy.
Ziehl-Neelsen. Method of staining the tubercle bacillus, named after Franz Ziehl (1859–1926), physician of Lübeck, and Friedrick Karl Adolph Neelsen (1854–94), pathologist of Dresden.
Zuckerkandl, Emil (1849–1910). Anatomist of Vienna.

Index

Page references in *italics* refer to figures or the legends accompanying them.